MRCP 2
PRACTICE PAPERS
Case Histories
Data Interpretations
and
Photographic Material

Third Edition

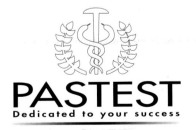

PASTEST
Dedicated to your success

For Immy – who is going to teach me a thing or two.

Cover Slides:

- 3RD Cranial nerve palsy
- Acute myocardial infarction
- Haemochromatosis
- Calcified pleural plaques and folded lung (asbestos)
- Barrett's oesophagus
- Acute lymphocytic leakaemia

MRCP 2
PRACTICE PAPERS
Case Histories
Data Interpretations
and
Photographic Material

Third Edition

Hans-Ulrich Laasch Dr.med, MRCP, FRCR
COOK Fellow in Interventional Radiology
Academic Department of GI-Radiology
South Manchester University Hospitals

© 2001 PASTEST
Egerton Court
Parkgate Estate
Knutsford
Cheshire WA16 8DX

Telephone: 01565 752000

First published 2000
Second edition 2001
Reprinted 2002
Third edition 2003

ISBN 1 901198 170

A catalogue record for this book is available from the British Library.

The information contained within this book was obtained by the author from reliable sources. However, while every effort has been made to ensure its accuracy, no responsibilty for loss, damage or injury occasioned to any person acting or refraining from action as a result of information contained herein can be accepted by the publishers or author.

PasTest Revision Books and Intensive Courses
PasTest has been established in the field of postgraduate medical education since 1972, providing revision books and intensive study courses for doctors preparing for their professional examinations.
Books and courses are available for the following specialties:
MRCP Part 1 and Part 2, MRCPCH Part 1 and Part 2, MRCOG, DRCOG, MRCGP, MRCPsych, DCH, FRCA, MRCS, PLAB.
For further details contact:
**PasTest, Freepost, Knutsford, Cheshire WA16 7BR
Tel: 01565 752000 Fax: 01565 650264
E-mail: enquiries@pastest.co.uk
Web site: www.pastest.co.uk**

Typeset by Saxon Graphics Ltd, Derby
Printed and bound in the UK by Page Bros Ltd, Norwich

CONTENTS

PREFACE TO THE THIRD EDITION

Further to the changes of the written parts of the MRCP exam, notably the removal of negative marking in Part 1 and the change to MCQ ('Best of Five') based questions in Part 2A, there has also been a change in the content of the MRCP 2A papers. The exam is increasingly orientated around evidence based medicine, up-to-date patient management and current guidelines. This is a move away from the esoteric questions seen in the past and it makes a more useful exam. Candidates have said that a large proportion of questions could now be answered with adequate clinical experience. That does however mean that preparation for Part 2A needs to include the *British Medical Journal*, the *Journal of the Royal College of Physicians* and the *Drugs and Therapeutics Bulletin*. The candidates need to be aware of the latest guidelines regarding the treatment of bread and butter entities such as hypertension, diabetes and chronic chest disease. The bodies involved in these guidelines besides the *National Institute of Clinical Excellence* (NICE) are the respective societies such as the *British Thoracic Society* and the *British Society of Gastroenterology*. Fortunately these are all now available on the internet and time is well invested in checking the headlines on the respective sites. A short list of these can be found on page ix.

The first few of the new papers for Part 2A contained 70–75 questions, most of which consisted of a single stem. For each possible correct answer there are 5 possible options i.e. if the question asks for two differential diagnoses there will be ten possible answers. Remember the exam is not negatively marked, therefore all questions must be answered, but do not tick more than requested.

If in doubt choose the answer that represents the logical next step in patient management as you would do with a patient in Accident and Emergency or the Outpatient department. Bear in mind this is an *entry* exam to higher medical training, and increasingly aiming to assess good patient management skills.

That does however not invalidate my motto from the previous editions: 'Übung macht den Meister!' So get practicing.

For this particular edition I am indebted to my friend Ed Gamble, stroke physician South Manchester University Hospitals for his efforts to keep my medicine up-to-date.

Good Luck

HUL

Many thanks also to those who have taken the trouble to send in comments. All feedback serves to improve the next edition.

PREFACE TO THE SECOND EDITION

In 2001, the exam for the membership of the Royal College of Physicians remains in a state of change. The College is concerned to produce a fairer and more transparent exam. From next year negative marking for wrong answers in MRCP Part 1 will be removed, and the papers will be criterion referenced rather than peer referenced, i.e. everybody of a certain standard will pass the exam, rather than a fixed fraction of the candidates. In Part 2, the written and the clinical section have been uncoupled. Once the written exam has been passed three attempts at the clinical part are allowed within a space of two years. Increasingly questions are of a modified multiple choice type. Particularly Case Histories are getting more complex and not only 'one-of-five' answers are seen, but several correct answers may be chosen from a selection of up to ten. More importantly, the number of questions in each section have increased. In the July 2001 paper the following number of questions were found in each section: 23 Slides, 14 Data Interpretations, 14 Case Histories. The time available for each section remained unchanged: Slides 50 minutes, Data Interpretations 45 minutes, Case Histories 55 minutes. As before each section carries approximately the same weight in the overall mark. In line with these changes the second edition has now been re-written and consists entirely of modified MCQ.

The clinical section of part II has now changed to PACES (Practical Assessment of Clinical Examination Skills). There will no longer be a Viva and a Long Case, but circuits of five stations with twenty minutes at each. The stations are 1. Short case chest and short case abdomen; 2. History taking; 3. Short case cardiovascular system and short case central nervous system; 4. Communications skills and ethics (e.g. obtaining consent and breaking bad news); 5. Short cases skin, locomotor system, eyes and endocrine.

The latest information regarding changes to the exam is available from the following websites:
MRCP website – www.mrcpuk.org
RCP website – www.rcplondon.ac.uk

Hopefully these changes will reduce the number of people failing the exam, however the most important factor in the preparation remains the same: Practice.

I wish to thank my wife Rebecca for her continued support and remain grateful to my teachers, who have coached me through more than one attempt at MRCP.

HUL

PREFACE

The second part of the MRCP examination has seen some interesting changes in 1999. Firstly, the number of attempts is no longer limited to six. Secondly, a multiple choice type format has been introduced in all three parts of the written exam (Slide, Data and Case History sections). We thought that this would make the questions easier to answer however, this is not so! Minor details in the history often only discriminate between the two best possible answers. It must, however, be remembered that the exam is **not** negatively marked and it is therefore foolish to leave any questions unanswered. Thirdly, a bare fail in the written part (9/20 marks) now only requires one extra mark to be gained in the clinical section, as opposed to the three marks previously required. In theory this should make the exam easier to pass, in practice the vast majority of candidates fail on the short cases. A bare fail in the shorts (5/10) or in the long case (4/8) still requires 3 additional marks from the other three parts, thus increasing the total pass mark to 27. The most important aspect for passing the exam is practice. This applies to the clinical part even more than for the written. First-timers do not usually realise that the 4–6 weeks between the written and clinical part is generally *insufficient time* to practise all the examination routines for heart, chest, abdomen, CNS, cranial nerves, legs… Reading material for the Viva, besides the BMJ editorials, should include Drugs and Therapeutics Bulletin, CMOS-update and the Sunday papers.

It must be remembered that the exam is set so that overall only 25–30% of all candidates pass. The most enthusiastic and knowledgeable teachers for MRCP often had three or four, or even all six attempts at the exam. Although the College is trying to make the exam more objective, a good portion of luck is required on the day. This book is an attempt to repay all the help I have received from my friends and consultants on my way to membership. A special thanks goes to Dr Datta-Chaudhuri and Dr Downton from the Care of the Elderly Department in Stockport. I also need to thank my wife for her patience as well as her continued input into this work. Finally, if there is one piece of advice that summarises my experience:

There is no substitute for having seen or done it before.

Best of luck

HUL

USEFUL WEBSITE ADDRESSES

MRCP-website
www.mrcpuk.org

The Royal College of Physicians, London
www.rcplondon.ac.uk

British Thoracic Society
www.brit-thoracic.org.uk

British Cardiac Society
www.bcs.com

British Society of Gastroenterology
www.bsg.org.uk

National Institute of Clinical Excellence
www.nice.org.uk

Department of Health (white papers and political issues)
www.doh.gov.uk

Chief Medical Officer (CMO guidelines)
www.doh.gov.uk/cmo

British National Formulary (Library of drugs and therapy)
www.bnf.org

Drugs and Therapeutics Bulletin (Evaluation of pharmacotherapy)
www.which.net/health/dtb

The Society of Radiologists in Training
www.thesrt.org.uk

Google search engine
www.google.com

INDEX OF NORMAL RANGES

These are for reference only, for clinical use check with the local laboratory as ranges as well as units used vary.

ACTH, supine	8–30 ng/l
Activated partial thromboplastin time (APTT)	20–35 s
Adrenaline, urine	<110 nmol/24h
Alanine amino transferase (ALT, GPT)	5–40 U/l
Aspartate amino transferase (AST, GOT)	5–40 U/l
Albumin	35–55 g/l
Aldosterone supine [standing]	0.08–0.27 [0.14–0.83] ng/l
Alpha-fetoprotein	<10 μmg/l
Aluminium	0.22–0.26 μmol/l
Aminolaevulanic acid, urine [serum]	11–57 [1.1–1.8] μmol/24h
Ammonia	11–32 μmol/l
Amylase (assay dependent)	<300 U/l
Angiotensin I, [Angiotensin II]	11–88 [10–60] ng/l
Anion gap	10–18
Antinuclear antibody	<1:20 dilution
Antitrypsin	0.82 g/l
Aspartate aminotransferase (AST)	10–40 U/l
Arterial blood gases	
● pH	7.36–7.44
● pO_2	11–13 kPa (80–100 mmHg)
● pCO_2	4.7–5.9 kPa (35–45 mmHg)
● Bicarbonate (HCO_3^-)	22–28 mmol/l
B_{12} serum	160–900 pmol/l
Bilirubin, total [conjugated]	2–17 [<5] μmol/l
Bleeding time	<7 min
C-reactive protein (CRP)	<10 mg/l
Caeruloplasmin	180–450 mg/l
Calcitonin	<19 ng/l
Calcium, total [ionised]	2.2–2.6 [1.1–1.4] mmol/l
Carboxyhaemoglobin, [smoker]	<5% [<15%]
Cardiac index	2.4–4.2 l/min/m²
Chloride, serum [CSF]	95–110 [120–130] mmol/l
Cholesterol	
● Total	3.65–5.5 mmol/l
● HDL	> 0.9 mmol/l
● LDL	< 4.0 mmol/l
Clotting time (platelet rich plasma)	100–150 sec
Coeruloplasmin	270–370 mg/l
Complement C_3 [C_4]	0.7–1.3 [0.12–0.27] g/l

Copper, serum [urine]	12.5–25 [0.05–0.5]
Coproporphyrin, urine	52–350 nmol/l
Cortisol, free, urine	28–276 nmol/l
Cortisol, total, serum, 9am	130–150 nmol/l
Creatinine	50–120 µmol/l
Creatinine phosphokinase (CPK)	20–140 U/l
CSF pressure	50–180 mm H_2O
D-Dimer	20–400 µg/l
Differential leucocyte count	
● Neutrophils	40–65%
● Lymphocytes	15–45%
● Monocytes	4–10%
● Eosinophils	<4%
● Basophils	<2%
Dopamine	425–2600 nmol/l
Erythrocyte sedimentation rate (ESR)	0–10 mm/h
Faecal fat, 3 day collection	<7 g/24h
Ferritin, male [female]	20–250 [10–120] µg/l
Fibrin degradation products (FDP)	<10 µg/ml
Fibrinogen	1.5–5 g/l
5-hydroxyindolacetic acid (HIAA), urine	5–75 µmol/24h
Folate, RBC [serum]	130–630 [4–18] nmol/l
FSH, follicular phase [ovulatory peak]	<8 [6–26] U/l
Gamma-GT	5–30 U/l
Gastrin	<100 pmol/l
Globulin	22–35 g/l
Glomerular filtration rate (GFR)	90–130ml/min
Glucose [CSF]	4.5–5.8 [2.2–3.9] mmol/l
Growth Hormone (GH), 9am	4–10 mU/l
Haematocrit (Hk=PCV), male [female]	40–55% [35–50%]
Haemoglobin	
● Total Hb, male [female]	130–180 [110–160] g/l
● Hb A1	95–98%
● HbA2	2–3%
● HbF	1–2%
● HbC	0%
● HbS	0%
Haptoglobin	40–200 mg/dl
HCG	<5 U/l
Homovanillic acid, urine	8–48 mmol/24h
Hydroxyproline, urine	5–25mg/24h/m²
Immunoglobulins	
● IgA	1–4 g/l
● IgD	0–0.08 g/l
● IgE	<0.00025 g/l
● IgG	7.5–15 g/l

- IgM   0.5–2.5 g/l
- Insulin, free [reactive]   <120 [40–170] pmol/l
- Insulin glucose ratio   <0.3
- Iron   13–32 µmol/l
- Iron saturation, male [female]   20–50% [15–50%]
- Lactate (lactic acid)   0.9–1.7 mmol/l
- Lactate dehydrogenase (LDH)   100–190 U/l
- Lead   <1 µmol/l
- Lipase   <160 U/l
- Luteinising hormone (LH), follicular phase [midcycle peak]   <6 [16–104] U/l
- Magnesium, fasting   0.65–1.05 mmol/l
- Mean corp. Volume (MCV)   80–95 fl
- Mean corp. Hb (MCH)   27–32 pg
- Mean corp. Hb concentratrion (MCHC = MCH/MCV)   32–36 g/dl
- Metanephrins, urine total   <5 µmol/l
- Methaemoglobnin   <3%
- Noradrenaline, urine   90–475 nmol/l
- Osmolality, serum   270–295 mOsm/kg
- Oestrogens, total male [female]   20–80 [60–400] ng/l
- Parathyroid hormone, intact   10–65 ng/l
- Packed cell volume (PCV=Hk), male [female]   40–55% [35–50%]
- Phosphatase, acid, male   0–5.5 U/l
- Phosphatase, alkaline (ALP)   25–100 U/l
- Phosphate   0.8–1.5 mmol/l
- Plasma viscosity (PV)   1.5–1.75 cp
- Plasma volume   40–50 ml/kg
- Plasminogen   100–300 mg/l
- Potassium (K^+)   3.5–5.0 mmol/l
- Porphobilinogen, 24h urine   0.9–8.8 µmol/24h
- Pressure, CSF   50–180 mmH$_2$O

Pressure cardiac, diastole/systole

- Right atrium   0/8 mmHg
- Right ventricle   0/12 mmHg
- Pulmonary artery [mean]   5/30 [9–17] mmHg
- Pulmonary capillary wedge pressure   5–15 mmHg
- Left atrium   0/12 mmHg
- Left ventricle   5–140 mmHg
- Progesteron, male [female]   <5 [15–77] nmol/l
- Prolactin, non-pregnant [pregnant]   0–20 [20–385] mg/l
- Protein, serum [CSF]   62–80 [0.15–0.4] g/l
- Prothrombine time (PT)   10–13 s
- Prostate specific antigen (PSA)   <1 mg/l
- Red cell volume (RCV)   20–30 ml/kg
- Renin, supine [standing]   3–19 [5–40] ng/l
- Renin activity, supine [standing]   0.5–1.6 [2–5x increase] µg/l/hr
- Rheumatoid factor   <1:16

Secretin	12–75 ng/l
Sex hormone binding globulin, male [female]	17–52 [35–104] nmol/l
Sodium (Na+), serum [urine]	132–144 [60–160] mmol/l
Testosterone, total, adult male [female]	12–30 [0.7–2.6] nmol/l
Thyrotopin (TSH)	0.5–5.5 mU/l
Thyroxoine (T_4), total [free]	75–150 nmol/l [10–29 pmol/l]
Total iron binding capacity	45–75 mmol/l
Total blood volume	60–80 ml/kg
Total red cell volume (^{51}CT or ^{99m}TC)	22–35 ml/kg
Total plasma volume (^{125}I-albumin)	40–50 ml/kg
Total protein	62–80 g/l
Triglycerides	<2.3 mmol/l
Triiodothyronine (T3), total [free]	1.5–3.0 nmol/l [4–7.4 pmol/l]
Troponin I / Troponin T	<0.1 ng/ml
Urea	2.5–7.5 mmol/l
Uric acid	<420 µmol/l
Urine microscopy	
• Red cells	<5 /µl
• White cells	<10 /µl
Urobilinogen, 24h urine	0.5–4.0 U/l
Uroporphyrine, 24h urine, male [female]	<55 [<26] nmol/24h
Vasoactive intestinal polypeptide (VIP)	<20 pmol/l
Vanillinmandelicacid, urine	10–35 µmol/24h

Paper 1 – Questions

1 (4 marks)

These are the feet of a 17-year-old hairdresser who complains of rapidly increasing dyspnoea on exercise.

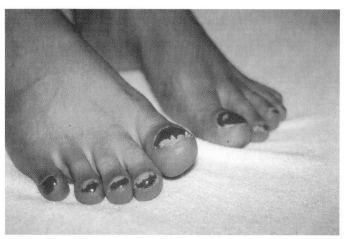

1. **What is the most likely diagnosis?**

☐ **A**   Bronchiectasis
☐ **B**   Cystic fibrosis
☐ **C**   Ventricular septal defect
☐ **D**   Kartagener's syndrome
☐ **E**   Primary pulmonary hypertension

2. **What is the likely cause for her recent symptoms?**

☐ **A**   Chest infection
☐ **B**   Shunt reversal
☐ **C**   Pneumothorax
☐ **D**   Bronchial carcinoma
☐ **E**   Pulmonary fibrosis

2 (9 marks)

A 59-year-old bachelor is admitted to the A&E Department with acute central abdominal pain. The pain came on while lifting a crate of beer out of the car and became worse over the following two hours. It is exacerbated by movement and deep inspiration. Over the last year he has noticed a decline in exercise tolerance, but has put this down to 'old age'. He has developed an irritating nocturnal cough, and a salbutamol inhaler prescribed by the GP has given no relief.

On examination he is pale and sweating and there is guarding and rebound tenderness in the umbilical region. No organomegaly is felt. Pulse 124/min, irregular; BP 105/60 mmHg. There is a right parasternal heave and a low-frequency diastolic murmur is auscultated over the apex. The chest is clear except for minimal crackles at the lung bases.

Investigations show:

Hb	121 g/l
WCC	11.3 × 10^9/l (83% granulocytes)
Plt	301 × 10^9/l
MCV	79 fl
ESR	41 mm/h

Na	138 mmol/l
K	5.0 mmol/l
Urea	10.3 mmol/l
Creatinine	156 µmol/l
Chloride	93 mmol/l
Bilirubin	21 U/l
AST	61 U/l
ALT	73 U/l

Arterial blood gases (on air):

pH	7.31
pO$_2$	10.9 kPa (82 mmHg)
pCO$_2$	4.1 kPa (31 mmHg)
Bicarbonate	18 mmol/l
O$_2$sat.	97%

Chest X-ray: Mild cardiomegaly, pulmonary congestion, left main bronchus elevated
ECG: Fast atrial fibrillation, 1-mm ST depression in V$_5$ and V$_6$.

1. **What is the cardiac abnormality?**

- [ ] **A** Mitral stenosis
- [ ] **B** Atrial septal defect
- [ ] **C** Atrial myxoma
- [ ] **D** Mitral regurgitation
- [ ] **E** Dressler's syndrome

2. **What is the cause for the acute presentation?**

- [ ] **A** Posterior myocardial infarction
- [ ] **B** Pulmonary embolus
- [ ] **C** Pericarditis
- [ ] **D** Hepatitis
- [ ] **E** Mesenteric infarction

3. **What is the cause of the acid–base abnormality?**

- [ ] **A** Acute hepatocellular injury
- [ ] **B** Alveolar hypoventilation
- [ ] **C** Acute renal failure
- [ ] **D** Lactic acidosis
- [ ] **E** Aspirin overdose

4. **Which of the following investigations is urgently indicated?**

- [ ] **A** Echocardiogram
- [ ] **B** Mesenteric angiogram
- [ ] **C** Barium enema
- [ ] **D** Ventilation–perfusion scan
- [ ] **E** Serology for atypical infection

3 (8 marks)

A 62-year-old man is admitted to Coronary Care with an acute anterior myocardial infarction. He is treated with rt-PA and makes an initially uneventful recovery. One week later he complains of increasing breathlessness and is found to be hypotensive.

On examination the venous pressure is raised and a new systolic murmur is heard through the precordium. Bilateral crackles are present at both bases, pulse 112/min, regular; BP 80/45 mmHg; respiratory rate 28/min.

The ECG shows no new changes and a chest X-ray shows bilateral peri-hilar oedema.

A right-sided cardiac catheter gives the following measurements for the pulmonary artery:

Pressure	43/14 mmHg
Capillary wedge pressure	10 mmHg
O_2 sat.	91%

1. What is the likely diagnosis?

- ☐ **A** Inferior extension of myocardial infarct
- ☐ **B** Pericardial haemorrhage
- ☐ **C** Ruptured chordae tendineae
- ☐ **D** Perforated ventricular septum
- ☐ **E** Aortic dissection

2. What is your next investigation?

- ☐ **A** Troponin T levels
- ☐ **B** Left-sided cardiac catheter
- ☐ **C** Spiral CT angiogram
- ☐ **D** Anti-myocardial antibodies
- ☐ **E** Transthoracic echocardiogram

3. What management would you recommend?

- ☐ **A** iv antibiotics
- ☐ **B** Cardiac surgery
- ☐ **C** Oral non-steroidal anti-inflammatory drugs
- ☐ **D** iv hydrocortisone
- ☐ **E** iv heparin

4 (5 marks)

A 66-year-old diabetic patient is admitted with a two-day history of pleuritic chest pain and exercise-induced dyspnoea. He had required a triple bypass eight months previously for worsening ischaemic heart disease. He had made an uneventful recovery, now only requiring glyceryl trinitrate spray two to three times per month. His current medication is enalapril for microalbuminuria and mild hypertension, 75 mg aspirin and intensified insulin therapy. On examination the patient has a temperature of 38.3 °C and the chest is clear. The heart sounds are quiet, no murmurs are heard. Pulse 92/min, regular; BP 125/70 mmHg. Sharp anterior central chest pain is provoked by deep inspiration. Examination of the abdomen is normal. Investigations reveal the following results:

Hb	134 g/l
WCC	8.8 × 10⁹/l (normal differential)
Plt	398 × 10⁹/l
ESR	43 mm/h

Na	140 mmol/l
K	4.0 mmol/l
Urea	12 mmol/l
Creatinine	153 µmol/l

ECG: Sinus rhythm 90/min, QRS axis 0°, concave ST elevation of 2–3 mm in the anterior chest leads
Chest X-ray: Mild cardiomegaly, moderate pulmonary congestion and small right pleural effusion

1. What is the likely diagnosis?

☐ **A** Silent myocardial infarction
☐ **B** Viral pericarditis
☐ **C** Left ventricular aneurysm
☐ **D** Autoimmune pericarditis
☐ **E** Myocarditis

2. What is the treatment?

☐ **A** Anticoagulation
☐ **B** Pericardial fenestration
☐ **C** Indometacin
☐ **D** Steroids
☐ **E** Streptokinase

5 (2 marks)

A 73-year-old retired postman presents with difficulties walking and intermittent confusion.

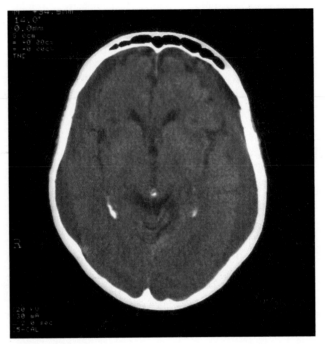

1. What is the diagnosis?

- ☐ **A**   Benign intracranial hypertension
- ☐ **B**   Extradural haematoma
- ☐ **C**   Normal-pressure hydrocephalus
- ☐ **D**   Stroke disease
- ☐ **E**   Subdural haematoma

6 (4 marks)

A 56-year-old man is under investigation for atypical chest pain. The following ECG was recorded during an exercise test. The patient has reached Stage II of the standard Bruce protocol.

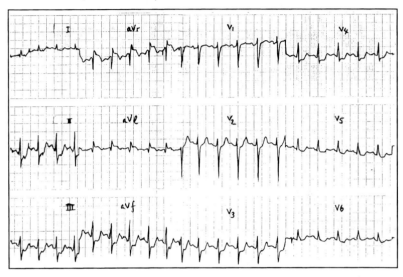

1. How do you interpret the ECG?

☐ **A**   Insignificant changes
☐ **B**   Significant ischaemia
☐ **C**   Acute myocardial infarction
☐ **D**   Old myocardial infarction
☐ **E**   Left ventricular hypertrophy

2. What further investigation would you recommend?

☐ **A**   Echocardiogram
☐ **B**   Barium swallow
☐ **C**   Thallium myocardial scintigraphy
☐ **D**   Gastroscopy
☐ **E**   Coronary angiography

7 (4 marks)

A 29-year-old woman is under investigation for renal colic. These are her blood results:

Na	139 mmol/l
K	2.8 mmol/l
Urea	6.3 mmol/l
Creatinine	131 µmol/l
Bicarbonate	13 mmol/l
Calcium	2.0 mmol/l
Phosphate	0.8 mmol/l
Albumin	29 mmol/l
Total protein	59 g/l
AST	95 U/l

1. What is the likely renal diagnosis?

- ☐ **A** Hyperoxaluria
- ☐ **B** Congenital hyperuricaemia
- ☐ **C** Renal tubular acidosis type I (distal)
- ☐ **D** Lactic acidosis type B
- ☐ **E** Cystinosis

2. Suggest an underlying cause.

- ☐ **A** Hypergammaglobulinaemia
- ☐ **B** Primary biliary cirrhosis
- ☐ **C** Wilson's disease
- ☐ **D** Chronic alcohol abuse
- ☐ **E** Multiple endocrine neoplasia type I

8 (4 marks)

The following ECG is recorded during an insurance medical from a 32-year-old builder.

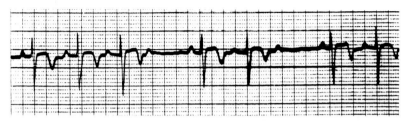

1. What is the diagnosis?

- ☐ **A** Sick sinus syndrome
- ☐ **B** First-degree heart block
- ☐ **C** Second-degree heart block
- ☐ **D** Third-degree heart block
- ☐ **E** Wandering pacemaker

2. What therapy would you recommend?

- ☐ **A** Observation only
- ☐ **B** Atropine
- ☐ **C** Verapamil
- ☐ **D** Sotalol
- ☐ **E** Pacemaker

9 (2 marks)

This is the endoscopic view of the lower oesophagus of a 42-year-old hospital manager with intermittent chest pain.

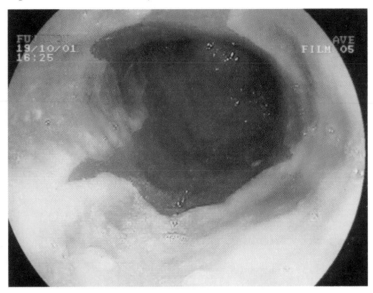

1. **Which of the following is *not* indicated?**

☐ **A**   Quadrantic biopsies
☐ **B**   Proton pump inhibitor therapy
☐ **C**   Barium swallow
☐ **D**   Repeat endoscopy
☐ **E**   Dietary advice

10 (6 marks)

A patient is admitted acutely ill. The following ECG is recorded on arrival:

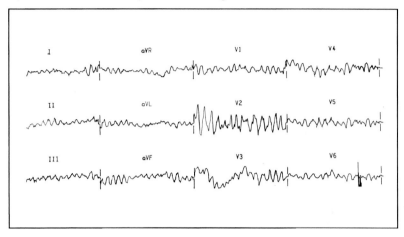

1. What does it show?

☐ **A**   Ventricular tachycardia
☐ **B**   Ventricular fibrillation
☐ **C**   Torsade de pointes
☐ **D**   Artefact
☐ **E**   Muscle tremor

2. What is your management?

☐ **A**   Check leads
☐ **B**   Precordial thump
☐ **C**   DC shock 200 J
☐ **D**   DC shock 360 J
☐ **E**   Synchronised cardioversion

The following ECG is recorded after admission to the Coronary Care Unit:

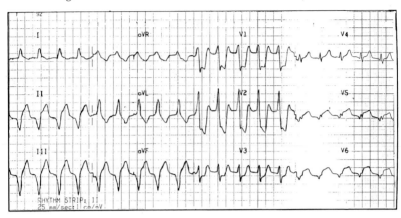

3. What is the underlying abnormality?

☐ **A** Romano-Ward syndrome
☐ **B** Lown-Ganong-Levine syndrome
☐ **C** Pericarditis
☐ **D** Myocardial infarction
☐ **E** Myocarditis

11 (5 marks)

A 22-year-old woman presents with amaurosis fugax and a heart murmur. The following are the results of her cardiac catheter study (ECG showed sinus rhythm 64/min, QRS axis +150°, incomplete right bundle branch block):

	Pressure [mmHg]	O$_2$ saturation
SVC	Mean 2	68%
RA	Mean 6	78%
RV	25/2	79%
PA	25/8	80%
LA	Mean 6	97%
LV	110/2	96%
Aorta	110/70	95%

1. What is the likely diagnosis?

☐ **A**   Ostium primum atrial septal defect
☐ **B**   Patent foramen ovale
☐ **C**   Ventricular septal defect
☐ **D**   Ostium secundum atrial septal defect
☐ **E**   Anomalous pulmonary venous drainage

2. Which of the following investigations is relatively contraindicated?

☐ **A**   Ventilation–perfusion lung scan
☐ **B**   Exercise tolerance test
☐ **C**   Coronary angiogram
☐ **D**   Cerebral angiogram
☐ **E**   Myocardial scintigraphy

12 (5 marks)

A 43-year-old diabetic is under investigation for deteriorating exercise tolerance. On examination he looks very well, pulse 68/min, regular; BP 160/90 mmHg.

The following results are obtained:

Hb	181 g/l
WCC	5.2 × 10⁹/l

U&Es	Normal
Bilirubin	43 mmol/l
AST	412 U/l
ALT	387 U/l

Echocardiogram: Left ventricular dilatation and dyskinesia, ejection fraction 23%

1. What is the cardiac diagnosis?

□ **A**   Ischaemic heart disease
□ **B**   Viral myocarditis
□ **C**   Toxic cardiomyopathy
□ **D**   Amyloidosis
□ **E**   Constrictive pericarditis

2. What therapy would you recommend?

□ **A**   Steroids
□ **B**   Venesection
□ **C**   Cyclophosphamide
□ **D**   α-interferon
□ **E**   Cardiac transplant

13 (2 marks)

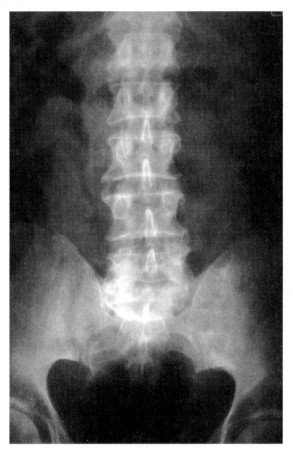

1. **Which of the following is *least* likely to cause the appearance on this abdominal X-ray?**

☐ **A** Diverticular disease
☐ **B** Carcinoma of the colon
☐ **C** Radiotherapy of the pelvis
☐ **D** Lymphoma
☐ **E** Crohn's disease

(Radiograph courtesy of Dr A J Bradley)

14 (9 marks)

A 35-year-old woman presents with a seven-month history of palpitations and intermittent diarrhoea. She describes episodes of 'feeling sweaty and hungry' but has lost 5 kg in weight. She smokes 10 cigarettes a day, drinks approximately 20 units of alcohol per week and her only medication is a low-dose oestrogen contraceptive pill. On examination, she has a pulse rate of 115/min, which is irregular in rate and volume, BP 150/95 mmHg. Examination of the abdomen is normal. Investigations show:

FBC	Normal
U&Es	Normal
Random blood glucose	4.2 mmol/l
Serum albumin	42 g/l
Bilirubin	18 µmol/l
ALT	28 U/l
Total serum thyroxine (tT4)	285 nmol/l (75–150 nmol/l)
3-tri-iodothyronine (fT3)	13.5 pmol/l (3–9 pmol/l)
Serum TSH	9.3 mU/l (0.5–5.5 mU/l)
Serum TRH	Not measurable

Ultrasound of the thyroid shows diffuse enlargement of both lobes and the isthmus, without focal abnormality.

1. What is the diagnosis?

- ☐ **A** Primary hyperthyroidism
- ☐ **B** Secondary hyperthyroidism
- ☐ **C** Tertiary hyperthyroidism
- ☐ **D** Self-administration of thyroxine
- ☐ **E** Subacute thyroiditis

2. Which examination is likely to be the most useful?

- ☐ **A** TRH test
- ☐ **B** Ultrasound of the pelvis
- ☐ **C** MR scan of the pituitary
- ☐ **D** Thyroid autoantibodies
- ☐ **E** Radio-isotope thyroid scan

The patient fails to attend follow-up, but is referred back to the clinic one year later with the following results:

Hb   95 g/l
WCC   1.8 × 10⁹/l (89% lymphocytes)
Plt   138 × 10⁹/l

Total T4   195 nmol/l (75–150 nmol/l)
Serum TSH   16.2 mU/l (0.5–5.5 mU/l)

3. What therapy has the patient had in the interim?

☐ **A**   Radioiodine therapy
☐ **B**   Subtotal thyroidectomy
☐ **C**   Partial hypophysectomy
☐ **D**   Carbimazole
☐ **E**   No treatment

4. What therapy is likely to be most effective?

☐ **A**   Carbimazole combined with thyroxine
☐ **B**   Total thyroidectomy
☐ **C**   Trans-sphenoidal hypophysectomy
☐ **D**   Radiotherapy of the pituitary fossa
☐ **E**   Propylthiouracil

15 (10 marks)

A 71-year-old retired carpenter is brought to the Casualty Department following a grand mal fit. In the resuscitation room the patient has two further generalised seizures without regaining consciousness between them. His past medical history includes hypertension, which has been well controlled over the last 15 years on Moduretic® (amiloride and hydrochlorothiazide). A year previously his diet-controlled diabetes worsened and he was started on chlorpropamide by his GP.

On examination, the patient has a Glasgow Coma Scale score of 7/15, only localising to pain. There is mild meningism but no focal neurology. Fundoscopy only shows some silver-wiring and AV-nipping. The chest is clear and examination of heart and abdomen are normal. The following results are obtained:

Hb	146 g/l
WCC	10.6 × 10⁹/l
Plt	285 × 10⁹/l
Na	110 mmol/l
K	3.5 mmol/l
Urea	4.0 mmol/l
Creatinine	168 µmol/l
Glucose	9 mmol/l
Urine osmolality	589 mOsm/kg
Chest X-ray	normal
CT brain	normal

1. What is the serum osmolality?

☐ **A**   230
☐ **B**   240
☐ **C**   253.5
☐ **D**   267
☐ **E**   270.5

2. What is the likely diagnosis?

☐ **A**   Water intoxication
☐ **B**   Peripheral diabetes insipidus
☐ **C**   Central diabetes insipidus
☐ **D**   Addisonian crisis
☐ **E**   Syndrome of inappropriate ADH secretion (SIADH)

3. What two treatments would you instigate?

- ☐ **A** iv saline and phenobarbitone
- ☐ **B** iv hydrocortisone and diazepam
- ☐ **C** im hydrocortisone and iv furosemide (frusemide)
- ☐ **D** Fluid restriction and iv diazepam
- ☐ **E** iv phenytoin and saline

No medical bed is available and the patient is treated by the A&E staff. The following morning the patient is transferred under your care. He has made an initial recovery, his Glasgow Coma Scale score returning to 14, with some remaining disorientation. However, over the following hours the patient deteriorates rapidly again and becomes hypotensive and unresponsive. There is generalised reduction in tone but both plantars are up-going.

Biochemical profile now reveals:

Na	129 mmol/l
K	2.8 mmol/l
Urea	2.2 mmol/l
Creatinine	151 μmol/l
Glucose	8 mmol/l

4. What is the likely cause?

- ☐ **A** Diazepam overdose
- ☐ **B** Central pontine myelinolysis
- ☐ **C** Cerebral oedema
- ☐ **D** Cerebral infarction
- ☐ **E** Brainstem haemorrhage

5. What examination is most likely to be diagnostic?

- ☐ **A** CT of the brain
- ☐ **B** MR scan of the brain
- ☐ **C** EEG
- ☐ **D** ADH levels
- ☐ **E** Urinary electrolytes

16 (2 marks)

A 14-year-old girl with short stature is under investigation for delayed skeletal maturation. The following results were obtained during an Ellsworth-Howard test.

	Baseline	After infusion of parathormone
Urinary phosphate [nmol/d]	4.8	5.0
Urinary cyclic-AMP [nmol/mmol creatinine]	0.31	0.29
Parathyroid hormone [pmol/l]	261(10–90)	
9am growth hormone [mU/l]	7 (4–8)	

1. What is the likely diagnosis?

- ☐ **A** Hypoparathyroidism
- ☐ **B** Hyperparathyroidism
- ☐ **C** Pseudohypoparathyroidism type I
- ☐ **D** Pseudohypoparathyroidism type II
- ☐ **E** Pseudo-pseudohypoparathyroidism

17 (2 marks)

These are the forearms of a 41-year-old woman with chest pain.

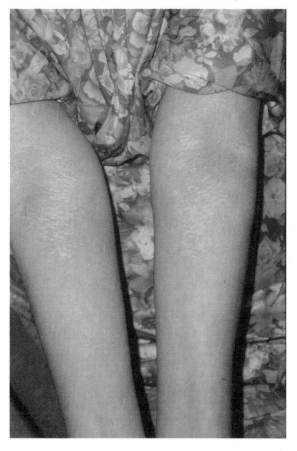

1. What is the likely cause of her symptoms?

- ☐ **A** Ischaemic heart disease
- ☐ **B** Oesophageal dysmotility
- ☐ **C** Pneumothorax
- ☐ **D** Pulmonary embolus
- ☐ **E** Pericarditis

18 (4 marks)

A 25-year-old woman presents with atrial fibrillation. The only medication she is taking is the oral contraceptive pill.

Investigations show:

Total T4   164 nmol/l (75–150 nmol/l)
Free T4   14.2 pmol/l (10–25 pmol/l)

A TRH test is performed.
TSH levels after 20 µg TRH iv:

0 minutes   < 0.1 U/l
30 minutes   < 0.1 U/l

1. What is the diagnosis?

☐ **A**   Autonomous adenoma
☐ **B**   Pregnancy
☐ **C**   T3 thyrotoxicosis
☐ **D**   Hashimoto's thyroiditis
☐ **E**   Self-medication with thyroxine

2. How do you interpret the total T4 levels?

☐ **A**   Increased thyroxine-binding globulin (TBG)
☐ **B**   Reactive increase
☐ **C**   Cell damage
☐ **D**   Increased fetal thyroxine
☐ **E**   Paraneoplastic phenomenon

19 (6 marks)

A 42-year-old woman presents with a tender neck swelling. The following results are obtained:

Hb	144 g/l
WCC	5.2 × 10⁹/l
ESR	99 mm/h
Total T4	192 nmol/l (75–150 nmol/l)
TSH	<0.1 mU/l (0.5–5.5 mU/l)

⁹⁹ᵐTechnetium thyroid scan shows diffuse reduction in uptake, no hot spots.

1. What is the most likely diagnosis?

- ☐ **A** Subacute thyroiditis
- ☐ **B** Acute bacterial thyroiditis
- ☐ **C** Autoimmune thyroiditis
- ☐ **D** Iodine deficiency
- ☐ **E** Toxic multinodular goitre

2. What management is most appropriate?

- ☐ **A** Ultrasound scan and antibiotics
- ☐ **B** Thyroid antibodies and oral thyroxine
- ☐ **C** Fine-needle aspiration and systemic steroids
- ☐ **D** Estimation of free T3 and T4 and carbimazole
- ☐ **E** Radioiodine therapy and oral thyroxine

3. What is the most likely complication without treatment?

- ☐ **A** Abscess formation
- ☐ **B** Established thyrotoxicosis
- ☐ **C** Malignant change
- ☐ **D** Hypothyroidism
- ☐ **E** Solid fibrosis of the thyroid

20 (5 marks)

A 61-year-old woman is under investigation for a six-month history of tiredness and weight loss. These are her blood results:

Na	132 mmol/l
K	5.8 mmol/l
Urea	5.7 mmol/l
Creatinine	138 µmol/l
Hb	107 g/l
MCV	105 fl
WCC	3.8×10^9/l
Plt	158×10^9/l
TSH	9.8 mU/l (0.5–5.5 mU/l)
9am cortisol	66 nmol/l
9am growth hormone	6 mU/l (4–10 mU/l)

1. What is the diagnosis?

☐ **A** Sheehan's syndrome
☐ **B** Addison's disease
☐ **C** Polyglandular failure (Schmidt's syndrome)
☐ **D** Hashimoto's thyroiditis
☐ **E** Acromegaly

2. Which of the following investigations would be the most useful?

☐ **A** Autoantibody screen
☐ **B** MR scan of the pituitary
☐ **C** Short Synacthen® test
☐ **D** TRH test
☐ **E** Ultrasound scan of the thyroid

21 (8 marks)

A 23-year-old male travel agent presents to his GP with a short history of increasing heartburn and dysphagia. He was treated with moderate success with anti-reflux medication, but over the following months developed recurring episodes of spasmodic abdominal pain associated with watery diarrhoea. He has lost 2 kg in weight, there is cervical lymphadenopathy, abdominal examination is unremarkable. Two dark nodules are present on his arm. The following results are obtained:

Hb	122 g/l
MCV	98/fl
WCC	3.8 × 10⁹/l
Plt	156 × 10⁹/l
ESR	18 mm/h

Electrolytes	Normal
LFTs	Normal
Albumin	28 g/l
Faecal occult blood × 3 –ve	

A Dicopac® test shows the following results:

Urinary excretion of vitamin B$_{12}$	15%
Urinary excretion of combined intrinsic factor and B$_{12}$	19%

1. **What do these results suggest?**

- [ ] **A** Normal vitamin B$_{12}$ metabolism
- [ ] **B** Pernicious anaemia
- [ ] **C** Terminal ileal disease
- [ ] **D** Atrophic gastritis
- [ ] **E** Bacterial overgrowth

The patient is admitted for investigations. A barium swallow shows fine confluent ulceration of the oesophagus. Colonoscopy shows small patches of inflammation in the large bowel. The ileocaecal junction shows nodular thickening of the bowel wall; the mucosa is intact except for a few small areas of aphthous ulceration.

2. **What is the likely cause for the patient's dysphagia?**

- [ ] **A** Barrett's oesophagus
- [ ] **B** *Candida* oesophagitis
- [ ] **C** Cytomegalovirus (CMV)
- [ ] **D** Plummer-Vinson syndrome
- [ ] **E** Gastro-oesophageal reflux

3. What is the likely underlying cause?

- ☐ **A** Ulcerative colitis
- ☐ **B** Crohn's disease
- ☐ **C** HIV infection
- ☐ **D** *Campylobacter* infection
- ☐ **E** Small bowel carcinoma

An ultrasound of the abdomen shows several hypoechoic foci in the liver and mild splenomegaly. An indolent mass is seen in the right iliac fossa.

4. What complication has occurred?

- ☐ **A** Haematogenic liver abscesses
- ☐ **B** Adenocarcinoma with liver metastases
- ☐ **C** Focal fatty change due to malabsorption
- ☐ **D** Hepatoma
- ☐ **E** Secondary lymphoma

22 (8 marks)

A 29-year-old Greek immigrant is admitted to the A&E Department with a severe episode of abdominal pain. In the past year she had three similar admissions to different hospitals, but was discharged after a few days with no specific diagnosis made. She was well until 15 months ago when she took an overdose of paracetamol and was started on fluoxetine by her GP. She is currently on no other medication. On examination she appears in pain. The abdomen is tender with some rebound pain and voluntary guarding. Bowel sounds are active. There is no hepatosplenomegaly or lymphadenopathy. The chest is clear. There is no focal neurology. Heart rate 104/min, sinus rhythm; BP 105/60 mmHg.

Hb	108 g/l
WCC	5.6 × 10⁹/l
Plt	322 × 10⁹/l
ESR	7 mm/h
Na	127 mmol/l
K	3.0 mmol/l
Urea	4.0 mmol/l
Glucose	5 mmol/l
Dipstix urinalysis:	Protein + +, Blood –, Bilirubin +
Urine osmolality	895 mOsm/kg

1. **Suggest two investigations.**

  ☐ **A**   Intravenous urogram
  ☐ **B**   Chest X-ray
  ☐ **C**   Faecal porphyrins
  ☐ **D**   Abdominal ultrasound
  ☐ **E**   Skin biopsy
  ☐ **F**   Urine microscopy and culture
  ☐ **G**   Abdominal X-ray
  ☐ **H**   Urinary porphyrins
  ☐ **I**   Lipid profile
  ☐ **J**   Amylase levels

2. **What is the likely diagnosis?**

  ☐ **A**   Primary amyloidosis
  ☐ **B**   Pancreatitis
  ☐ **C**   Acute intermittent porphyria
  ☐ **D**   Familial Mediterranean fever
  ☐ **E**   Lesch-Nyhan syndrome

The patient recovers spontaneously over the following two days.

3. Suggest two steps in the further management.

- ☐ **A** Psychiatry assessment
- ☐ **B** Regular venesection
- ☐ **C** Stop fluoxetine
- ☐ **D** Sun avoidance
- ☐ **E** Prophylactic colchicine
- ☐ **F** Monitor white blood cell differential
- ☐ **G** Splenectomy
- ☐ **H** Colonic screening
- ☐ **I** Iron therapy
- ☐ **J** Low-dose aspirin

23 (5 marks)

A 56-year-old veterinary surgeon is under investigation for recurrent chest and upper respiratory tract infections. He also gives a history of episodic diarrhoea over the last 18 months. Clinical examination is normal. His blood results show:

Full blood count	Normal
Electrolytes	Normal
Total protein	59 g/l
Albumin	51 g/l
IgG	4.5 g/l (7.5–15 g/l)
IgA	0.3 g/l (1.2–4.0 g/l)
IgM	0.3 g/l (0.5–1.5 g/l)

1. What is the likely diagnosis?

- ☐ **A** Hodgkin's disease
- ☐ **B** Non-Hodgkin's lymphoma
- ☐ **C** Acquired hypogammaglobinaemia
- ☐ **D** Kartagener's syndrome
- ☐ **E** Yellow nail syndrome

2. What is the most likely cause for the diarrhoea?

- ☐ **A** Villous atrophy
- ☐ **B** Maldigestion
- ☐ **C** Lymphoma of the terminal ileum
- ☐ **D** Chronic *Giardia* infection
- ☐ **E** Steatorrhoea

24 (2 marks)

A 42-year-old patient has collapsed on the ward.

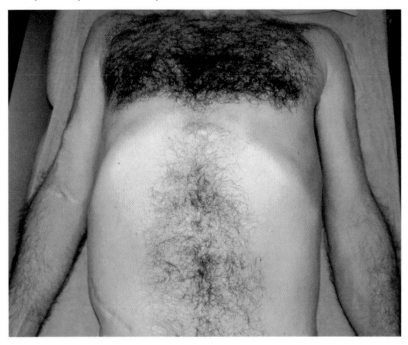

1. Which of the following is the *least* likely precipitating cause?

☐ **A**   Cerebral haemorrhage
☐ **B**   Aortic dissection
☐ **C**   Cerebral abscess
☐ **D**   Ventricular arrhythmia
☐ **E**   Viral encephalitis

25 (6 marks)

A 26-year-old woman is under investigation at the infertility clinic for malaise and secondary amenorrhoea. On examination she is moderately obese with abdominal striae and spider naevi. A firm tender liver edge can just be palpated under the right costal margin. Investigations show:

Hb	113 g/l
WBC	4.8×10^9/l
Plt	128×10^9/l

Electrolytes	Normal
Albumin	32 g/l
Total protein	86 g/l
Bilirubin	92 µmol/l
AST	512 U/l

1. What is the most likely diagnosis?

- ☐ **A** Haemochromatosis
- ☐ **B** Autoimmune chronic active hepatitis
- ☐ **C** Wilson's disease
- ☐ **D** α_1-antitrypsin deficiency
- ☐ **E** Hepatitis E

2. Which of the following is the most important investigation?

- ☐ **A** Liver ultrasound
- ☐ **B** ERCP
- ☐ **C** Hepatitis serology
- ☐ **D** Coeruloplasmin level
- ☐ **E** Liver biopsy

3. What treatment would you recommend?

- ☐ **A** Azathioprine
- ☐ **B** Immunoglobulins
- ☐ **C** Liver transplant
- ☐ **D** Repeated venesection
- ☐ **E** D-penicillamine

26 (6 marks)

A 16-year-old boy is admitted after an episode of haematemesis. The only past history of note is a premature delivery at 30 weeks followed by hyaline membrane disease. The spleen is enlarged, the liver is not palpable. Gastroscopy shows oesophageal varices which are successfully injected and sclerosed. Ascites is found which shows the following biochemistry:

Specific gravity	1025
Protein	28 g/l
Glucose	5.8 mmol/l
Blood glucose	6.2 mmol/l

1. What do these results suggest?

- ☐ **A** Septic peritonitis
- ☐ **B** Portal vein thrombosis
- ☐ **C** Tuberculous peritonitis
- ☐ **D** End-stage liver cirrhosis
- ☐ **E** Budd-Chiari syndrome

2. What is the likely underlying cause?

- ☐ **A** Prolonged severe illness in the neonatal period
- ☐ **B** Umbilical vein catheterisation
- ☐ **C** Hepatitis C following transfusion
- ☐ **D** Hypogammaglobulinaemia
- ☐ **E** α_1-antitrypsin deficiency

After two days the patient has a further episode of haematemesis.

3. What is the likely cause?

- ☐ **A** Mucosal necrosis following sclerotherapy
- ☐ **B** Boerhaave's syndrome
- ☐ **C** Fundal varices
- ☐ **D** Recanalisation of the oesophageal varices
- ☐ **E** Acute on chronic liver failure due to GI haemorrhage

27 (5 marks)

A 42-year-old woman is admitted for investigation of nocturnal fits. Her weight has increased by 3 kg over the last six months. Three separate early morning glucose samples were obtained with the following results:

Monday	4.6 mmol/l
Tuesday	2.3 mmol/l
Wednesday	7.8 mmol/l

C-peptide after 24-hour fast 1.8 nmol/l (normal range 0.2–0.6 nmol/l)

1. **What diagnosis do these results suggest?**

- [ ] **A**   Glucagonoma
- [ ] **B**   Self-administration of insulin
- [ ] **C**   Multiple endocrine neoplasia type I
- [ ] **D**   Insulinoma
- [ ] **E**   Maturity onset of diabetes in the young (MODY)

2. **What is the next investigation?**

- [ ] **A**   Repeat C-peptide after 72-hour fast
- [ ] **B**   Estimation of pro-insulin
- [ ] **C**   Oral glucose tolerance test
- [ ] **D**   CT pancreas
- [ ] **E**   Insulin stress test

28 (1 mark)

This is a sigmoid spot view from a barium enema in a 58-year-old patient with abdominal pain.

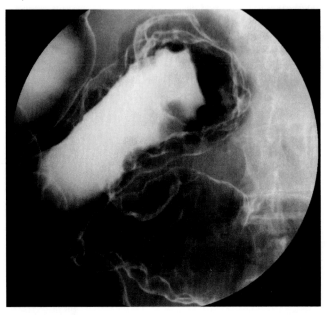

1. What does it show?

☐ **A** Polyposis coli
☐ **B** Carcinoma
☐ **C** Pneumatosis coli
☐ **D** Crohn's disease
☐ **E** Ischaemic colitis

29 (9 marks)

A 59-year-old woman is being referred for investigation of amaurosis fugax. She was started on enalapril and low-dose aspirin six months previously by her GP for newly diagnosed hypertension and one TIA affecting her left arm.

She has been previously well, smokes 15 cigarettes per day and drinks two glasses of sherry per night.

On examination she looks extremely well; BP 165/95 mmHg; pulse 68/min, regular; on auscultation 2/6 ejection systolic murmur over the aorta.

The lungs are clear. A mass is palpable in the left upper quadrant and no enlarged lymph nodes are found. Examination of the CNS is unremarkable.

The following blood results are obtained:

Hb	158 g/l
MCV	67 fl
MCHC	26 g/dl
WCC	14.2×10^9/l
Differential: neutrophils 83%, lymphocytes 11%, monocytes 5%	
Plt	489×10^9/l
PCV	0.58
Blood film	Hypochromia, polychromasia
Biochemical profile	Normal

1. What examination is *least* likely to be useful?

- ☐ **A** Chest X-ray
- ☐ **B** Erythrocyte sedimentation rate
- ☐ **C** Ultrasound abdomen
- ☐ **D** Arterial blood gases
- ☐ **E** Bone marrow biopsy

While on the ward, the patient has a severe episode of epistaxis.

2. Which of the following tests is likely to be *normal*?

- ☐ **A** Bleeding time
- ☐ **B** Uric acid levels
- ☐ **C** Free iron binding capacity
- ☐ **D** Erythropoietin
- ☐ **E** Prothrombin time

3. What is the treatment?

- [ ] **A** 5-hydroxyurea
- [ ] **B** Aspirin
- [ ] **C** Venesection
- [ ] **D** Methotrexate
- [ ] **E** Splenectomy

The patient is treated successfully and makes a good recovery. Seven years later, however, she is re-admitted with the following results:

Hb   91 g/l
WCC $2.8 \times 10^9/l$
Plt $93 \times 10^9/l$
Blood film: Multiple nucleated red cells, myeloblasts and megakaryocytes
ESR   52 mm/h

On examination, the patient is pale and several ecchymoses are present over her arms and trunk. A firm mass is occupying the whole of the abdomen.

4. What complication has arisen?

- [ ] **A** Chronic myeloid leukaemia
- [ ] **B** Aplastic anaemia
- [ ] **C** Iron depletion
- [ ] **D** Myelofibrosis
- [ ] **E** Acute myelomonocytic leukaemia

30 (7 marks)

A 10-year-old boy is under investigation for suspected bilateral Perthes' disease of the hip. While on bed rest, awaiting investigation, he develops painful swelling of the right leg.

Examination of the abdomen shows no enlargement of liver or spleen, and there is no adenopathy. The chest is clear. The circumference of the mid-thigh on the right is increased by 2 cm when compared with the left. No cellulitis is seen.

The following results are obtained:

Hb	142 g/l
WCC	6.7×10^9/l
Plt	338×10^9/l
ESR	31mm/h
Biochemical profile	Normal
PT	12 s (control 12–14 s)
APTT	31 s (control 32–34 s)
Bleeding time	5.5 min (5–8 min)
D-dimer	960 μg/l (20–400 μg/l)

1. Which of the following examinations is likely to be *least* useful?

- ☐ **A** Thrombin time
- ☐ **B** Doppler ultrasound
- ☐ **C** Protein C levels
- ☐ **D** Protein S levels
- ☐ **E** Antithrombin levels

The patient is fully anticoagulated with low molecular weight heparin. Two days later, whilst still on bed rest, he develops a tender swelling of the left calf. A venogram is performed which demonstrates thrombosis of two pairs of calf veins but patent popliteal and femoral veins.

2. What is the most likely diagnosis?

- ☐ **A** Protein C deficiency
- ☐ **B** Protein S deficiency
- ☐ **C** Disseminated intravascular coagulation
- ☐ **D** Antithrombin III deficiency
- ☐ **E** Haemoglobin C disease

An ultrasound scan of the abdomen and a chest X-ray are normal. While awaiting the results of further investigations, oral anticoagulants are withheld.

One week later the patient develops bruising over the extensor surfaces and has a severe episode of epistaxis.

The following results are obtained:

Hb	138 g/l
WCC	6.2×10^9/l
Plt	32×10^9/l
Prothrombin time	13 s (control 12–14 s)

3. What is the likely cause for the haemorrhage?

☐ **A**   Disseminated intravascular coagulation
☐ **B**   Heparin overdose
☐ **C**   Hypersplenism
☐ **D**   Heparin side-effect
☐ **E**   Factor VIII depletion

31 (6 marks)

A 21-year-old woman is brought to the Accident & Emergency Department by her mother with a three-day history of fevers to 39 °C with associated rigors and increasing confusion.

The blood results show:

Hb	89 g/l
MCV	76 fl
RCC	2.6×10^{12}/l (0.2% reticulocytes)
WCC	1.1×10^9/l (95% lymphocytes, no blasts)
Plt	23×10^9/l

1. What investigation would you perform?

- ☐ **A** Epstein-Barr virus antibody titres
- ☐ **B** Throat swab
- ☐ **C** Bone marrow biopsy
- ☐ **D** Lumbar puncture
- ☐ **E** Serum and urine drug screen

2. Which of the following diagnoses is *least* likely?

- ☐ **A** Acute myeloid leukaemia
- ☐ **B** Hodgkin's disease
- ☐ **C** Drug-induced aplastic anaemia
- ☐ **D** Postviral aplastic anaemia
- ☐ **E** Idiopathic aplastic anaemia

3. What is the immediate management?

- ☐ **A** iv immunoglobulins
- ☐ **B** Transfusion of granulocytes
- ☐ **C** Stimulators of granulopoiesis (GM-CSF)
- ☐ **D** iv antibiotics
- ☐ **E** iv hydrocortisone

32 (1 mark)

This is the hand of a 28-year-old pianist who has increasing difficulties playing his instrument.

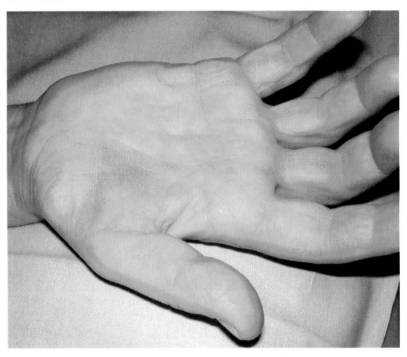

1. **Which is the likely level of the lesion demonstrated?**

☐ **A** Cerebral cortex
☐ **B** Internal capsule
☐ **C** Medulla oblongata
☐ **D** Brachial plexus
☐ **E** Carpal tunnel

33 (4 marks)

A 37-year-old Hindu woman presents with tiredness and menorrhagia. The following results are obtained:

Hb	91 g/l
MCV	108 fl
WCC	3.1×10^9/l
Plt	128×10^9/l
Biochemical profile	Normal
Serum gastrin	31 pmol/l (20–100 pmol/l)

1. What is the most likely diagnosis?

☐ **A** Dietary deficiency
☐ **B** Aplastic anaemia
☐ **C** Organophosphate poisoning
☐ **D** Pernicious anaemia
☐ **E** Hookworm infection

2. Suggest two further investigations.

☐ **A** Schilling test
☐ **B** Vitamin B_{12} levels
☐ **C** Bone marrow biopsy
☐ **D** Blood film
☐ **E** Gastroscopy and biopsy

34 (4 marks)

A 28-year-old Asian man is investigated for night sweats and low-grade pyrexia. He has also developed an intolerance to alcohol. Clinical examination is normal. Blood samples show the following results:

Hb   132 g/l
WCC   4.7 × 10⁹/l (87% neutrophils,
                        7% eosinophils)
Plt   218 × 10⁹/l
ESR   56 mm/h

Ultrasound abdomen   Normal

1. What is the likely diagnosis?

☐ A   Pulmonary aspergillosis
☐ B   Non-Hodgkin's lymphoma
☐ C   Hodgkin's disease
☐ D   Hydatid disease
☐ E   Pulmonary eosinophilia

2. Which of the following treatments would you recommend?

☐ A   Radiotherapy
☐ B   Chemotherapy
☐ C   Amphotericin B
☐ D   Surgical excision
☐ E   Oral prednisolone

35 (6 marks)

A 15-year-old Israeli boy is returned to the UK by air ambulance from a holiday in Kenya. He had not felt particularly ill, but on the second day he developed jaundice and frank haematuria. His pulse rate is 100/min, regular; BP 110/60 mmHg. His blood results show:

Hb	87 g/l
MCV	101 fl
WCC	$5.9 \times 10^9/l$
Plt	$329 \times 10^9/l$
ESR	34 mm/h
Haptoglobin	12 mg/dl (50–200 mg/dl)

Blood film: Bite cells, extensive Heinz body formation, 11% reticulocytes

1. **What is the most important step in the management?**

☐ **A** Intravenous hydrocortisone
☐ **B** Discontinue any medication
☐ **C** Administration of two units O rhesus-negative blood
☐ **D** Plasmapheresis
☐ **E** Continue malaria prophylaxis

2. **What is the likely diagnosis?**

☐ **A** Glucose-6-phosphate-dehydrogenase deficiency
☐ **B** Rotor syndrome
☐ **C** Hereditary spherocytosis
☐ **D** Haemoglobin C disease
☐ **E** Hereditary elliptocytosis

3. **What is the inheritance of this condition?**

☐ **A** Sporadic
☐ **B** Autosomal dominant
☐ **C** Autosomal recessive
☐ **D** X-linked dominant
☐ **E** X-linked recessive

36 (1 mark)

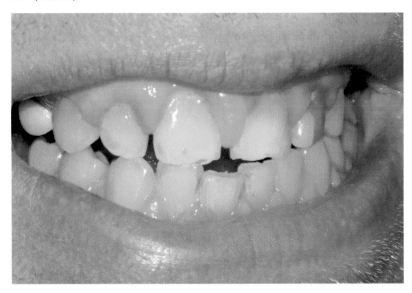

1. Which of the following is *not* a recognised cause of this appearance?

☐ **A**   Amiodarone
☐ **B**   Ciclosporin
☐ **C**   Acute myelomonocytic leukaemia
☐ **D**   Phenytoin
☐ **E**   Nifedipine

37 (9 marks)

A 66-year-old man is under investigation for backache, weight loss and intermittent low-grade temperature. In the past he had a Polya gastrectomy at the age of 39 for recurrent ulcers, and a right-sided renal colic ten years previously. His current medication is lisinopril and bumetanide K for moderate hypertension and warfarin which was started three years previously for transient ischaemic attacks. He is an ex-smoker and drinks approximately 25 units of alcohol per week.

Clinical examination reveals an emphysematous chest; BP 160/90 mmHg; pulse 80–85/min, atrial fibrillation; 1/6 ejection systolic murmur in the aortic area; and a soft right-sided carotid bruit. The liver edge is just palpable but non-tender, the spleen is not enlarged. The left testicle is tender with a moderate varicocele. No lymphadenopathy is present and the CNS shows no deficit.

The following results are obtained:

Hb	179 g/l
WCC	4.7×10^9/l
Plt	210×10^9/l
PCV	0.68
ESR	70 mm/h
INR	3.4

Na	147 mmol/l
K	3.2 mmol/l
Creatinine	178 µmol/l
Random glucose	6.8 mmol/l
Dipstix urinalysis	Glucose –, Bilirubin –, Blood + +, Protein +
Urinary Na	48 mmol/l (60–160 mmol/l)

1. What is the likely diagnosis?

☐ A   Renal artery stenosis
☐ B   Renal infarction
☐ C   Adrenal carcinoma
☐ D   Conn's syndrome
☐ E   Hypernephroma

2. What is the likely cause for the electrolyte disturbance?

☐ A   Diuretic therapy
☐ B   ACE-inhibitor therapy
☐ C   Hyperaldosteronaemia
☐ D   Hyperreninaemia
☐ E   Reduced renal blood flow

3. What complication has apparently arisen?

☐ **A**   Renal artery occlusion
☐ **B**   Renal vein thrombosis
☐ **C**   Renal embolisation
☐ **D**   Chronic renal hypoxia
☐ **E**   Secondary hyperaldosteronism

While awaiting further investigations, the patient collapses with a right-sided weakness and up-going plantar. An immediate CT brain is reported as normal.

4. What cause has to be considered?

☐ **A**   Hypertensive stroke
☐ **B**   Significant hypotensive episode
☐ **C**   Vascular occlusion due to polycythaemia
☐ **D**   Embolism from right carotid plaque
☐ **E**   Over-anticoagulation

38 (5 marks)

A 23-year-old medical student on holiday in Greece became unwell with a sore throat, cervical lymphadenopathy and a low-grade pyrexia. He started himself on oral amoxicillin, but three days later noticed a dark discoloration of his urine. This improved slightly with increased fluid intake, but he went to consult a local GP as there was no improvement in his symptoms after five days. He was given oral clarithromycin and after a further two days he developed abdominal pain and diarrhoea. He returned to the United Kingdom and presented to Casualty.

On examination, he has some small lymph nodes in the anterior cervical triangle. Both tonsils and Waldeyer's ring are mildly erythematous, but no pus is seen. There is tenderness in both loins but no hepatosplenomegaly. BP 175/95; mmHg, pulse 88/min, regular; no peripheral oedema; normal fundoscopy.

The following results were obtained:

Hb	151 g/l
WCC	8.5 × 10⁹/l (58% lymphocytes)
Plt	158 × 10⁹/l
ESR	24 mm/h

Na	142 mmol/l
K	4.1 mmol/l
Urea	9.8 mmol/l
Creatinine	134 μmol/l

Urinary Na	85 mmol/l (60–160 mmol/l)
Dipstix urinalysis	Blood + + +, Protein +, Glucose +

Urine microscopy: Numerous red cells, some red cell casts

Serum C3 complement	1.25 g/l (0.55–1.20 g/l)
Serum C4 complement	0.38 g/l (0.20–0.50 g/l)

1. What is the likely diagnosis?

☐ **A** Poststreptococcal glomerulonephritis
☐ **B** Henoch-Schönlein purpura
☐ **C** Wegener's granulomatosis
☐ **D** Acute tubular necrosis
☐ **E** IgA nephropathy

2. How would you confirm the diagnosis?

☐ **A** Culture of a throat swab
☐ **B** ASO titre
☐ **C** Renal biopsy
☐ **D** Autoantibody screen
☐ **E** Serum IgA levels

39 (3 marks)

A diet-controlled type II diabetic is admitted with blunt abdominal trauma following a road traffic accident. He is stabilised with conservative management, but a day later shows the following blood results:

Na	142 mmol/l
K	5.5 mmol/l
Chloride	98 mmol/l
Bicarbonate	19.5 mmol/l
Urea	16 mmol/l
Creatinine	196 µmol/l
Glucose	13 mmol/l
Dipstix urinalysis	Blood + +, Protein –, Ketones + Glucose + +

1. What is the likely cause for these results?

- ☐ **A**   Renal contusion
- ☐ **B**   Ketoacidosis
- ☐ **C**   Lactic acidosis type A
- ☐ **D**   Lactic acidosis type B
- ☐ **E**   Rhabdomyolysis

40 (2 marks)

A 23-year-old man who had been fostered as a child is under investigation for abdominal pain and hypertension.

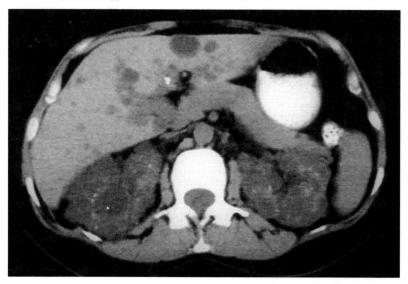

1. **What is the diagnosis?**

☐ **A** Phaeochromocytoma
☐ **B** Von Hippel-Lindau syndrome
☐ **C** Conn's syndrome
☐ **D** Adult polycystic kidney disease
☐ **E** Infantile polycystic kidney disease

41 (4 marks)

A 46-year-old woman had a pan-proctocolectomy for ulcerative colitis at the age of 38. She now presents with symptoms of an acute left renal colic. A plain abdominal radiograph shows no evidence of stones. Ultrasound of the kidneys shows no evidence of hydronephrosis. The following blood results are obtained:

Na	141 mmol/l
K	3.6 mmol/l
Urea	7.8 mmol/l
Bicarbonate	18 mmol/l
Albumin	31 g/l
Calcium	2.2 mmol/l
Phosphate	0.85 mmol/l

1. What is the most likely diagnosis?

- ☐ **A** Renal papillary necrosis
- ☐ **B** Urate stones
- ☐ **C** Oxalate stones
- ☐ **D** Retroperitoneal fibrosis
- ☐ **E** Ureteric stricture

2. What treatment would you suggest?

- ☐ **A** Ureteric stent
- ☐ **B** Extracorporeal lithotripsy
- ☐ **C** Balloon dilatation
- ☐ **D** Bicarbonate supplements
- ☐ **E** Urine acidification

42 (4 marks)

A medical referral is made from the psychiatric unit about a 23-year-old man with deteriorating renal function and acute arthritis in the right foot. The only family history of note is schizophrenia in the maternal grandfather, who committed suicide at the age of 29. The following results are obtained:

Na	138 mmol/l
K	4.9 mmol/l
Urea	16.3 mmol/l
Creatinine	437 µmol/l
Bicarbonate	20 mmol/l

An X-ray of his foot shows areas of soft tissue calcification and punched out juxta-articular erosions around the interphalangeal joints.

1. What is the likely diagnosis?

☐ **A** Variegate porphyria
☐ **B** Gout nephropathy
☐ **C** Lithium toxicity
☐ **D** Lesch-Nyhan syndrome
☐ **E** Exacerbation of psoriatic arthropathy

2. What is the underlying mechanism?

☐ **A** Increased cell turnover
☐ **B** X-linked recessive enzyme defect
☐ **C** Autosomal recessive liver defect
☐ **D** Chronic haemolytic anaemia
☐ **E** Familial tubular defect

43 (4 marks)

A 32-year-old woman is under investigation for dysuria and secondary infertility. She also complains of polyarthralgia and sharp pains in the right upper quadrant. The following results are obtained:

Hb	129 g/l
WCC	8.9×10^9/l
Plt	328×10^9/l
ESR	56 mm/h

Na	138 mmol/l
K	4.1 mmol/l
Creatinine	92 µmol/l
Albumin	42 g/l
Dipstix urinalysis	Blood +, white cells + +
Mid-stream urine culture	Negative

1. What is your next investigation?

☐ **A**   Pelvic ultrasound
☐ **B**   Hysterosalpingography
☐ **C**   Blood culture
☐ **D**   Cervical swab
☐ **E**   Liver function tests

2. What is the likely diagnosis?

☐ **A**   Gonorrhoea
☐ **B**   *Chlamydia* infection
☐ **C**   Endometriosis
☐ **D**   Reiter's syndrome
☐ **E**   Behçet's disease

44 (2 marks)

These are the legs of a 43-year-old gentleman with increasing difficulties walking.

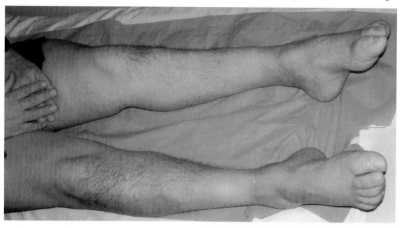

1. What is the likely diagnosis?

- ☐ **A** Friedreich's ataxia
- ☐ **B** Subacute combined degeneration of the cord
- ☐ **C** Poliomyelitis
- ☐ **D** Syringomyelia
- ☐ **E** Hereditary sensorimotor neuropathy

45 (7 marks)

A 73-year-old man is brought to the A&E Department with weakness of his left arm and leg. He has a history of atrial fibrillation and was anticoagulated two years previously after several TIAs affecting his right arm. Three weeks prior to admission, his General Practitioner was called to see him because he had become unrousable. He had recovered by the time the GP arrived and had no residual neurological signs. Since then, however, he has been experiencing difficulties in concentrating and has become unsteady on his feet. His current medication is digoxin 125 µg, enalapril 10 mg and warfarin.

On examination he is alert but disorientated to time and place. BP 185/100 mmHg; pulse 88/min, irregular. There is a soft, left-sided carotid bruit and a flow murmur in the aortic area. He has a 4/5 pyramidal weakness affecting the left arm and leg with extensor response in both plantars. There is no papilloedema; examination of chest and abdomen are unremarkable.

While recording an ECG, a nurse observes the patient becoming drowsy and unresponsive to speech. However when re-examined by the House Officer 10 minutes later he is fully alert again with no change in clinical signs. During that episode he has been incontinent of urine.

Investigations reveal:

Hb	142 g/l
WCC	5.3 × 10⁹/l
Plt	177 × 10⁹/l
ESR	16 mm/h
Na	130 mmol/l
K	3.5 mmol/l
Urea	3.0 mmol/l
Creatinine	127 µmol/l

ECG: controlled atrial fibrillation, 1-mm ST depression in lateral chest leads

1. Which of the following investigations is *unlikely* to be helpful?

- ☐ **A**   Prothrombin time
- ☐ **B**   Blood glucose
- ☐ **C**   Carotid Doppler
- ☐ **D**   Serum and urine osmolality
- ☐ **E**   Brain CT

2. What is the likely diagnosis?

☐ **A** Vertebro-basilar insufficiency
☐ **B** Right middle cerebral artery emboli
☐ **C** Cerebral metastases
☐ **D** Colloid cyst of third ventricle
☐ **E** Chronic subdural haematoma

3. Which of the following management options would be the most appropriate?

☐ **A** Neurosurgical referral
☐ **B** iv dexamethasone
☐ **C** Radiotherapy
☐ **D** Add oral aspirin
☐ **E** Increase warfarin

46 (7 marks)

The 49-year-old wife of a publican presents to the Outpatient Department with a history of difficulty with walking over several weeks. She also complains of annoying paraesthesiae of the toes and fingertips which has been worse at night. She also gives a six-month history of tiredness and finding it difficult to cope with her daily tasks. At the age of 28 she had been successfully treated for lymphoma. Her current medication consists of bezafibrate for a raised cholesterol and folate prescribed by her GP. She smokes 20 cigarettes per day and suffers from a chronic, productive cough. Alcohol intake is 15–20 units per week.

On examination she is pale with a blood pressure of 155/90 mmHg. No murmurs. There are bibasal crackles on auscultation, improved after coughing. In the abdomen a smooth liver edge is palpable without splenomegaly or lymphadenopathy.

In the legs there is a 4/5 weakness at the knees and ankles. Both knee jerks are brisk and several beats of clonus can be elicited at the patellae. However, there is reduced tone at the ankles and the ankle jerks are absent. Both plantar responses are extensor. Vibration sense is absent at the ankle and reduced at the knee; there is reduced sensation to pinprick below the ankle. Slight sensory loss was found in the fingertips but no significant abnormality is found otherwise in the upper limbs. No cerebellar signs can be elicited.

The following results are obtained:

Hb	102 g/l
WCC	3.8 × 10⁹/l
Plt	106 × 10⁹/l
ESR	23 mm/h

Na	139 mmol/l
K	4.1 mmol/l
Creatinine	138 µmol/l
Albumin	44 g/l
AST	26 U/l

Nerve conduction studies:

Sural sensory action potential	4 µV (> 50 µV)
Peroneal nerve conduction velocity	49 m/s (> 45 m/s)

1. **Which of the following investigations is likely to be of diagnostic value?**

- ☐ **A**   Chest X-ray
- ☐ **B**   Blood film
- ☐ **C**   Red cell transketolase
- ☐ **D**   MR scan of the brain
- ☐ **E**   MR scan of the spine

2. What is the diagnosis?

- ☐ **A** Subacute combined degeneration of the cord
- ☐ **B** Tabes dorsalis
- ☐ **C** Hereditary sensorimotor neuropathy
- ☐ **D** Eaton-Lambert syndrome
- ☐ **E** Toxic neuropathy

3. Which of the following may worsen the condition?

- ☐ **A** Alcohol withdrawal
- ☐ **B** Bedrest
- ☐ **C** Folate replacement
- ☐ **D** Antibiotic therapy
- ☐ **E** Physiotherapy

47 (4 marks)

A Polish tourist presents to the A&E Department with headache, ataxia and diplopia on left lateral gaze. The following results are obtained:

Hb	135 g/l
WCC	10 × 10⁹/l (59% granulocytes)
Plt	277 × 10⁹/l
Glucose	5.6 mmol/l

A lumbar puncture is performed with the following results:

Opening pressure	29 cmH₂O
Protein	2.1 g/l
Glucose	0.7 mmol/l
Microscopy	125 cells/mm³
	(90% lymphocytes)

1. What is the likely diagnosis?

- ☐ **A** Viral meningitis
- ☐ **B** Herpes encephalitis
- ☐ **C** Cerebral toxoplasmosis
- ☐ **D** Tuberculous meningitis
- ☐ **E** Cerebral cysticercosis

2. What complication has arisen?

- ☐ **A** Sinus cavernosus thrombosis
- ☐ **B** Subdural empyema
- ☐ **C** Brainstem abscess
- ☐ **D** Communicating hydrocephalus
- ☐ **E** Obstructive hydrocephalus

48 (2 marks)

This is a sagittal section from a T$_2$-weighted MR scan of a 34-year-old woman. Her CT brain scan was normal.

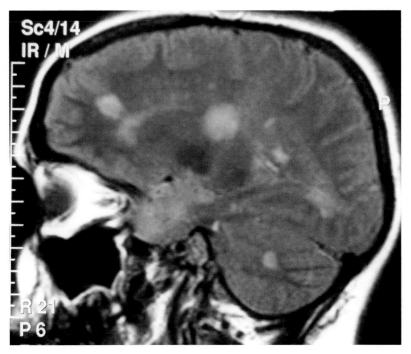

1. What is the likely diagnosis?

- ☐ **A** Tuberose sclerosis
- ☐ **B** Metastatic disease
- ☐ **C** Multiple sclerosis
- ☐ **D** Toxoplasmosis
- ☐ **E** Cerebral abscesses

49 (5 marks)

A 32-year-old man has come to the A&E Department insisting that he has eaten 'forbidden food' and that 'the evil spirits are trying to explode his bowel'. He has peritonism with increased bowel sounds and he seems oblivious to pinprick below mid-calf. Despite fierce resistance, he is fairly easily restrained and blood samples show the following results:

Hb	151 g/l
WCC	12.2 × 10⁹/l (88% neutrophils)
Plt	253 × 10⁹/l
Na	127 mmol/l
K	4.8 mmol/l
Creatinine	99 μmol/l
CRP	3 mg/l

1. **What is the likely diagnosis?**

☐ **A**   Familial Mediterranean fever
☐ **B**   Amphetamine overdose
☐ **C**   Hypoglycaemia
☐ **D**   General paralysis of the insane
☐ **E**   Acute intermittent porphyria

2. **What drug would you use for sedation?**

☐ **A**   Midazolam
☐ **B**   Nalbuphine
☐ **C**   Phenobarbitone
☐ **D**   Chlorpromazine
☐ **E**   Diazemuls®

50 (5 marks)

A 63-year-old woman is brought into Casualty having been found wandering the streets. She is confused and punches the House Officer during venesection. No focal weakness is found, but the tendon reflexes are reduced.

The following results are obtained:

Hb	106 g/l
WCC	3.3×10^9/l
Plt	107×10^9/l
Na	129 mmol/l
K	4.6 mmol/l
Urea	3.8 mmol/l
Bilirubin	15 μmol/l
Albumin	42 g/l
Gamma-GT	26 U/l
Creatinine kinase	385 U/l
Total cholesterol	7.9 mmol/l

1. What is the most important investigation?

- □ **A** Chest X-ray
- □ **B** Blood film
- □ **C** Thyroid function tests
- □ **D** Urine osmolality
- □ **E** Enhanced CT of the brain

2. What combination of pathologies is most likely to explain the results?

- □ **A** Carcinoma of lung with bone marrow invasion
- □ **B** Alcohol abuse and malnutrition
- □ **C** Drug overdose and aplastic anaemia
- □ **D** Carcinoma of stomach and brain metastases
- □ **E** Hypothyroidism and pernicious anaemia

51 (4 marks)

A 46-year-old woman presents with the following neurological signs:

Wasting of the small muscles of the hands, reduced biceps reflexes and multiple scars and burns over both hands. Sensation to soft touch and vibration is preserved. Fasciculations are seen within the tongue and both legs show increased tone and brisk reflexes.

1. **Which of the following diagnoses explains the findings?**

☐ **A** Rheumatoid arthritis
☐ **B** Syringobulbia
☐ **C** Motor neurone disease
☐ **D** Multiple sclerosis
☐ **E** Cervical spondylosis

2. **Which of the following investigations is indicated?**

☐ **A** ESR
☐ **B** Nerve conduction studies
☐ **C** Flexion views of cervical spine
☐ **D** MR scan of the cervical spine
☐ **E** MR scan of the brain

52 (2 marks)

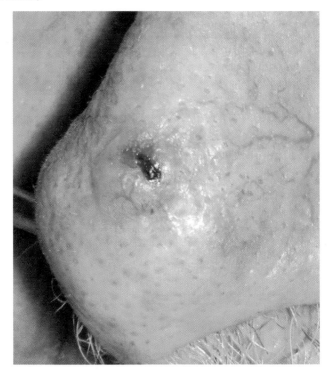

1. **What is the lesion on the tip of the nose of an 83-year-old pensioner?**

- ☐ **A** Basal cell carcinoma
- ☐ **B** Squamous cell carcinoma
- ☐ **C** Discoid lupus
- ☐ **D** Secondary syphilis
- ☐ **E** Porphyria cutanea tarda

53 (9 marks)

A 61-year-old housewife is referred by her GP following an 18-month history of slowly worsening shortness of breath on exercise. She was well until six months ago when she started to find it difficult helping her husband with the family-run plumbing business. She smokes 10 cigarettes per day, but is on no regular medication. Her 32-year-old son keeps racing pigeons in the garden, and the couple own two cats.

On examination there is finger clubbing and bilateral fine inspiratory crackles are heard at both lung bases. Examination of heart and abdomen is normal.

A chest X-ray shows lateral pleural thickening in both mid-zones and a small left pleural effusion.

Investigations show:

Hb	138 g/l
WCC	5.9 × 10⁹/l (normal differential)
Plt	179 × 10⁹/l
ESR	23 mm/h
U&Es	Normal

Arterial blood gases (on air):

pH	7.36
pO_2	8.3 kPa (62 mmHg)
pCO_2	4.1 kPa (31 mmHg)
Bicarbonate	21 mmol/l

FEV_1	1.9 l (2.0–3.3 l)
FVC	2.4 l (2.8–4.5 l)
FEV_1/FVC	79%

1. What is the correct description of her biochemical state?

- [ ] **A** Respiratory alkalosis
- [ ] **B** Metabolic alkalosis
- [ ] **C** Mixed respiratory and metabolic alkalosis
- [ ] **D** Compensated respiratory alkalosis
- [ ] **E** Compensated metabolic acidosis

2. Which of the following investigations is indicated?

- [ ] **A** Estimation of transfer factor
- [ ] **B** Autoantibody screen
- [ ] **C** High-resolution CT scan
- [ ] **D** Bronchoscopy and alveolar lavage
- [ ] **E** Transbronchial lung biopsy

3. What is the likely diagnosis?

☐ **A** Cryptogenic fibrosing alveolitis
☐ **B** Rheumatoid lung
☐ **C** Sarcoidosis
☐ **D** Chronic extrinsic allergic alveolitis
☐ **E** Asbestosis

Two years later she is referred back to clinic with a deterioration of her symptoms, and the following results are obtained:

FEV_1	1.7 l
FVC	2.0 l
FEV_1/FVC	85%
Transfer factor (DLCO)	59%
Transfer coefficient (KCO)	98%

4. What complication has arisen?

☐ **A** Adenocarcinoma
☐ **B** Tuberculosis
☐ **C** Pleural encasement
☐ **D** Bronchiectasis
☐ **E** Bullous emphysema

54 (8 marks)

A 59-year-old Turkish blacksmith presents with increasing episodes of haemoptysis. He smokes 25 cigarettes a day and gives a long-standing history of cough, producing sputum on most days first thing in the morning. Initially he only produced small amounts of bloodstained sputum but, over the last two weeks, coughed up a cupful of blood on three occasions.

On examination he is not cyanosed. He has a barrel-shaped chest and there is early finger clubbing. Respiratory rate 20/min. There are crackles at the right base which improve after coughing; no wheeze is heard. There is a slight right ventricular heave and a pronounced second heart sound, but no cardiac murmurs are heard. BP 160/95 mmHg; pulse 88/min, regular.

The liver edge is palpable 5 cm under the costal margin; spleen and kidneys cannot be palpated.

Blood samples reveal the following results:

Hb	131 g/l
WCC	8.6×10^9/l
Differential: 76% neutrophils, 20% lymphocytes, 3% eosinophils	
Plt	268×10^9/l
ESR	16 mm/h
U&Es	Normal
FEV_1	2.0 l (predicted 2.4–3.5 l)
FVC	3.2 l (predicted 3.4–4.9 l)
FEV_1/FVC	63%

Chest X-ray: Overinflated lungs, right apical consolidation containing calcification and some air

Bronchoscopy shows no abnormality, bronchial washings are negative for acid-fast bacilli. Cytology shows no evidence of malignancy.

1. What is the likely cause for the patient's symptoms?

- ☐ **A** Adenocarcinoma
- ☐ **B** Polyarteritis nodosa
- ☐ **C** Squamous cell carcinoma
- ☐ **D** Aspergilloma
- ☐ **E** Histoplasmosis

2. How is the diagnosis confirmed?

- ☐ **A** Transbronchial lung biopsy
- ☐ **B** Transthoracic lung biopsy
- ☐ **C** CT scan
- ☐ **D** Autoantibody screen
- ☐ **E** Fungal serology

3. What is the background pulmonary pathology?

- ☐ **A** Emphysema
- ☐ **B** Bronchiectasis
- ☐ **C** Cryptogenic fibrosing alveolitis
- ☐ **D** Pneumoconiosis
- ☐ **E** Chronic extrinsic allergic alveolitis

4. What is the treatment of choice?

- ☐ **A** Direct injection of antibiotics
- ☐ **B** iv antibiotics
- ☐ **C** Radiotherapy
- ☐ **D** Surgery
- ☐ **E** Steroids

55 (5 marks)

A 27-year-old woman presents with a three-day history of painful swallowing and sore throat. Over the last 24-hours she has become breathless on exercise and she has noticed her breathing becoming noisy. She has been given amoxicillin by her GP. Her only other medication is the oral contraceptive pill. She suffered from asthma up to the age of 17 and there is a family history of asthma.

On examination she is anxious and sweating. Respiratory rate 28/min, temperature 38.3 °C. Normal appearances of mouth and fauces. Breath sounds are normal on auscultation, but there is an audible loud inspiratory wheeze. Several lymph nodes are palpable in the anterior cervical triangle. No organomegaly is present in the abdomen.

Investigations reveal:

Hb	136 g/l
WCC	16.2 × 10⁹/l
Differential: 77% granulocytes, 15% lymphocytes, 6% monocytes	
Plt	371 × 10⁹/l
ESR	51 mm/h
U&Es	Normal
Peak expiratory flow rate	385 l/min
	(predicted 440–600 l/min)

Arterial blood gases on air:

pH	7.52
pO_2	11.6 kPa (87 mmHg)
pCO_2	3.5 kPa (26 mmHg)
Bicarbonate	23 mmol/l

Chest X-ray: Overinflated lungs without consolidation

1. What is the most likely diagnosis?

☐ **A** Acute epiglottitis
☐ **B** Hereditary angio-oedema
☐ **C** Infective exacerbation of asthma
☐ **D** Whooping cough
☐ **E** Acute laryngitis (croup)

2. Which of the following is the most appropriate management?

- ☐ **A** Urgent ENT referral and intubation
- ☐ **B** Inhaled salbutamol and iv hydrocortisone
- ☐ **C** im adrenaline and iv midazolam
- ☐ **D** iv aminophylline and tracheostomy
- ☐ **E** iv benzylpenicillin and sc salbutamol

56 (2 marks)

This 17-year-old lady was referred to her GP after her pre-employment visit prior to nurse training. Dipstix testing of her urine was normal.

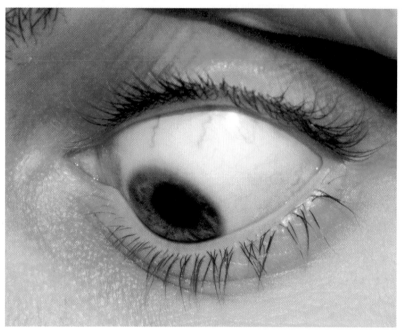

What is the most like diagnosis?

- ☐ **A**   Rotor syndrome
- ☐ **B**   Thalassaemia minor
- ☐ **C**   Sclerosing cholangitis
- ☐ **D**   Primary biliary cirrhosis
- ☐ **E**   Gilbert's syndrome

57 (4 marks)

An obese 43-year-old woman complains of morning headaches and malaise.

The following results are obtained:

Hb	154 g/l
MCV	101 fl
WCC	6.2 × 10⁹/l (normal differential)

Arterial blood gases (on air):

pO_2	10.4 kPa (78 mmHg)
pCO_2	5.6 kPa (42 mmHg)
Total cholesterol	6.2 mmol/l

1. **What is the likely cause for her symptoms?**

☐ **A**   Type I respiratory failure
☐ **B**   Sleep apnoea
☐ **C**   Type II respiratory failure
☐ **D**   Nocturnal asthma
☐ **E**   Diaphragmatic weakness

2. **What underlying cause has to be considered?**

☐ **A**   Cushing's disease
☐ **B**   Pernicious anaemia
☐ **C**   Cerebrovascular disease
☐ **D**   Cushing's syndrome
☐ **E**   Hypothyroidism

58 (4 marks)

A patient in her twenties is brought unconscious to the A&E Department. She is tachycardic and tachypnoeic, but haemodynamically stable.

The following results are obtained:

Na	144 mmol/l
K	6.0 mmol/l
Urea	13.6 mmol/l
Chloride	101 mmol/l
Glucose	4.3 mmol/l

Arterial blood gases (room air):

pH	6.96
pO_2	14.1 kPa (106 mmHg)
pCO_2	1.9 kPa (14 mmHg)
Bicarbonate	9 mmol/l

1. What is the most accurate description of the metabolic abnormality?

☐ **A** Respiratory acidosis
☐ **B** Azotaemia
☐ **C** Combined respiratory/metabolic acidosis
☐ **D** Partially compensated metabolic acidosis
☐ **E** High anion gap acidosis

2. What is the likely cause?

☐ **A** Alveolar hypoventilation
☐ **B** Rhabdomyolysis
☐ **C** Salicylate overdose
☐ **D** Lactic acidosis type A
☐ **E** Lactic acidosis type B

59 (4 marks)

A 16-year-old asthmatic patient is admitted with breathlessness. There is only minimal wheeze on auscultation. The patient receives two doses of oxygen-driven nebulised bronchodilators and a subsequent arterial blood sample shows the following results:

pH	7.35
pO_2	8.1 kPa (61 mmHg)
pCO_2	5.7 kPa (43 mmHg)

Chest X-ray   Clear lungs, no pneumothorax

1. Which of the following would be the most appropriate management?

☐ **A**   iv hydrocortisone and 60% O_2
☐ **B**   iv aminophylline and 28% O_2
☐ **C**   iv doxapram and 95% O_2
☐ **D**   Nebulised adrenaline on air
☐ **E**   Subcutaneous salbutamol injections and anaesthetic assessment

60 (2 marks)

A 56-year-old renal patient is found collapsed at home.

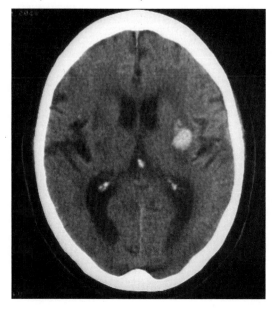

1. **What is the likely underlying cause for the finding on the CT?**

□ **A**   Hypertension
□ **B**   Warfarin therapy
□ **C**   Immune suppressant therapy
□ **D**   Metastatic disease
□ **E**   Infection

61 (5 marks)

A 68-year-old woman presents with polyarthritis, low-grade fever and exercise-induced dyspnoea.

The following results are obtained:

Hb	103 g/l
WCC	7.1×10^9/l (normal differential)
Plt	528×10^9/l
CRP	43 mg/l (< 10 mg/l)

FEV_1/FVC	58%
Total lung capacity	5.0 l (predicted 4–5.2 l)
Residual capacity	0.7 l (predicted 0.5–0.9 l)
Transfer coefficient (KCO)	99%
Pulse oximetry (on air)	99% O_2 saturation

1. What is the likely diagnosis?

☐ **A** Rheumatoid arthritis
☐ **B** Systemic sclerosis
☐ **C** Relapsing polychondritis
☐ **D** Extrinsic allergic alveolitis
☐ **E** Churg-Strauss syndrome

2. What would you expect to find on the chest X-ray?

☐ **A** Normal appearances
☐ **B** Basal fibrosis
☐ **C** Apical fibrosis
☐ **D** Pleural effusion
☐ **E** Alveolar shadowing

62 (4 marks)

A 37-year-old female secretary presents with acute onset of dyspnoea. Clinical examination and a chest radiograph are normal.

Investigations show:

FEV$_1$	2.7 l (predicted 2.5–3.8 l)
FVC	3.8 l (predicted 3.2–5.9 l)

Arterial blood gases (room air):

pH	7.45
pO$_2$	9.5 kPa (71 mmHg)
pCO$_2$	4.1 kPa (31 mmHg)

Ventilation–perfusion scan: two subsegmental mismatched defects, intermediate probability for embolus

1. Which of the following is the most appropriate investigation?

- ☐ **A** CT angiogram
- ☐ **B** Chest X-ray in expiration
- ☐ **C** D-dimer levels
- ☐ **D** Serology for atypical infection
- ☐ **E** Full blood count

2. What is the likely diagnosis?

- ☐ **A** Hyperventilation
- ☐ **B** Pulmonary embolus
- ☐ **C** Pneumothorax
- ☐ **D** *Mycoplasma* infection
- ☐ **E** Macleod's syndrome

63 (2 marks)

Following a holiday in Mexico, a 41-year-old rock-climber presents with pyrexia, dry cough and polyarthralgia. Erythema nodosum is present on his shins.

Examinations reveal:

Hb   153 g/l
WCC   10.1 × 10⁹/l
Differential: 62% neutrophils, 31% lymphocytes, 4% eosinophils
Plt   309 × 10⁹/l
ESR   41 mm/h

Chest X-ray: Diffuse micronodular infiltrates; hilar and mediastinal adenopathy

1. What is the likely diagnosis?

☐ **A**   Varicella pneumonia
☐ **B**   Acute sarcoidosis
☐ **C**   Tuberculosis
☐ **D**   Non-Hodgkin's lymphoma
☐ **E**   Histoplasmosis

64 (10 marks)

A 37-year-old man presents to his GP with a painful penile ulcer. A swab is taken for culture and the patient started on oral amoxicillin. Ten days later he is admitted with photophobia and neck stiffness. On examination there is no focal neurology and both plantars are down-going. Over his right shin several purple, coalescent nodules are seen and he has a pustular rash over his trunk. In addition, he has painful swelling of both knees and the left elbow. Examination of chest and cardiovascular system is unremarkable. Fundoscopy is normal, but both eyes are red with ciliary injection.

The following results are obtained:

Hb	142 g/l
WCC	9.8 × 10⁹/l
Differential: 64% neutrophils, 31% lymphocytes, 4% eosinophils	
Plt	476 × 10⁹/l
ESR	38 mm/h

Biochemical profile	Normal
Bilirubin	19 μmol/l
AST	18 U/l
Glucose	5.9 mmol/l

One day later pustules have formed at the venepuncture sites.

1. Which of the following investigations would you recommend?

- ☐ **A** HLA-B27
- ☐ **B** Joint aspiration
- ☐ **C** CT brain scan
- ☐ **D** Blood cultures
- ☐ **E** Skin biopsy

A lumbar puncture is performed with the following results:

CSF bloodstained, no xanthochromia

Opening pressure	14 cmH$_2$O
Protein	0.45 g/l
Glucose	3.1 g/l
Microscopy [/mm³]	18 mononuclear cells
	12 red cells

2. What do these results suggest?

- ☐ **A** Viral meningitis
- ☐ **B** Bacterial meningitis
- ☐ **C** Subarachnoid haemorrhage
- ☐ **D** Traumatic tap
- ☐ **E** Brain abscess

3. What is the likely diagnosis?

- ☐ **A** Gonorrhoea
- ☐ **B** Reiter's syndrome
- ☐ **C** Behçet's disease
- ☐ **D** Lymphogranuloma venereum
- ☐ **E** Syphilis

4. What treatment would you recommend?

- ☐ **A** iv gentamicin
- ☐ **B** Systemic steroids
- ☐ **C** im penicillin
- ☐ **D** Oral doxycycline
- ☐ **E** iv ciclosporin

After an initial recovery, the patient becomes severely obtunded with a Glasgow Coma Scale score of 5/15. A CT scan shows bilateral deep white matter haemorrhage.

5. What complication has occurred?

- ☐ **A** Superior sagittal sinus thrombosis
- ☐ **B** Cerebral vasculitis
- ☐ **C** Disseminated intravascular coagulation
- ☐ **D** Autoimmune thrombocytopenia
- ☐ **E** Over-anticoagulation

65 (6 marks)

A 42-year-old Egyptian travel agent presents with an 18-month history of back pain and intermittent arthritis of both knees and elbows. Lately he has also noticed a decrease in exercise tolerance and has had intermittent right-sided pleuritic chest pains. He also gives a history of episodic diarrhoea, but a colonoscopy and small bowel enema performed six months previously showed no abnormalities. He is on no current medication, drinks 25 units of alcohol per week and does not smoke.

Small effusions are present in both knees, examination of the spine reveals a full range of movements, but there is tenderness over the right sacroiliac joint. Chest examination shows dullness on percussion at the right base, but no crackles. Cardiovascular system is unremarkable.

The following blood results are obtained:

Hb	105 g/l
WCC	4.8 × 10⁹/l
Plt	193 × 10⁹/l
MCV	103 fl
MCHC	22 g/dl
ESR	47 mm/h
Na	139 mmol/l
K	4.2 mmol/l
Urea	5.2 mmol/l
Albumin	31 g/l
Calcium	2.0 mmol/l
Bilirubin	15 μmol/l
Gamma-GT	19 U/l

X-rays show a small right-sided pleural effusion and a globular heart. Sclerosis around both SI joints is present, worse on the right.

A radio-labelled white cell scan shows normal appearance of the abdomen, but some increased activity at the pleural surfaces and the mediastinum.

1. **What investigation would you recommend?**

   □ **A**   Joint aspirate
   □ **B**   Small bowel biopsy
   □ **C**   Pleural aspirate
   □ **D**   Gliadin antibodies
   □ **E**   Autoantibody screen

2. What is the likely diagnosis?

☐ **A** Coeliac disease
☐ **B** Crohn's disease
☐ **C** Tropical sprue
☐ **D** Whipple's disease
☐ **E** Familial Mediterranean fever (FMF)

3. What is the appropriate therapy?

☐ **A** Tetracycline
☐ **B** Mesalazine
☐ **C** Oral steroids
☐ **D** Colchicine
☐ **E** Diclofenac

66 (5 marks)

A 32-year-old farmer presents to the Neurology Department with a left-sided facial weakness. Over the previous six weeks he had developed aches and pains in muscles and joints and intermittently had to stop working.

On examination, Bell's phenomenon is positive, but he is able to wrinkle his forehead normally.

Hb	119 g/l
WCC	6.1 × 10⁹/l (65% neutrophils)
Plt	375 × 10⁹/l
ESR	58 mm/h
Biochemical profile	Normal
Autoantibody screen	Negative

1. What is the likely diagnosis?

☐ **A**   Reiter's syndrome
☐ **B**   Bell's palsy
☐ **C**   Heerfordt's syndrome
☐ **D**   Lyme disease
☐ **E**   Behçet's disease

2. What investigation is likely to be most useful?

☐ **A**   Chest X-ray
☐ **B**   HLA-B27
☐ **C**   *Borrelia* serology
☐ **D**   Joint aspirate
☐ **E**   Skin biopsy

67 (2 marks)

This is the blood film of a 69-year-old with a four-month history of malaise and shortness of breath.

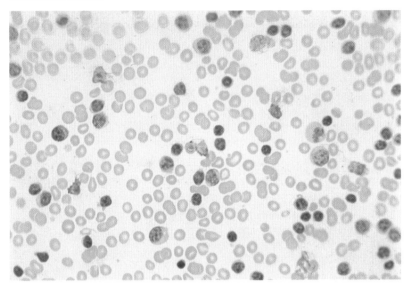

1. **What is the diagnosis?**

☐ **A**   Myeloma
☐ **B**   Chronic myeloid leukaemia
☐ **C**   Vitamin B$_{12}$ deficiency
☐ **D**   Chronic lymphocytic leukaemia
☐ **E**   Iron deficiency

68 (4 marks)

A 28-year-old woman with tuberose sclerosis presents with left-side pleuritic chest pain. Over the previous three months she has also developed an asymmetric polyarthropathy. On examination there is a fine pleural rub on the left and dullness to percussion at the right base. Mild synovitis is present in the joints of both hands. An autoantibody screen reveals:

ANA	1:640
Anti-dsDNA	1:1
Anti-histone	1:320
Anti-Sm	1:10
Rheumatoid factor	Negative
CRP	28 mg/l

1. What is the likely diagnosis?

- ☐ **A** Drug-induced lupus
- ☐ **B** Systemic lupus erythematosus
- ☐ **C** Paraneoplastic syndrome
- ☐ **D** Mixed connective tissue disease
- ☐ **E** Systemic sclerosis

2. What management would you recommend?

- ☐ **A** Aspirin
- ☐ **B** Chloroquine
- ☐ **C** Alter current medication
- ☐ **D** Oral steroids
- ☐ **E** Methotrexate

69 (4 marks)

A 56-year-old man is being assessed for a total knee replacement. The following results are obtained in the Orthopaedic Outpatient Department:

U&Es	Normal
Glucose	14.7 mmol/l
AST	51 U/l
ALT	72 U/l
Gamma-GT	53 U/l
Bilirubin	16 µmol/l
Calcium	2.3 mmol/l
Ferritin	295 nmol/l (6–120 nmol/l)
Transferrin saturation	99%

Radiographs show advanced degenerative changes and chondrocalcinosis in both knees.

1. What is the likely diagnosis?

- ☐ **A** Acromegaly
- ☐ **B** Calcium pyrophosphate deposition disease
- ☐ **C** Chronic hepatic porphyria
- ☐ **D** Haemochromatosis
- ☐ **E** Neuropathic joint disease

2. Which of the following investigations is likely to be diagnostic?

- ☐ **A** Haemoglobin A$_{1c}$
- ☐ **B** Liver biopsy
- ☐ **C** Joint aspirate
- ☐ **D** Oral glucose tolerance test
- ☐ **E** Faecal porphyrins

70 (4 marks)

A 56-year-old vagrant presents to Casualty complaining of pain in his right hip and difficulties getting up from lying and squatting positions. On examination he is cachectic with palmar erythema.

Investigations show:

Hb	106 g/l
WCC	3.2 × 10⁹/l
Plt	142 × 10⁹/l
MCV	102 fl
ESR	73 mm/h

Na	132 mmol/l
K	3.1 mmol/l
Urea	2.8 mmol/l
Creatinine	153 µmol/l
Calcium	1.9 mmol/l
Phosphate	0.7 mmol/l
Albumin	28 g/l
ALT	116 U/l
Gamma-GT	186 U/l
Bilirubin	21 µmol/l
Alkaline phosphatase	563 U/l

1. **What is the likely cause of the presenting symptoms?**

☐ **A** Pathological fracture
☐ **B** Paraneoplastic syndrome
☐ **C** Myositis ossificans
☐ **D** Subacute combined degeneration of the cord
☐ **E** Osteomalacia

2. **What is your next investigation?**

☐ **A** C-reactive protein
☐ **B** Blood cultures
☐ **C** Lumbar puncture
☐ **D** Echocardiogram
☐ **E** Chest X-ray

Paper 2 – Questions

1 (2 marks)

This is the tongue of a 47-year-old with dysphagia.

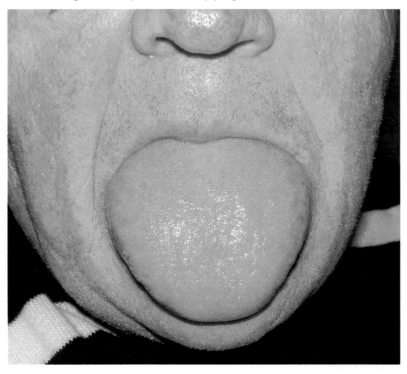

1. Which of the following is *not* a cause of this appearance?

☐ **A** Amyloidosis
☐ **B** Acromegaly
☐ **C** Down's syndrome
☐ **D** Mucopolysaccharidosis
☐ **E** Glycogen storage disease

2 (8 marks)

A 24-year-old patient with learning difficulties is referred for investigation of hypertension. He works as a helper in the local garden centre with a particular interest in herbs. There is a family history of hypertension and heart disease.

On examination he is of short stature with underdeveloped secondary sexual characteristics. He has mild dyspnoea at rest, but is not cyanosed. Pulse 96/min, regular; BP 195/100 mmHg in both arms. The apex beat is thrusting and a loud mid-systolic murmur is heard throughout the precordium radiating into the neck and back. Crackles are audible at both lung bases; examination of the abdomen is unremarkable.

The following results are obtained:

Hb	143 g/l
WCC	5.5 × 10⁹/l (normal differential)
Plt	183 × 10⁹/l
ESR	8 mm/h

Na	138 mmol/l
K	4.1 mmol/l
Creatinine	92 µmol/l
Dipstix urinalysis	Protein +, Blood −

ECG: QRS axis −15°, sinus rhythm 98/min, QRS 0.11 s
$S_{V2} + R_{V5} = 51$ mm

A chest X-ray of poor quality could only be obtained as the patient was frightened by the X-ray machine, but cardiomegaly is present and there is dilatation of the ascending aorta.

1. What is the cardiac diagnosis?

☐ **A** Hypertrophic obstructive cardiomyopathy
☐ **B** Sub-valvular aortic stenosis
☐ **C** Coarctation
☐ **D** Patent ductus arteriosus
☐ **E** Ventricular septum defect

2. Which of the following is the *least* useful investigation?

☐ **A** Echocardiogram
☐ **B** MR scanning
☐ **C** Cardiac scintigraphy
☐ **D** Cardiac catheterisation
☐ **E** Angiography

3. What is the likely underlying condition?

- ☐ **A** Turner's syndrome
- ☐ **B** Noonan's syndrome
- ☐ **C** Klinefelter's syndrome
- ☐ **D** Hurler's syndrome
- ☐ **E** Homocysteinuria

4. What treatment would you recommend?

- ☐ **A** Balloon dilatation
- ☐ **B** ACE inhibitors
- ☐ **C** Calcium antagonists
- ☐ **D** Indometacin
- ☐ **E** Surgery

3 (6 marks)

A 21-year-old woman is under investigation for hypertension. She also gives a history of malaise and dizzy spells over several months. On examination she looks well, without evidence of anaemia or jaundice. Her right radial pulse is weak; the left radial pulse is absent. Blood pressure measurements give the following results:

Right arm 185/125 mmHg   Left arm unrecordable
Right leg 180/100 mmHg   Left leg 175/105 mmHg

The following blood results are obtained:

Hb	133 g/l
WCC	6.2×10^9/l (normal differential)
Plt	343×10^9/l
ESR	56 mm/h

Na	136 mmol/l
K	5.1 mmol/l
Urea	7.9 mmol/l
Creatinine	171 µmol/l
Dipstix urinalysis	Blood + +, Protein –, Glucose –

A carotid Doppler shows occlusion of the right internal carotid artery.

1. What is the likely cause for the hypertension?

- ☐ **A** Aortic aneurysm
- ☐ **B** Aortic occlusion
- ☐ **C** Coarctation
- ☐ **D** Renal artery stenosis
- ☐ **E** Chronic renal failure

2. What is the likely diagnosis?

- ☐ **A** Marfan's syndrome
- ☐ **B** Takayasu's arteritis
- ☐ **C** Pseudoxanthoma elasticum
- ☐ **D** Conn's syndrome
- ☐ **E** Kawasaki disease

4 (7 marks)

A 17-year-old boy complains of rapid palpitations associated with dizziness and shortness of breath. The episodes are self-limiting and not clearly related to exercise. There is no previous history of note. On examination he is thin with mild central cyanosis and a raised venous pressure with a prominent systolic wave. Pulse 80/min, regular; BP 115/75 mmHg. A pan-systolic murmur is heard at the left sternal edge, accentuated on inspiration. There is mild, pulsatile hepatomegaly. Examinations reveal:

Full blood count	Normal
U&Es	Normal
ESR	5 mm/h

ECG: Sinus rhythm 80/min, PR 0.10 s. A Δ-wave and an incomplete right bundle branch block pattern are present in keeping with Wolff-Parkinson-White (WPW) syndrome type A

1. What is the most important investigation?

☐ **A** Chest X-ray
☐ **B** Blood cultures
☐ **C** Echocardiogram
☐ **D** Cardiac catheterisation
☐ **E** 24-hour cardiac monitoring

2. What is the likely diagnosis?

☐ **A** Corrected transposition of the great arteries
☐ **B** Fallot's tetralogy
☐ **C** Ostium primum atrial septal defect
☐ **D** Patent ductus arteriosus
☐ **E** Ebstein's anomaly

3. What is the likely form of his arrhythmias?

☐ **A** Sinus tachycardia
☐ **B** AV re-entrant tachycardia
☐ **C** Paroxysmal atrial fibrillation
☐ **D** Intermittent AV block
☐ **E** Ventricular tachycardia

5 (2 marks)

A 34-year-old vagrant is brought into Casualty profoundly intoxicated and has the following chest X-ray.

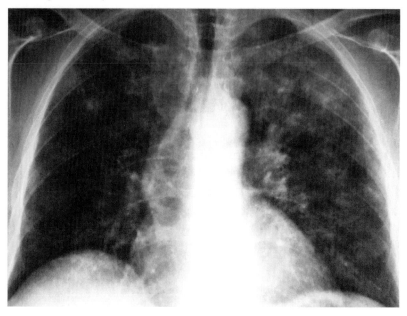

1. What is the appropriate management?

- ☐ **A** Oral erythromycin and oral thiamine
- ☐ **B** Sputum microscopy and barrier nursing
- ☐ **C** Full blood count and inhaled pentamidine
- ☐ **D** Bronchoscopy and transbronchial lung biopsy
- ☐ **E** iv ampicillin and iv vitamin B complex

6 (3 marks)

This is a ST-segment analysis from a 24-hour tape in a man complaining of intermittent central chest pain at rest.

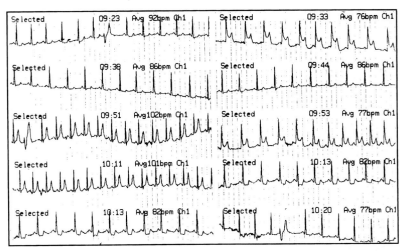

1. **What is the diagnosis?**

☐ **A** Unstable angina
☐ **B** Crescendo angina
☐ **C** Prinzmetal (variant) angina
☐ **D** Subendocardial infarction
☐ **E** Transmural infarction

7 (5 marks)

A 65-year-old pensioner with known ischaemic heart disease is brought to hospital having been found collapsed by the warden. Tablets from his bedside table are presented by the ambulance driver and include aspirin, lisinopril, glyceryl trinitrate spray, amiloride and phenytoin.

Investigations show:

Na	134 mmol/l
K	5.6 mmol/l
Creatinine	159 μmol/l
Creatinine kinase	8300 U/l
AST	230 U/l
ALT	56 U/l

ECG: Sinus rhythm 76/min, QRS axis +0°, 2-mm antero-lateral ST depression

1. What is the most likely explanation for these findings?

- ☐ **A** Stroke
- ☐ **B** Subarachnoid haemorrhage
- ☐ **C** Salicylate overdose
- ☐ **D** Myocardial infarction
- ☐ **E** Epileptic fit

2. Which of the following investigations is *not* indicated?

- ☐ **A** Serial electrocardiograms
- ☐ **B** Electroencephalogram
- ☐ **C** CT brain scan
- ☐ **D** Dipstix urinalysis
- ☐ **E** Blood glucose

8 **(3 marks)**

This is the ECG of a 41-year-old man with chest pain.

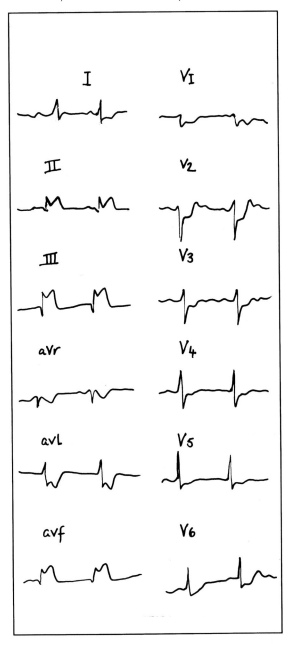

1. What does it show?

- ☐ **A** Inferior MI
- ☐ **B** Septal MI
- ☐ **C** Pericarditis
- ☐ **D** Myocarditis
- ☐ **E** Postero-inferior MI

9 (3 marks)

This is the ECG of a 49-year-old woman who has experienced several blackouts over the last 18 months. Pulse 72/min regular; BP 105/85 mmHg in both arms.

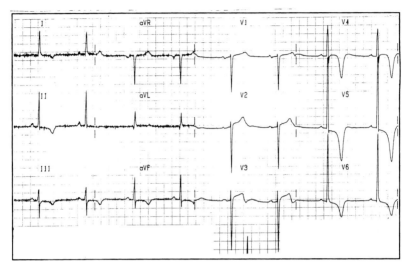

1. **What is the most likely diagnosis?**

- ☐ **A** Aortic incompetence
- ☐ **B** Restrictive cardiomyopathy
- ☐ **C** Coarctation
- ☐ **D** Aortic stenosis
- ☐ **E** Ventricular septal defect

10 (4 marks)

A 41-year-old man is admitted cold and sweating. The following ECG is taken in the A&E Department.

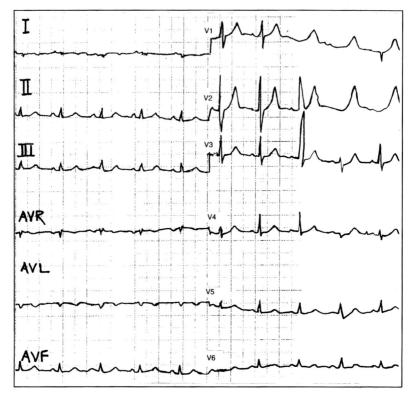

1. **Which part of the coronary artery system is affected?**

☐ **A**   Left anterior descending artery
☐ **B**   Left circumflex artery
☐ **C**   Posterior descending artery
☐ **D**   Left obtuse marginal branch
☐ **E**   Left main stem

2. What is the therapy of choice?

☐ **A**   Streptokinase and beta-blocker
☐ **B**   Urokinase and GTN spray
☐ **C**   Aspirin and GTN infusion
☐ **D**   Aspirin and rt-PA
☐ **E**   iv heparin and GTN spray

11 (4 marks)

A 31-year-old Jamaican chef is referred with an 18-month history of shortness of breath. More recently he complained of increased thirst and recurring palpitations. The following rhythm strip is obtained.

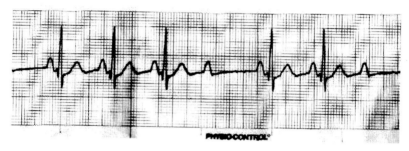

1. **What does it show?**

- ☐ **A** Atrial standstill
- ☐ **B** Sick sinus syndrome
- ☐ **C** Mobitz type 1 heart block
- ☐ **D** Ectopic atrial pacemaker
- ☐ **E** Mobitz type 2 heart block

2. **What underlying diagnosis has to be considered?**

- ☐ **A** Kawasaki disease
- ☐ **B** Amyloidosis
- ☐ **C** Sarcoidosis
- ☐ **D** Rheumatoid arthritis
- ☐ **E** Diabetes mellitus

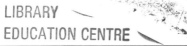
12 **(4 marks)**

These are the hands of a 42-year-old teacher with breathlessness.

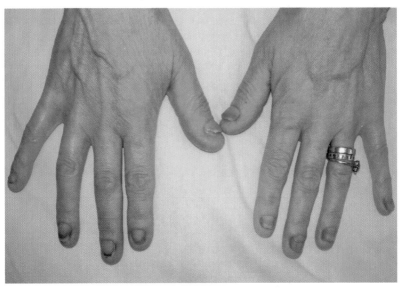

1. **What is the likely diagnosis?**

☐ **A**   Fungal infection
☐ **B**   Yellow nail syndrome
☐ **C**   Psoriasis
☐ **D**   Tetracycline therapy
☐ **E**   Tylosis

2. **Which of the following is *not* a recognised association?**

☐ **A**   Lymphoma
☐ **B**   Bronchiectasis
☐ **C**   Pleural effusion
☐ **D**   Lymphoedema
☐ **E**   Hypoalbuminaemia

13 (10 marks)

A 43-year-old diabetic man is referred for investigation of nocturnal epigastric pain which has been present, on and off, for the last 18 months. He had a good initial response to ranitidine but has relapsed after seven months. There is a strong family history of diabetes, his father died of carcinoma of the pancreas and his brother has renal stones. The patient is well controlled on intensified insulin therapy and, other than H_2-antagonists, he is on no medication. He does not smoke and does not drink alcohol.

A gastroscopy shows a scarred duodenal cap with some active ulceration.

The following blood results are obtained:

Hb	132 g/l
MCV	73 fl
WCC	5.4 × 10⁹/l (normal differential)
Plt	231 × 10⁹/l
ESR	16 mm/h
Na	141 mmol/l
K	4.7 mmol/l
Calcium	3.63 mmol/l
Albumin	38 g/l
Liver function tests	Normal
Dipstix urinalysis	Normal

An abdominal X-ray shows no evidence of perforation, but bilateral medullary nephrocalcinosis. There are also some erosions in both sacroiliac joints.

1. What is the likely underlying cause?

☐ **A** Milk-alkali syndrome
☐ **B** Crohn's disease of terminal ileum
☐ **C** Primary hyperparathyroidism
☐ **D** Zollinger-Ellison syndrome
☐ **E** Sarcoidosis

2. What investigation would be the most useful?

☐ **A** Secretin-suppression test
☐ **B** Urease test for *Campylobacter*
☐ **C** Chest X-ray
☐ **D** Technetium-MIBI-subtraction scan
☐ **E** Small bowel enema

The patient improves initially on proton pump inhibitors, but over the following months develops profuse watery diarrhoea as well as a migrating, scarring rash over the trunk and upper arms. His diabetic control is worsening, he is also complaining of headaches and, on examination, a bi-temporal hemianopia is found.

3. Suggest two further tests.

☐ **A**   MR scan of the pituitary and CT of the pancreas
☐ **B**   CT of the brain and small bowel enema
☐ **C**   Combined pituitary function tests and radio-labelled white cell scan
☐ **D**   Stool cultures and lumbar puncture
☐ **E**   Small bowel biopsy and visual-evoked potentials

4. What is the unifying diagnosis?

☐ **A**   Gardner's syndrome
☐ **B**   Peutz-Jeghers' syndrome
☐ **C**   Wermer's syndrome (multiple endocrine neoplasia type I)
☐ **D**   Verner-Morrison syndrome (pancreatic VIPoma)
☐ **E**   Sipple's syndrome (multiple endocrine neoplasia type IIa)

5. What is the association with the skin rash?

☐ **A**   Pancreatic VIPoma
☐ **B**   Small bowel adenocarcinoma
☐ **C**   Phaeochromocytoma
☐ **D**   Glucagonoma
☐ **E**   Parathyroid adenoma

14 (8 marks)

A 35-year-old woman presents with malaise and increasing shortness of breath. Since the birth of her second child three years ago her periods have been irregular with intermittent menorrhagia and she has gained 5 kg in weight. She has been diagnosed as having postnatal depression and she has lost her job as a secretary. On examination, she is pale and mildly tachypnoeic. Her heart sounds are quiet, without any murmurs; her chest is clear. Pulse 56/min; BP 115/60 mmHg.

Examination of the CNS reveals a mild reduction in the lateral visual field of the right eye. Both ankle jerks are sluggish.

Investigations:

Hb	103 g/l
MCV	100 fl
WCC	4.1 × 10⁹/l (normal differential)
Plt	273 × 10⁹/l

Na	141 mmol/l
K	4.2 mmol/l
Creatinine	88 μmol/l

Total T4	34 nmol/l (75–150 nmol/l)
Free T3	1.5 pmol/l (3–9 pmol/l)
Serum TSH	58 mU/l (0.5–5.5 mU/l)
9am plasma cortisol	280 nmol/l (200–700 nmol/l)
Prolactin	3750 U/l (< 700 U/l)
Gonadotrophins	Normal

Thyroid, microsomal and thyroglobulin autoantibodies positive

ECG: Sinus bradycardia with low-voltage complexes

1. What is the diagnosis?

- ☐ **A** Sheehan's syndrome (pituitary infarction)
- ☐ **B** Primary hypothyroidism
- ☐ **C** Prolactinoma
- ☐ **D** Non-functioning pituitary adenoma
- ☐ **E** Subacute thyroiditis

2. What investigation would you perform next?

- ☐ **A** Combined pituitary function tests
- ☐ **B** Chest X-ray
- ☐ **C** Viral serology
- ☐ **D** Ultrasound of the thyroid
- ☐ **E** MR scan of the pituitary

3. What is the cause of the raised prolactin levels?

- ☐ **A** Increased TRH production
- ☐ **B** Pituitary tumour
- ☐ **C** Pituitary failure
- ☐ **D** Hypothalamic failure
- ☐ **E** Pregnancy

4. What is the treatment?

- ☐ **A** Oral steroids
- ☐ **B** Radio-iodine therapy
- ☐ **C** Oral thyroxine
- ☐ **D** Trans-sphenoidal hypophysectomy
- ☐ **E** Oral bromocriptine

15 (2 marks)

A 34-year-old nurse is under investigation for weight loss, episodes of early morning dizziness and faints. The following results were obtained after an overnight fast:

Plasma glucose   2.3 mmol/l
Plasma insulin   460 pmol/l (35–150 pmol/l)
C-peptide   0.15 nmol/l (0.2–0.6 nmol/l)

1. **What is the likely diagnosis?**

☐ **A**   Insulinoma
☐ **B**   Glucagonoma
☐ **C**   Self-administration of insulin
☐ **D**   Self-administration of sulphonylureas
☐ **E**   Acromegaly

16 (1 mark)

This is the spot review of a barium enema of a 58-year-old man presenting with constipation and weight loss.

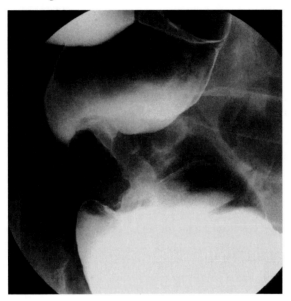

1. **Which of the following is *not* a significant risk factor?**

☐ **A**   Familial polyposis coli
☐ **B**   Peutz-Jeghers' syndrome
☐ **C**   Ulcerative colitis
☐ **D**   Pelvic radiotherapy
☐ **E**   Villous adenoma

17 (4 marks)

A 38-year-old inpatient on a psychiatric unit is investigated for polydipsia and polyuria. A water deprivation test is performed.

Time [hours]	0	2	5	8
Plasma osmolality [mOsm/kg]	289	302	307	309
Urine osmolality [mOsm/kg]	121	134	159	188

1. What is the likely underlying diagnosis?

☐ **A**   Psychogenic polydipsia
☐ **B**   Central diabetes insipidus
☐ **C**   Psychogenic water deprivation
☐ **D**   Peripheral diabetes insipidus
☐ **E**   Renal tubular acidosis type II

2. What would you expect after the im injection of DDAVP (Vasopressin)?

☐ **A**   No change
☐ **B**   Increase in urine osmolality > 15%
☐ **C**   Drop in plasma osmolality > 10 mOsm/kg
☐ **D**   Increase in plasma osmolality > 10%
☐ **E**   Rise in urine osmolality > 500 mOsm/kg

18 (5 marks)

A 42-year-old woman presents with secondary amenorrhoea, malaise and anaemia. The following are the results after the combined administration of 0.15 µ/kg of insulin, 200 µg TRH and 100 µg GN-releasing hormone.

Time [min]	0	30	60	120
Glucose [mmol/l]	4.4	1.9	2.1	6.8
GH [mU/l]	2.5 (< 10)	4.8	9.2 (>20)	7.9
TSH [mU/l]	4.2 (5–20)	5.7	4.1	
Prolactin [mU/l]	5320 (100–550)	5820	5950	
LH [mU/l]	1.5 (2–4)	13.8 (15–30)	3.2	

1. What two diagnoses can be made from these results?

- ☐ **A** Pituitary infarction
- ☐ **B** Prolactinoma
- ☐ **C** Primary hypoparathyroidism
- ☐ **D** Tertiary hypoparathyroidism
- ☐ **E** Diabetes Mellitus
- ☐ **F** Panhypopituitarism
- ☐ **G** Hypothalamic dysfunction
- ☐ **H** Raised intracranial pressure
- ☐ **I** Craniopharyngioma
- ☐ **J** Turner's syndrome

2. Which two investigations would be the most useful?

- ☐ **A** Neck ultrasound
- ☐ **B** Dopamine levels
- ☐ **C** Synacthen® test
- ☐ **D** Autoantibody screen
- ☐ **E** Insulin levels
- ☐ **F** MR scan of the pituitary
- ☐ **G** Antidiuretic Hormone (ADH) levels
- ☐ **H** Radionuclide parathyroid scan
- ☐ **I** CT scan of the neck
- ☐ **J** TSH levels

19 (6 marks)

A 54-year-old publican presents with a hoarse voice and an increasing inability to climb stairs and get out of his chair. The weakness worsens throughout the day. Investigations show:

Na	144 mmol/l
K	2.9 mmol/l
Urea	3.7 mmol/l
Glucose	13.2 mmol/l
Bicarbonate	34 mmol/l
Random cortisol	985 nmol/l

1. **Suggest two further investigations.**

☐ **A**   Fasting glucose levels
☐ **B**   ACTH levels
☐ **C**   Muscle biopsy
☐ **D**   Acetylcholine-receptor antibodies
☐ **E**   Nerve conduction studies
☐ **F**   Tensilon® test
☐ **G**   Temporal artery biopsy
☐ **H**   Chest X-ray
☐ **I**   Bronchoscopy
☐ **J**   Creatinine kinase levels

2. **Give two possible reasons for the myopathy.**

☐ **A**   Hypokalaemia
☐ **B**   Eaton-Lambert syndrome
☐ **C**   Myasthenia gravis
☐ **D**   Demyelination
☐ **E**   Hypercortisolism
☐ **F**   Motor neurone disease
☐ **G**   Polymyositis
☐ **H**   Mononeuritis multiplex
☐ **I**   Polymyositis
☐ **J**   Anaemia

20 (6 marks)

A 38-year-old man living in shared accommodation is brought to the A&E Department pyrexial and obtunded. Over the last ten days he has complained of malaise, headaches and 'pains all over'. He has become confused and has been incontinent, with several episodes of diarrhoea. He is a smoker of 30 cigarettes per day, drinks 40–50 units of alcohol per week and works part-time for the local water company.

On examination the patient is jaundiced, with a temperature of 39.2 °C. He has a regular tachycardia of 116/min, blood pressure of 105/65 mmHg and normal heart sounds. There is two fingers of tender hepatomegaly; the tip of the spleen can just be palpated under the left costal margin. The patient shows mild photophobia and neck stiffness but Kernig's sign is negative and there is no focal neurology. Fundoscopy is normal. Some petechial haemorrhages are present over the trunk and the thighs.

The following results are obtained:

Hb	119 g/l
MCV	96 fl
WBC	19 × 10⁹/l (95% neutrophils)
Plt	98 × 10⁸/l
Prothrombin time	19 s (control 13 s)
APTT	46 s (control < 34 s)
Na	133 mmol/l
K	5.1 mmol/l
Urea	19.5 mmol/l
Creatinine	205 μmol/l
Bilirubin	92 μmol/l
Albumin	32 g/l
Dipstix urinalysis	Blood + + +, Bilirubin + + +, Protein + +

1. Which pair of investigations would be most useful?

☐ **A**   ECG and chest X-ray
☐ **B**   Ultrasound of the abdomen and liver biopsy
☐ **C**   Blood cultures and urine antibody studies
☐ **D**   CT of the brain and lumbar puncture
☐ **E**   CT of the abdomen and renal biopsy

2. What is the likely diagnosis?

☐ **A**   Leptospirosis
☐ **B**   Bacterial meningitis
☐ **C**   Herpes simplex encephalitis
☐ **D**   Brucellosis
☐ **E**   Shigellosis

21 (10 marks)

A 24-year-old man is admitted to hospital with right loin pain. He was diagnosed as suffering from severe haemophilia A at the age of three. His brother is also affected. He has advanced secondary degenerative changes of his knees, elbows and hips, but there is no other significant past medical history. On examination he is extremely tender in the right flank and has an extension deficit in the right hip of 20°. No haematoma is evident on inspection. There is some guarding in the right iliac fossa; bowel sounds are present. No organomegaly. Pulse rate 96/min, regular. BP 100/50 mmHg. An ejection systolic murmur is heard in the aortic region.

Hb	108 g/l
MCV	76 fl
WCC	8.2 × 10⁹/l (63% neutrophils)
Plt	236 × 10⁹/l

Electrolytes	Normal
Bilirubin	20 μmol/l
ALT	640 U/l
Albumin	34 g/l
INR	1.8
APTT	68 seconds
Dipstix urinalysis	Blood + +, Protein +, Ketones −

1. What is the mode of inheritance?

☐ **A** Autosomal dominant
☐ **B** Autosomal recessive
☐ **C** X-linked dominant
☐ **D** X-linked recessive
☐ **E** Y-linked

2. What is the likely cause for the patient's acute presentation?

☐ **A** Renal haemorrhage
☐ **B** Psoas haematoma
☐ **C** Haemobilia
☐ **D** Variceal haemorrhage
☐ **E** Ileocaecal tuberculosis

3. What is the likely underlying cause for the deranged liver function?

☐ **A**   Haemolysis
☐ **B**   Clot obstruction
☐ **C**   Hepatitis B
☐ **D**   Cholangitis
☐ **E**   Liver cirrhosis

4. Suggest two investigations to confirm this.

☐ **A**   Abdominal ultrasound
☐ **B**   Liver biopsy
☐ **C**   Hepatitis serology
☐ **D**   Gastroscopy
☐ **E**   CT of the abdomen
☐ **F**   Alkaline phosphatase
☐ **G**   ERCP
☐ **H**   MRCP
☐ **I**   Autoantibody screen

22 (6 marks)

A 19-year-old blood donor has the following blood results:

Bilirubin   36 µmol/l
Alkaline phosphatase   96 U/l
ALT   28 U/l
Haptoglobin   78 mg/dl (40–220 mg/dl)
Dipstix urinalysis   Normal

1. What is the likely diagnosis?

- ☐ **A** Hereditary spherocytosis
- ☐ **B** Dubin-Johnson syndrome
- ☐ **C** Gilbert's syndrome
- ☐ **D** Rotor syndrome
- ☐ **E** Budd-Chiari syndrome

2. How is the condition transmitted?

- ☐ **A** Autosomal dominant
- ☐ **B** Autosomal recessive
- ☐ **C** X-linked dominant
- ☐ **D** X-linked recessive
- ☐ **E** Sporadic

3. What test is confirmatory?

- ☐ **A** Liver biopsy
- ☐ **B** Autoantibody profile
- ☐ **C** Red cell membrane electrophoresis
- ☐ **D** Hepatic angiogram
- ☐ **E** Nicotinic acid test

23 (2 marks)

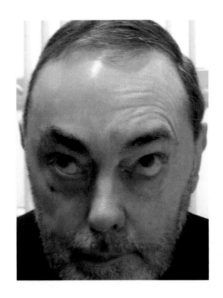

1. Which of the following is *not* a recognised cause?

☐ **A**   Neurofibromatosis type II
☐ **B**   Herpes zoster
☐ **C**   Sarcoidosis
☐ **D**   Paget's disease
☐ **E**   Systemic lupus erythematosus

24 (6 marks)

A 56-year-old man gives a four-month history of abdominal pain, diarrhoea and weight loss of 2 kg. He had a partial gastrectomy at the age of 40. The following results are obtained:

Full blood count   Normal
Bilirubin   20 µmol/l
Albumin   34 g/l
ALT   59 U/l
3-day faecal fat excretion   18 g per day/54 g total

Urinary xylose excretion after 25 g oral D-xylose: 8 g/5 h (normal > 6 g/5 h)

1. What is the most likely diagnosis?

- ☐ **A**   Malabsorption
- ☐ **B**   Chronic pancreatitis
- ☐ **C**   Bacterial overgrowth
- ☐ **D**   Terminal ileal disease
- ☐ **E**   Liver cirrhosis

2. What are the two most likely underlying causes?

- ☐ **A**   Whipple's disease
- ☐ **B**   Alcohol abuse
- ☐ **C**   Gallstones
- ☐ **D**   Coeliac disease
- ☐ **E**   Crohn's disease
- ☐ **F**   Gastric carcinoma
- ☐ **G**   Blind loop syndrome
- ☐ **H**   Chronic haemolysis
- ☐ **I**   Autoimmune hepatitis
- ☐ **J**   Sclerosing cholangitis

3. Suggest two further tests.

- ☐ **A**   Amylase
- ☐ **B**   Small bowel biopsy
- ☐ **C**   Barium meal
- ☐ **D**   ERCP
- ☐ **E**   Gastroscopy
- ☐ **F**   Lipase
- ☐ **G**   Nicotinic acid test
- ☐ **H**   Gastrin levels
- ☐ **I**   MR of the pancreas
- ☐ **J**   Barium follow-through

25 (5 marks)

A 23-year-old woman who is 33 weeks pregnant is referred to the clinic for investigation of hypertension and proteinuria. Investigations show:

Hb	99 g/l
WCC	6.4 × 10⁹/l
Plt	58 × 10⁹/l
Blood film	Spherocytes and 'bite cells'
Bilirubin	196 μmol/l
ALT	350 mmol/l
Total protein	68 g/l
Dipstix urinalysis	Blood + +, Urobilinogen + +, Protein + + +
INR	1.0

1. **What is the diagnosis based on these results?**

☐ **A**   HELLP syndrome
☐ **B**   Rhesus incompatibility
☐ **C**   Acute fatty liver of pregnancy
☐ **D**   Cholestasis of pregnancy
☐ **E**   Eclampsia

2. **What is the treatment?**

☐ **A**   Anti-rhesus immunoglobulins
☐ **B**   High-dose methylprednisolone
☐ **C**   Exchange transfusion
☐ **D**   Beta-blockers
☐ **E**   Delivery of the baby

26 (5 marks)

A 71-year-old woman is investigated, with the following results:

Hb	94 g/l
MCV	71 fl
WCC	4.8×10^9/l
Plt	134×10^9/l
ESR	52 mm/h
Normal electrolytes	

She had a partial gastrectomy three years previously for a 'growth'. Clinical examination demonstrates ascites. On aspiration, clear, gelatinous fluid is obtained. A chest X-ray shows right hilar adenopathy and pleural effusion.

1. How do you explain the appearance of the ascites?

☐ **A**   Tuberculous peritonitis
☐ **B**   Pseudomyxoma peritonei
☐ **C**   Aspiration of giant ovarian cyst
☐ **D**   Infected ascites
☐ **E**   Diffuse lymphoma

2. What is the likely diagnosis?

☐ **A**   Disseminated tuberculosis
☐ **B**   Ovarian teratodermoid
☐ **C**   Peritoneal mesothelioma
☐ **D**   Krukenberg metastases
☐ **E**   Non-Hodgkin's lymphoma

27 (3 marks)

This patient was admitted unconscious to Casualty.

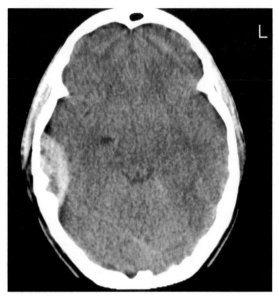

1. What is the treatment?

☐ **A**   Steroids
☐ **B**   Lumbar puncture
☐ **C**   Surgery
☐ **D**   Mannitol
☐ **E**   Intravenous cefotaxime

28 (9 marks)

A 9-year-old black foster child is brought into hospital extremely unwell. He is complaining of severe abdominal pain and is unable to lie still.

On examination the patient has a pyrexia of 38.9 °C. He is pale with a sinus tachycardia of 132/min. Respiratory rate is 40/min and the right lung base is dull on percussion with increased vocal resonance.

The abdomen is tender to palpation, with peritonism. However, rebound is negative and the bowel sounds are hyperactive but of normal quality. A blood sample taken in the resuscitation room yields the following results:

Hb	89 g/l
MCV	100 fl
WCC	14.1 × 10⁹/l
Plt	439 × 10⁹/l

Na	141 mmol/l
K	5.2 mmol/l
Urea	10.8 mmol/l
Creatinine	88 µmol/l
Dipstix urinalysis	Blood + +, Protein –, Ketones –

Arterial blood gases (on air):

pH	7.51
pO_2	8.6 kPa
pCO_2	3.8 kPa
Bicarbonate	21 mmol/l

An abdominal X-ray shows a normal bowel gas pattern but sclerotic areas within the pelvic bones.

A chest X-ray shows right lower lobe consolidation.

1. Which combination of investigations would you request?

- ☐ **A** White cell differential and bone marrow biopsy
- ☐ **B** Sputum culture and ultrasound of the abdomen
- ☐ **C** Blood cultures and standard blood film
- ☐ **D** Urine antibody studies and blood clotting
- ☐ **E** Thick-film microscopy and Gram stain of sputum

2. What immediate management would you advise?

☐ **A** Resuscitation and iv penicillin
☐ **B** iv morphine and iv doxycycline
☐ **C** Blood transfusion and iv hydrocortisone
☐ **D** High-dose oxygen and iv gentamicin
☐ **E** Forced diuresis and iv heparin

Over the next two weeks, the patient makes a good recovery and is about to be discharged.

3. What further treatment is important?

☐ **A** Prolonged course of antibiotics
☐ **B** Pneumococcal vaccination
☐ **C** Prophylactic antibiotics
☐ **D** Monitoring of blood film
☐ **E** Monitoring of renal function

Two years later, the patient is re-admitted to hospital two weeks after a febrile illness. He is pale and short of breath at rest. There is evidence of a bilateral, asymmetrical arthropathy affecting the elbows, wrists and knees.

The following results are obtained:

Hb   42 g/l
MCV   91 fl
WCC $3.1 \times 10^9/l$
Plt $102 \times 10^9/l$

Blood film: Profound anaemia, numerous Howell-Jolly bodies, multiple hyper-segmented neutrophils

4. What is the likely cause for these results?

☐ **A** Idiosyncratic drug reaction
☐ **B** Acute leukaemia
☐ **C** Drug toxicity
☐ **D** Secondary lymphoma
☐ **E** Viral infection

29 (9 marks)

A 53-year-old widower is referred by his GP because of easy bruising and malaise. He has recently had recurrent upper respiratory tract infections but is otherwise well.

He takes ibuprofen for arthritis and peppermint oil for irritable bowel syndrome. On examination he is pale with no palpable organomegaly and no lymphadenopathy. Examination of chest and cardiovascular system is unremarkable.

The following results are obtained:

Hb	98 g/l
MCV	81 fl
WCC	4.1×10^9/l
Plt	108×10^9/l
ESR	53 mm/h

Blood film: Target cells, < 0.5% reticulocytes, 2% blasts, occasional ring sideroblast

Na	136 mmol/l
K	3.8 mmol/l
Creatinine	136 µmol/l
Albumin	41 g/l
Total protein	75 g/l
Liver function tests	Normal

Chest X-ray	Normal

1. Suggest one further investigation.

- [ ] **A** Haematinics
- [ ] **B** Urinary δ-aminolaevulinic acid
- [ ] **C** Schilling test
- [ ] **D** Bone marrow biopsy
- [ ] **E** Abdominal ultrasound

2. What is the likely diagnosis?

- [ ] **A** Chronic lymphocytic leukaemia
- [ ] **B** Myelodysplastic syndrome
- [ ] **C** Lead poisoning
- [ ] **D** Chronic myeloid leukaemia
- [ ] **E** Polycythaemia rubra vera

The patient remains well but 18 months later is admitted with a cough and shortness of breath. His full blood count shows:

Hb	69 g/l
WCC	$8.9 \times 10^9/l$
Plt	$83 \times 10^9/l$
Blood film	12% blasts, multiple Auer rods

Chest X-ray shows a small area of consolidation in right upper lobe with central cavitation; no pleural effusion; no adenopathy.

3. What are the two most likely causes for the respiratory symptoms?

☐ **A** Adenocarcinoma of lung
☐ **B** Tuberculosis
☐ **C** Pulmonary infarct
☐ **D** Pulmonary haemorrhage
☐ **E** *Pneumocystis carinii* pneumonia
☐ **F** Squamous carcinoma
☐ **G** Staphylococcal pneumonia
☐ **H** Mycetoma
☐ **I** Invasive aspergillosis
☐ **J** Wegener's granulomatosis

4. What do the blood results suggest?

☐ **A** Acute myeloid leukaemia
☐ **B** Hepatitis C
☐ **C** Multiple myeloma
☐ **D** Vitamin B_{12} deficiency
☐ **E** HIV infection

30 (6 marks)

A 7-year-old boy suffers excessive haemorrhage during appendicectomy. His mother has noticed small petechial skin haemorrhages in the past. Investigations show:

Hb	119 g/l
WCC	7.9 × 10⁹/l, normal differential
Plt	357 × 10⁹/l

Hb   119 g/l
WCC   7.9 × 10^9/l, normal differential
Plt   357 × 10^9/l
Blood film: Normal except for mild reticulocytosis of 3%
PT   14 s (control 12–14 s)
APTT   35 s (control 31–33 s)
Factor VIII activity   79%
Factor IX activity   99%

1. What further investigation would you perform?

- ☐ **A** Bleeding time
- ☐ **B** Thrombin time
- ☐ **C** Platelet antibodies
- ☐ **D** Red cell sequestration studies
- ☐ **E** Factor XI activity

2. What therapy would you recommend?

- ☐ **A** Plasmapheresis
- ☐ **B** Oral prednisolone
- ☐ **C** Splenectomy
- ☐ **D** Symptomatic therapy only
- ☐ **E** Dipyridamole

3. What is the aetiology of the condition?

- ☐ **A** Idiopathic
- ☐ **B** Post-infectious
- ☐ **C** X-linked recessive
- ☐ **D** Autosomal dominant
- ☐ **E** Autosomal recessive

31 (4 marks)

This is the ECG of a 24-year-old insulin-dependent diabetic under investigation for 'panic attacks'.

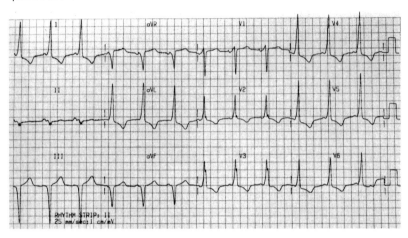

1. **What is the likely cause for his symptoms?**

☐ **A** Hyperventilation
☐ **B** Ketoacidosis
☐ **C** Sinus tachycardia
☐ **D** AV re-entrant tachycardia
☐ **E** R-on-T phenomenon

2. **What is the most appropriate management at this stage?**

☐ **A** Reassurance
☐ **B** 24 h ECG
☐ **C** Change insulin
☐ **D** Cardioselective beta-blockers
☐ **E** Amiodarone

32 (4 marks)

A 72-year-old woman is under investigation for back pain. It is noted that she passes 2.5 litres of urine per day.

A radio-isotope bone scan shows no abnormal areas of increased activity.

The following blood results are obtained:

Hb	94 g/l
WCC	$4.1 \times 10^9/l$
Plt	$128 \times 10^9/l$
MCV	85 fl
MCHC	31 g/dl

Blood film: Normocytic anaemia, rouleaux formation + +
Urinary protein electrophoresis   Normal

1. **What is the likely diagnosis?**

☐ **A**   Spinal tuberculosis
☐ **B**   Chronic lymphocytic leukaemia
☐ **C**   Multiple myeloma
☐ **D**   Waldenström's macroglobulinaemia
☐ **E**   Metastasised carcinoma of the breast

2. **Which of the following tests is going to be *least* useful?**

☐ **A**   Biochemical profile
☐ **B**   ESR
☐ **C**   Chest X-ray
☐ **D**   Serum protein electrophoresis
☐ **E**   Bone marrow aspiration

33 (5 marks)

A 30-year-old Nigerian woman requires a four-unit blood transfusion for post-partum haemorrhage after the birth of her second child.

Five days later she is noted to have scleral icterus and the following blood results are obtained:

Hb	83 g/l
MCV	101 fl
WCC	10.9 × 10^9/l (76% neutrophils)
Plt	604 × 10^9/l
Blood film	Dimorphic, 8% reticulocytes
Dipstix urinalysis	Protein –, Blood + + +, Glucose –

1. Which of the following tests would you perform?

- ☐ **A** Indirect Coombs' test
- ☐ **B** Direct Coombs' test
- ☐ **C** Osmotic resistance
- ☐ **D** Donath-Landsteiner test
- ☐ **E** Ham's test

2. What is the likely diagnosis?

- ☐ **A** Rhesus incompatibility between mother and child
- ☐ **B** ABO incompatibility between mother and child
- ☐ **C** Delayed transfusion reaction
- ☐ **D** Acquired autoimmune haemolysis
- ☐ **E** Postpartum sepsis

34 (4 marks)

A 56-year-old labourer complains of headaches and episodes of dizziness. He is on bumetanide and smokes 40 cigarettes a day.

On examination he has evidence of chronic airways disease, blood pressure 170/95 mmHg. Investigations show:

Hb	183 g/l
WCC	6.6 × 10^9/l
RBC	6.1 × 10^{12}/l
Plt	317 × 10^9/l
MCV	88 fl
MCH	30.5 pg
MCHC	31.5 g/dl
PCV	0.48

1. Which of the following tests is likely to be *normal*?

- ☐ **A** Arterial blood gases
- ☐ **B** FEV$_1$
- ☐ **C** Red cell mass
- ☐ **D** Carboxyhaemoglobin
- ☐ **E** Erythropoietin

2. What is the most important step in the management?

- ☐ **A** Stop diuretic
- ☐ **B** Stop smoking
- ☐ **C** Venesection
- ☐ **D** Tight blood pressure control
- ☐ **E** Commence low-dose aspirin

35 (2 marks)

A 22-year-old flight attendant is under investigation for 'cramps'. Outpatient investigations show:

Na	134 mmol/l
K	4.1 mmol/l
Ca	1.85 mmol/l
Creatinine	89 µmol/l
Total protein	68 g/l
Albumin	41 g/l
Alkaline phosphatase	80 U/l
PTH	0.3 pmol/l (1.5–6.5 pmol/l)

1. Which is the most appropriate investigation?

- ☐ **A** Autoantibody screen
- ☐ **B** MIBI-parathyroid scan
- ☐ **C** Ellsworth-Howard test
- ☐ **D** Small bowel biopsy
- ☐ **E** Hand X-ray

36 (5 marks)

A 16-year-old boy presents with increasing shortness of breath and bilateral ankle oedema. He has previously been fit and well, except for a severe lower respiratory tract infection six months previously. On examination there is mild ankle oedema. The lungs are clear; abdomen is unremarkable. The following results are obtained:

Hb	146 g/l
WCC	5.8×10^9/l
Plt	318×10^9/l
ESR	18 mm/h

Na	134 mmol/l
K	3.9 mmol/l
Urea	9.8 mmol/l
Creatinine	95 µmol/l
Albumin	27 g/l
Urinary protein	4.2 g/24 h
Dipstix urinalysis	Blood –, Protein + + +

A renal biopsy is normal on light microscopy, immune fluorescence is normal.

1. What is the likely diagnosis?

- ☐ **A** IgA nephropathy
- ☐ **B** Minimal change nephropathy
- ☐ **C** Immune complex nephritis
- ☐ **D** Goodpasture's syndrome
- ☐ **E** Crescentic glomuleronephritis

2. What therapy would you recommend?

- ☐ **A** Corticosteroids
- ☐ **B** Methotrexate
- ☐ **C** Ciclosporin
- ☐ **D** Cyclophosphamide
- ☐ **E** Protein supplements only

37 (6 marks)

A 53-year-old man presents with several weeks' history of malaise and exercise dyspnoea. He returned to the UK six months previously after having spent three years on agricultural development in Kenya. He is referred by the GP following two episodes of haemoptysis. Other than for exercise-induced episodes of asthma during adolescence, the only history of note is a cholecystectomy for gallstones at the age of 42.

He is on no current medication, smokes 25 cigarettes per day but does not drink any alcohol.

On examination, he is pale with bilateral ankle oedema. Auscultation reveals bilateral basal crackles, but no heart murmur. BP 185/100 mmHg; pulse 84/min, sinus rhythm. Examination of the abdomen and CNS are unremarkable.

The following results are obtained:

Hb	137 g/l
WCC	5.2×10^9/l
Plt	109×10^9/l
ESR	93 mm/h
Na	134 mmol/l
K	5.2 mmol/l
Creatinine	563 µmol/l
Total protein	53 g/l
Dipstix urinalysis	Blood +, Protein + + +, Glucose +

Renal Ultrasound: Bilaterally enlarged kidneys, without evidence of scars or hydronephrosis
Chest X-ray: Multiple ill-defined opacities in both lungs, bilateral septal lines and small pleural effusions

1. What diagnosis is *least* likely?

- ☐ **A** Polyarteritis nodosa
- ☐ **B** Medullary sponge kidney
- ☐ **C** Churg-Strauss syndrome
- ☐ **D** Goodpasture's syndrome
- ☐ **E** Membranous glomerulonephritis

A renal biopsy shows crescent formation in most glomeruli. The patient has a further episode of haemoptysis and a repeat chest X-ray shows deterioration of the previous appearances with several thick-walled cavities in both lungs. Renal angiography shows no vascular abnormality.

2. **What is the likely underlying diagnosis?**

☐ **A**   Wegener's granulomatosis
☐ **B**   Polyarteritis nodosa
☐ **C**   Churg-Strauss syndrome
☐ **D**   Alveolar cell carcinoma
☐ **E**   Goodpasture's syndrome

3. **What further investigation is likely to be diagnostic?**

☐ **A**   Anti-glomerular basement membrane antibodies
☐ **B**   Anti-neutrophil cytoplasmic antibodies
☐ **C**   Bronchoscopy and pulmonary lavage
☐ **D**   Pulmonary angiography
☐ **E**   Pulmonary transfer factor (DLCO)

38 (4 marks)

Following an episode of gastroenteritis, a 7-year-old child is admitted extremely unwell with the following blood results:

Hb   132 g/l
MCV   99 fl
WCC   7.2 × 10⁹/l
Plt   87 × 10⁹/l
Blood film: 9% reticulocytes, multiple schistocytes and fragmentocytes

Na   138 mmol/l
K   5.2 mmol/l
Creatinine   216 μmol/l

1. What is the likely diagnosis?

- ☐ **A**   Reiter's syndrome
- ☐ **B**   Henoch-Schönlein purpura
- ☐ **C**   Idiopathic thrombocytopenic purpura
- ☐ **D**   Acute sickle cell crisis
- ☐ **E**   Haemolytic uraemic syndrome

2. What is the likely precipitating cause?

- ☐ **A**   Dehydration
- ☐ **B**   Hypoxia
- ☐ **C**   Escherichia coli infection
- ☐ **D**   Parvovirus B19 infection
- ☐ **E**   Methanol ingestion

39 (2 marks)

A 23-year-old marathon runner presents with worsening dyspnoea.

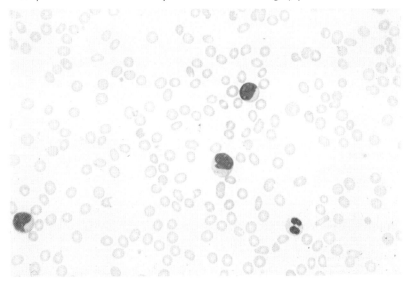

1. What does the blood film suggest?

☐ **A** Acute myeloid leukaemia
☐ **B** Iron deficiency anaemia
☐ **C** Sideroblastic anaemia
☐ **D** Aplastic anaemia
☐ **E** Vitamin B_{12} deficiency

40 (3 marks)

A two-year-old child is being investigated for irritability associated with a low-grade pyrexia. On examination, the patient has a right upper quadrant mass. The following blood results are obtained:

Hb	107 g/l
WCC	5.9 × 10⁹/l
Plt	241 × 10⁹/l
ESR	12 mm/h

Na	143 mmol/l
K	3.8 mmol/l
Creatinine	65 μmol/l
Dipstix urinalysis	Blood +, Protein −, Glucose −

Urine microscopy:

Red cells	15/μl (< 5/μl)
White cells	8/μl (< 10/μl)
Several granular casts	

1. What is the likely diagnosis?

- ☐ **A** Wilms' tumour
- ☐ **B** Horseshoe kidney
- ☐ **C** Crossed fused ectopia
- ☐ **D** Vesico-ureteric reflux
- ☐ **E** Infantile polycystic disease

41 (6 marks)

A 49-year-old woman with systemic lupus erythematosus (SLE) is under follow-up for membranous glomerulonephritis. Her previously impaired, but stable, renal function has deteriorated rapidly over the space of a week. Investigations reveal:

Na	138 mmol/l
K	5.8 mmol/l
Urea	38 mmol/l
Creatinine	1000 μmol/l
Albumin	19 g/l
Urinary protein	18 g/24 h
Dipstix urinalysis	Blood + +, Protein + + +

1. **What is the most likely diagnosis?**

☐ **A**   Acute cortical necrosis
☐ **B**   Acute exacerbation of SLE
☐ **C**   Bilateral renal vein thrombosis
☐ **D**   Renal artery occlusion
☐ **E**   Aortic thrombosis

2. **What treatment would you suggest?**

☐ **A**   Warfarin
☐ **B**   High-dose steroids
☐ **C**   Azathioprine
☐ **D**   Interferon
☐ **E**   Gammaglobulins

42 (4 marks)

A retired chemical worker presents with intermittent right loin pain. Clinical examination is unremarkable. He is on enalapril 10 mg and aspirin 150 mg. Blood results show:

Na	139 mmol/l
K	4.0 mmol/l
Urea	9.3 mmol/l
Creatinine	165 µmol/l
Calcium	2.6 mmol/l
Albumin	41 g/l
Bilirubin	18 µmol/l
Alkaline phosphatase	320 U/l

Urine microscopy:

Red cells	15/µl (< 5/µl)
White cells	8/µl (< 10/µl)
No casts	

1. What two investigations would you perform next?

- [ ] **A** Uric acid levels and cystoscopy
- [ ] **B** Captopril test and chest X-ray
- [ ] **C** DMSA renogram and serum bicarbonate
- [ ] **D** Urine electrolytes and renal angiography
- [ ] **E** Urine cytology and radio-isotope bone scan

2. What is the likely underlying cause?

- [ ] **A** Transitional cell carcinoma
- [ ] **B** Hemangioblastoma
- [ ] **C** Renal artery stenosis
- [ ] **D** Retroperitoneal fibrosis
- [ ] **E** Prostatic carcinoma

43 (2 marks)

This is the chest X-ray of a 56-year-old man with palpitations and dizziness.

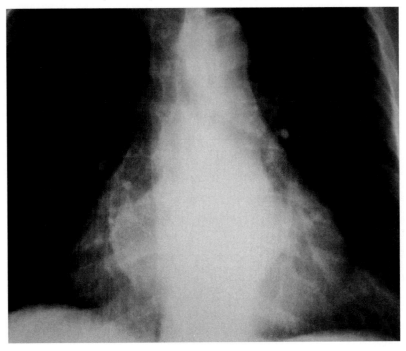

1. **What is the likely diagnosis?**

☐ **A**   Aortic regurgitation
☐ **B**   Mixed mitral valve disease
☐ **C**   Atrial septal defect
☐ **D**   Pulmonary hypertension
☐ **E**   Tricuspid incompetence

44 (8 marks)

A 23-year-old architecture student from Morocco is referred by his GP. Over the last six weeks he has become unsteady on his feet and now finds it impossible to keep his balance in the dark. The only past medical history of note is enucleation of his right eye at the age of 12 for a 'growth'.

On examination he is ataxic with a positive Romberg's test. Nystagmus is present which is not affected by posture and there is no definite associated vertigo. There is mild dysdiadochokinesis in the right hand. Examination of the cranial nerves and the remainder of the peripheral nervous system reveals no further abnormalities. The blood pressure is elevated at 190/110 mmHg with an ejection murmur over the aortic area.

The liver is not enlarged but a mass can be ballotted in the left upper quadrant.

The following results are obtained:

Hb	186 g/l
WCC	6.1×10^9/l
Plt	216×10^9/l
ESR	2 mm/hr
MCV	73 fl
Hct	61%

Na	136 mmol/l
K	4.1 mmol/l
Urea	6.2 mmol/l
Creatinine	81 µmol/l
Albumin	42 g/l
Dipstix urinalysis	Blood + +, Protein –, Bilirubin –

Ultrasound abdomen: 8-cm inhomogeneous mass, left kidney; 2-cm nodule, lower pole, right kidney; several liver cysts

1. What is your next investigation?

- ☐ **A** Chest X-ray
- ☐ **B** Intravenous urogram
- ☐ **C** Urinary catecholamine levels
- ☐ **D** Erythropoietin levels
- ☐ **E** CT of the abdomen

A CT scan of the brain shows two cystic nodules within the cerebellum. No supratentorial lesions are identified.

PAPER 2 – QUESTIONS

2. What is the underlying diagnosis?

- [ ] **A**   Malignant melanoma of the uvea
- [ ] **B**   Rhabdomyosarcoma of the orbit
- [ ] **C**   Von Hippel-Lindau syndrome
- [ ] **D**   Tuberose sclerosis
- [ ] **E**   Neurofibromatosis type II

3. What are the renal lesions?

- [ ] **A**   Metastases
- [ ] **B**   Haematomata
- [ ] **C**   Bilateral phaeochromocytoma
- [ ] **D**   Bilateral renal cell carcinoma
- [ ] **E**   Neurofibromata

The patient enquires whether there is a particular risk of his two-month-old son developing the same problem.

4. How do you estimate the risk?

- [ ] **A**   No increased risk
- [ ] **B**   25%
- [ ] **C**   40–50%
- [ ] **D**   66%
- [ ] **E**   92–100%

1

45 (8 marks)

A 53-year-old female office manager is referred by the GP for investigation of diplopia and a proximal muscle weakness. Her symptoms are worst in the morning and tend to improve through the day. In addition she complains of a three-month history of malaise and a weight gain of 1.5 kg.

On examination there is wasting of both thighs and upper arms with reduction of power at the hip flexors of 3/5 and at the deltoid of 4/5. She is unable to stand up from a squatting position, biceps and knee jerks are reduced and the ankle jerks are only present with reinforcement. Plantars are down-going. No motor deficit can be identified in the cranial nerves, but a mild dysarthria is present. There is a general reduction in tone. Co-ordination and sensation are normal.

The chest is clear; no heart murmurs; BP 180/105 mmHg; pulse 84/min, regular. Examination of the abdomen is difficult due to adiposity, but no organomegaly can be identified.

The following results are obtained:

Hb	109 g/l
WCC	5.7 × 10⁹/l
Plt	247 × 10⁹/l
MCV	73 fl
ESR	31 mm/h
Na	146 mmol/l
K	3.1 mmol/l
Urea	8.1 mmol/l
Creatinine	139 µmol/l
Random glucose	10.8 mmol/l

1. What is the likely cause for the neurological deficit?

- ☐ **A** Motor neurone disease
- ☐ **B** Myasthenia gravis
- ☐ **C** Polymyositis
- ☐ **D** Endocrine myopathy
- ☐ **E** Paraneoplastic syndrome

2. How would you confirm this?

- ☐ **A** Muscle biopsy
- ☐ **B** Electromyography
- ☐ **C** Sural nerve biopsy
- ☐ **D** Response to exercise
- ☐ **E** Tensilon® test

3. **What is the likely underlying cause for the abnormal biochemistry results?**

☐ **A**   Nelson's syndrome
☐ **B**   Islet cell tumour
☐ **C**   Ectopic ACTH secretion
☐ **D**   Multiple endocrine neoplasia type I
☐ **E**   Thrombosis of the inferior vena cava

4. **What is the most important next investigation?**

☐ **A**   Chest X-ray
☐ **B**   Muscle biopsy
☐ **C**   Early morning cortisol
☐ **D**   Autoantibody screen
☐ **E**   CT of the abdomen

46 (4 marks)

Following a night on the town, a 15-year-old boy is admitted with speech impairment and difficulty swallowing. There is a generalised reduction in tone, power and reflexes. Sensation is normal. The following results are obtained:

Na	142 mmol/l
K	2.7 mmol/l
Urea	6.1 mmol/l
Creatinine	85 μmol/l
Glucose	6.2 mmol/l

ECG	Normal
Chest X-ray	Normal
Dipstix urinalysis	Protein +, Glucose –, Blood –

1. Which of the following investigations would you recommend?

- ☐ **A**   Electromyography
- ☐ **B**   Nerve conduction studies
- ☐ **C**   CT of the brain
- ☐ **D**   Lumbar puncture
- ☐ **E**   Drug screen

2. What is the likely diagnosis?

- ☐ **A**   Ecstasy overdose
- ☐ **B**   Periodic paralysis
- ☐ **C**   McArdle's syndrome
- ☐ **D**   Cocaine overdose
- ☐ **E**   Myasthenia gravis

47 (2 marks)

This is the audiogram of a 43-year-old HGV driver under investigation for vertigo. Weber's test is lateralising to the right.

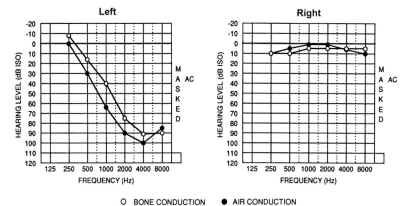

O BONE CONDUCTION   ● AIR CONDUCTION

1. Which of the following is the most likely diagnosis?

☐ **A** Ramsay-Hunt syndrome
☐ **B** Vestibular neuronitis
☐ **C** Vestibular schwannoma (acoustic neuroma)
☐ **D** Multiple sclerosis
☐ **E** Mononeuritis multiplex

48 (5 marks)

A 17-year-old African student presents with confusion, pyrexia and severe bone pain. There are no focal signs. The following results are obtained:

Hb	136 g/l
WCC	17 × 10⁹/l (12% lymphocytes)
Plt	561 × 10⁹/l
ESR	79 mm/h
Glucose	6.2 mmol/l

A lumbar puncture reveals:

Opening pressure	29 cmH$_2$O, turbid fluid
Protein	1.3 g/l
Glucose	2.6 mmol/l
Microscopy	230 cells/mm³
	(86% polymorphonuclear cells)
Gram stain	Gram-positive diplococci

1. What two diagnoses would you consider?

- ☐ **A** Staphylococcal meningitis
- ☐ **B** Meningococcal meningitis
- ☐ **C** Rabies
- ☐ **D** Malaria
- ☐ **E** Pneumococcal meningitis
- ☐ **F** Listeriosis
- ☐ **G** TB meningitis
- ☐ **H** Sickle cell disease
- ☐ **I** Tetanus
- ☐ **J** Cerebral abscess

2. What is the immediate treatment?

- ☐ **A** Cefotaxime + 100% O$_2$
- ☐ **B** Antitoxin + admission to ICU
- ☐ **C** Penicillin V + morphine
- ☐ **D** Penicillin G + midazolam
- ☐ **E** Gammaglobulins + steroids

3. **Give two further important steps in the late management.**

☐ **A** Barrier nursing
☐ **B** Family screening
☐ **C** Pneumococcal vaccination
☐ **D** Nasal swab
☐ **E** Notification of Public Health
☐ **F** Liver biopsy
☐ **G** CSF culture
☐ **H** Physiotherapy
☐ **I** Antibiotic prophylaxis

49 (6 marks)

A medical consultation is requested from the labour ward where a 26-year-old Greek woman has become confused after a spontaneous abortion at 9 weeks gestation. She has ataxia, dysarthria and a pyrexia of 38.2 °C.

A CT scan of the brain is normal but the CSF shows the following changes:

Pressure	21 cmH$_2$O
Colour	Clear
Protein	0.75 g/l
Glucose	2.0 mmol/l
	(blood glucose 4.1 mmol/l)
Microscopy	83 cells/mm^3,
	81% polymorphonuclear cells

1. What is the likely diagnosis?

- ☐ **A** Systemic lupus erythematosus (SLE)
- ☐ **B** Viral meningitis
- ☐ **C** Embolic brain abscess
- ☐ **D** Listeriosis
- ☐ **E** Sinus cavernosus thrombosis

2. How is the diagnosis confirmed?

- ☐ **A** Blood cultures
- ☐ **B** Autoantibody screen
- ☐ **C** Lupus anticoagulant estimation
- ☐ **D** MR scan of brain
- ☐ **E** Polymerase chain reaction

3. Which of the following treatments would you recommend?

- ☐ **A** iv hydrocortisone
- ☐ **B** iv erythromycin
- ☐ **C** iv benzylpenicillin
- ☐ **D** Warfarin
- ☐ **E** Low molecular weight heparin

50 (5 marks)

A 28-year-old woman with difficulties walking is admitted for investigation. The House Officer notices abnormal pupillary reflexes.

	Direct light reaction	Consensual light reaction
Right pupil	Absent	Present
Left pupil	Present	Absent

Both eyes show normal reflex on accommodation.

1. What abnormality is consistent with these findings?

- ☐ **A** Left optic neuritis
- ☐ **B** Right optic atrophy
- ☐ **C** Left retinal phacoma
- ☐ **D** Right Holmes-Adie pupil
- ☐ **E** Left optic glioma

2. What is the likely underlying diagnosis?

- ☐ **A** Neurosyphilis
- ☐ **B** Neurofibromatosis type II
- ☐ **C** Tuberose sclerosis
- ☐ **D** Tobacco amblyopia
- ☐ **E** Multiple sclerosis

51 **(2 marks)**

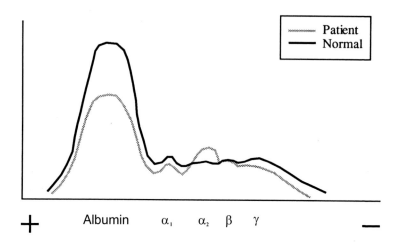

1. Which of the following diseases is the *least* likely to produce the changes seen on the protein electrophoresis?

- ☐ **A** Minimal change glomerulonephritis
- ☐ **B** Multiple myeloma
- ☐ **C** Penicillamine therapy
- ☐ **D** Membranous glomerulonephritis
- ☐ **E** Amyloidosis

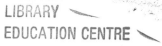

52 (9 marks)

A 36-year-old travelling businessman presents with dyspnoea after returning from a trip to the Far East. He has previously been fit and well, but on closer questioning admits to a four-month history of malaise.

On examination he is pale and some small lymph nodes are palpable in the neck. There is hyperresonant percussion at the right lung apex but clinical examination is otherwise unremarkable. Respiratory rate is 24/min; BP 120/70 mmHg; pulse 108/min, regular. He has an axillary temperature of 38.4 °C.

Investigations show:

Hb	119 g/l
WCC	3.3×10^9/l (70% lymphocytes)
Plt	108×10^9/l

Na	136 mmol/l
K	4.1 mmol/l
Urea	10.1 mmol/l
Creatinine	108 µmol/l

Arterial blood gases (room air):

pH	7.39
pO_2	9.0 kPa (68 mmHg)
pCO_2	3.9 kPa (29 mmHg)

Chest X-ray: Small right apical pneumothorax of 5–10%, no consolidation

1. What is the likely cause for the acute chest symptoms?

- ☐ **A** Tuberculosis
- ☐ **B** Leg vein thrombosis
- ☐ **C** Aircraft cabin pressure
- ☐ **D** *Mycoplasma* pneumonia
- ☐ **E** *Pneumocystis carinii* pneumonia

2. What is the likely underlying diagnosis?

- ☐ **A** Non-Hodgkin's lymphoma
- ☐ **B** Acute lymphocytic leukaemia
- ☐ **C** HIV infection
- ☐ **D** Pulmonary eosinophilia
- ☐ **E** Hodgkin's disease

3. Suggest two further investigations.

- ☐ **A** Sputum microscopy
- ☐ **B** Transthoracic lung biopsy
- ☐ **C** Bronchoscopy and lavage
- ☐ **D** Pulmonary transfer factor
- ☐ **E** AIDS test
- ☐ **F** Bone marrow biopsy
- ☐ **G** Blood cultures
- ☐ **H** Atypical serology screen
- ☐ **I** Mantoux test
- ☐ **J** High-resolution CT scan

4. What is the immediate treatment?

- ☐ **A** iv erythromycin
- ☐ **B** iv cotrimoxazole
- ☐ **C** Rifampicin plus isoniazid
- ☐ **D** 100% oxygen
- ☐ **E** iv amphotericin B

53 (7 marks)

A 20-year-old man is referred to the chest clinic for investigation of recurrent lower respiratory tract infection. He has been on repeated courses of antibiotics over the last year, but he is still producing yellow sputum most mornings. He can no longer manage to climb the three flights of stairs to his flat in one go, and he has lost 5 kg in weight over the last year.

On examination he is pale but not clubbed. Respiratory rate 22/min. Auscultation reveals bilateral early inspiratory crackles and a moderate wheeze. Examination of cardiovascular system and abdomen are unremarkable.

Investigations show:

Hb	138 g/l
WCC	10.3×10^9/l (89% neutrophils)
Plt	385×10^9/l
ESR	32 mm/h
Na	136 mmol/l
K	4.1 mmol/l
Urea	8.8 mmol/l
Creatinine	101 μmol/l

Bronchoscopy: Purulent secretions in both lower lobes, no endobronchial lesions
ECG: Sinus rhythm 88 bpm, QRS axis $+145°$, low voltage in lateral chest leads

Sweat Na content	21 mmol/l (20–40 mmol/l)

1. Which of the following is the most useful investigation?

- ☐ **A** Blood culture
- ☐ **B** Sputum culture
- ☐ **C** Chromosomal analysis
- ☐ **D** α_1-antitrypsin levels
- ☐ **E** Chest X-ray

2. What is the likely diagnosis?

- ☐ **A** Cystic fibrosis
- ☐ **B** Post-infective bronchiectasis
- ☐ **C** α_1-antitrypsin deficiency
- ☐ **D** Kartagener's syndrome
- ☐ **E** Macleod's syndrome (Swyer-James syndrome)

3. What is the likelihood of this patient having a son with the same condition?

- ☐ **A**   0%
- ☐ **B**   25%
- ☐ **C**   50%
- ☐ **D**   66%
- ☐ **E**   100%

54 (6 marks)

A 53-year-old steelworker is referred with malaise, dry cough and exercise-induced dyspnoea. He smokes 20 cigarettes/day but stopped drinking alcohol eight months ago after being told by his GP that he was damaging his liver. One year ago he suffered a severe episode of pyelonephritis which was treated with nitrofurantoin due to a penicillin allergy.

On examination he is clubbed with palmar erythema. Inspiratory crackles are present in both lungs. Respiratory rate 24/min; BP 170/90 mmHg; pulse 92/min, regular. In the abdomen there is 4-cm tender, smooth hepatomegaly, no splenomegaly or lymphadenopathy.

Investigations show:

Hb	151g/l
WCC	5.9 × 10⁹/l
Differential: 61% granulocytes, 33% lymphocytes, 3% monocytes	
Plt	347 × 10⁹/l
ESR	32 mm/h

Na	142 mmol/l
K	3.8 mmol/l
Urea	9.1 mmol/l
Creatinine	137 μmol/l
Albumin	39 g/l
Total protein	99 g/l
Bilirubin	57 U/l
AST	320 U/l
ALT	270 U/l

A liver biopsy shows areas of piecemeal necrosis.

A high resolution CT scan shows reduced lung volumes, septal thickening and multiple areas of ground-glass change.

Pulmonary function tests reveal:

TLC	3.8 l (predicted 5.7–7.5 l)
FEV_1/FVC	91%

1. Which of the following investigations would be most helpful?

- ☐ **A** Transbronchial lung biopsy
- ☐ **B** Autoantibody screen
- ☐ **C** Chest X-ray
- ☐ **D** Lupus anticoagulant
- ☐ **E** CO transfer coefficient (KCO)

2. What is the likely respiratory diagnosis?

☐ **A**   Occupational asthma
☐ **B**   Hypersensitivity pneumonitis
☐ **C**   Extrinsic allergic alveolitis
☐ **D**   Systemic lupus erythematosus
☐ **E**   Cryptogenic fibrosing alveolitis

3. What is the pathology affecting the liver?

☐ **A**   Autoimmune chronic active hepatitis
☐ **B**   Sclerosing cholangitis
☐ **C**   Primary biliary cirrhosis
☐ **D**   Heavy metal poisoning
☐ **E**   Viral hepatitis

55 (2 marks)

This is the hand of a 33-year-old male patient (P) under investigation for infertility.

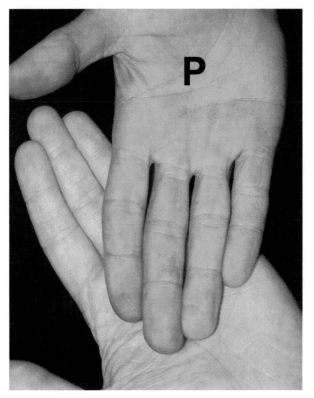

1. **Which of the following investigations is *not* indicated?**

☐ **A** Ultrasound scan of the liver
☐ **B** Serum gonadotrophin levels
☐ **C** Short Synacthen® test
☐ **D** Clotting screen
☐ **E** Family screening

56 (4 marks)

A 45-year-old man with chronic back pain is found to have an early diastolic murmur. Chest X-ray shows apical interstitial shadowing with a small cavity on the right.

Pulmonary function tests reveal:

FEV_1	2.0 l (predicted 2.1–3.1)
FVC	2.4 l (predicted 3.0–4.4)
TLC	4.8 (predicted 5.0–7.5)
Transfer factor (DLCO)	92%
Transfer coefficient (KCO)	105%

1. What type of abnormality is indicated by the results?

☐ **A**   Small airways obstruction
☐ **B**   Tracheal compression
☐ **C**   Bronchial collapse
☐ **D**   Pulmonary restrictive defect
☐ **E**   Extrapulmonary restriction

2. What is the likely diagnosis?

☐ **A**   Silicosis
☐ **B**   Ankylosing spondylitis
☐ **C**   Sarcoidosis
☐ **D**   Tuberculosis
☐ **E**   Extrinsic allergic alveolitis

57 (4 marks)

A 75-year-old woman presents with a six-week history of malaise and weakness. There is hepatosplenomegaly and a pleural effusion.

Hb	108 g/l
WCC	44 × 10⁹/l
Differential: 94% lymphocytes, 2% neutrophils, 2% eosinophils	
Plt	93 × 10⁹/l
ESR	> 120 mm/h

A pleural tap shows the following results:

Protein	48 g/l
Glucose	1.8 mmol/l
Microscopy: Lymphocytes + + +, no bacteria on Gram stain, no AAFB seen	

1. What is your next investigation?

☐ **A**   Silver stain of pleural fluid
☐ **B**   Serial blood cultures
☐ **C**   Sputum culture and microscopy
☐ **D**   Bone marrow biopsy
☐ **E**   Abdominal ultrasound scan

2. What is the diagnosis?

☐ **A**   Non-Hodgkin's lymphoma
☐ **B**   Chronic lymphocytic leukaemia
☐ **C**   TB empyema
☐ **D**   Histoplasmosis
☐ **E**   Sézary syndrome

58 (4 marks)

A 32-year-old foundry worker with long-standing mild asthma develops productive cough, fever and wheeze resistant to inhaled salbutamol.

Blood results reveal:

Hb	142 g/l
WCC	9.2×10^9/l
Differential: 61% neutrophils, 23% lymphocytes, 11% eosinophils, 4% monocytes	
Plt	217×10^9/l
ESR	59 mm/h

Three sputum samples and three early morning urines are negative for acid-fast bacilli.

1. What is the likely diagnosis?

- ☐ **A**   Occupational asthma
- ☐ **B**   Allergic bronchopulmonary aspergillosis
- ☐ **C**   Extrinsic allergic alveolitis
- ☐ **D**   Churg-Strauss syndrome
- ☐ **E**   Goodpasture's syndrome

2. Which investigation would confirm the diagnosis?

- ☐ **A**   Sputum microscopy
- ☐ **B**   Mantoux test
- ☐ **C**   High-resolution CT scan
- ☐ **D**   Autoantibody screen
- ☐ **E**   Renal biopsy

59 (4 marks)

This is the barium swallow of a patient with worsening dysphagia.

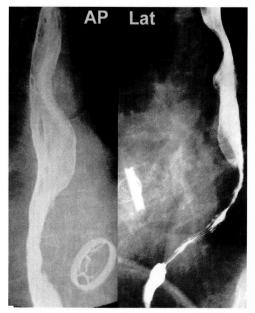

1. **What is the likely cause for the patient's symptoms?**

☐ **A** Achalasia
☐ **B** Oesophageal carcinoma
☐ **C** Left atrial enlargement
☐ **D** Peptic stricture
☐ **E** Left ventricular enlargement

2. **Which of the following blood parameters is likely to be abnormal?**

☐ **A** Haemoglobin
☐ **B** Potassium
☐ **C** Platelets
☐ **D** Creatinine
☐ **E** Prothrombin time

60 (3 marks)

A 55-year-old smoker presents with abdominal pain and confusion. Biopsy shows a small-vessel necrotising vasculitis.

A chest X-ray shows bilateral lower zone alveolar shadowing and small pleural effusions.

Investigations show:

Na	125 mmol/l
K	3.9 mmol/l
Urea	10.1 mmol/l
Creatinine	162 µmol/l
Bilirubin	28 µmol/l
AST	61 U/l
Albumin	29 g/l

Sputum: Negative Gram stain, negative culture
O_2 sat.   93% on air

1. What is your management?

- ☐ **A** Insertion of central line and 60% O_2 administration
- ☐ **B** iv diuretics and cardiac enzyme levels
- ☐ **C** Blood cultures and iv amoxicillin
- ☐ **D** ECG and iv albumin
- ☐ **E** Arterial blood gases and iv erythromycin

61 (3 marks)

A 29-year-old woman with antiphospholipid syndrome presents with a dry cough and mild wheeze. In the past she had two miscarriages.

The following results are obtained:

Hb	113 g/l
MCV	79 fl
WCC	7.3×10^9/l
Differential: 51% neutrophils, 37% lymphocytes, 8% eosinophils	
Plt	258×10^9/l
ESR	33 mm/h
PT	13 s (11–13 s)
APTT	58 s (28–4 s)
Bleeding time	11 s (control 6–9 s)

A chest X-ray shows ill-defined infiltrates in the periphery of both lungs.

1. What is the likely diagnosis?

- ☐ **A** Fungal infection
- ☐ **B** Loeffler's syndrome
- ☐ **C** Churg-Strauss syndrome
- ☐ **D** Drug side-effects
- ☐ **E** Polyarteritis nodosa

62 (5 marks)

A 23-year-old student is admitted unconscious to the A&E Department. A friend indicates that he has been suffering from headaches and malaise for several weeks. He is tachypnoeic, hyper-reflexic and pyrexial but not cyanosed.

Investigations reveal:

Arterial gases (on air):

pH	6.72
pO_2	6.8 kPa (51 mmHg)
pCO_2	2.4 kPa (18 mmHg)
Bicarbonate	23 mmol/l
O_2 sat.	61%

Chest X-ray: Normal

1. What is the likely diagnosis?

☐ **A**   Aspirin overdose
☐ **B**   Carbon monoxide poisoning
☐ **C**   Paracetamol overdose
☐ **D**   Methanol poisoning
☐ **E**   Ecstasy overdose

2. What is the immediate treatment?

☐ **A**   iv acetylcysteine
☐ **B**   Exchange transfusion
☐ **C**   iv bicarbonate
☐ **D**   iv ethanol
☐ **E**   Hyperbaric oxygen

63 (2 marks)

A 43-year-old man is admitted profoundly confused to the Accident and Emergency Department with the following results:

Hb	176 g/l
WCC	9.8 × 10⁹/l
Plt	405 × 10⁹/l
Na	143 mmol/l
K	4.5 mmol/l
Urea	10.8 mmol/l
Creatinine	153 μmol/l
Glucose	6.2 mmol/l

1. Which of the following has to be considered?

☐ **A** Rhabdomyolysis
☐ **B** Diabetes insipidus
☐ **C** Hyperosmolar non-ketotic coma
☐ **D** Furosemide (frusemide) overdose
☐ **E** Salicylate overdose

64 (7 marks)

A 61-year-old woman is referred for investigation with a three-month history of malaise and difficulties climbing the stairs to her first-floor flat. She also complains of difficulties swallowing, particularly with solids, which cause retrosternal pain. On examination she is pale with no lymphadenopathy. CNS and respiratory systems are unremarkable. The liver edge is firm and irregular, the spleen is not palpable and there is no adenopathy.

The following results are obtained:

Hb	98 g/l
MCV	69 fl
WCC	5.8 × 10⁹/l
Plt	219 × 10⁹/l
ESR	66 mm/h
MCHC	25 g/dl

U&Es	Normal
Bilirubin	22 μmol/l
AST	520 U/l
Gamma-GT	29 U/l
Alkaline phosphatase	112 U/l
Anti-nuclear antibodies	1:1024

A gastroscopy shows normal oesophagus and stomach.

1. Which of the following investigations would you perform next?

- ☐ **A** Temporal artery biopsy
- ☐ **B** Creatinine kinase
- ☐ **C** Fundoscopy
- ☐ **D** Anti-dsDNA antibodies
- ☐ **E** Acetylcholine-receptor antibodies

An EMG shows evidence of fibrillation and polyphasic bursts.

2. What is the diagnosis?

- ☐ **A** Polymyalgia rheumatica
- ☐ **B** Motor neurone disease
- ☐ **C** Myasthenia gravis
- ☐ **D** Systemic lupus erythematosus
- ☐ **E** Polymyositis

3. **What further investigation would you perform?**

☐ **A** Muscle biopsy
☐ **B** Barium enema
☐ **C** Tensilon® test
☐ **D** Electrocardiogram
☐ **E** Oesophageal manometry

65 (6 marks)

A 53-year-old man is referred for investigation of low-grade pyrexia and night sweats. He has lost 5 kg in weight over six months. More recently he has become breathless, and has experienced some relief with a salbutamol inhaler. He has a two-year history of angina which is controlled on oral nitrates and aspirin.

On examination there is some tenderness of the wrists and knees, but no active synovitis.

Mild pitting oedema is seen around both ankles; BP 175/100 mmHg; pulse 80/min, regular. Fine crackles are auscultated at the bases and there is a generalised wheeze. Investigations reveal:

Hb	138 g/l
WCC	10.5×10^9/l
Differential: 81% granulocytes, 6% eosinophils, 12% lymphocytes	
Plt	482×10^9/l
ESR	53 mm/h
MCV	81 fl
MCH	29 pg

Na	136 mmol/l
K	5.1 mmol/l
Urea	14.2 mmol/l
Creatinine	261 µmol/l
Albumin	36 g/l
LFTs	Normal

1. What is the likely diagnosis?

- ☐ **A** Polyarteritis nodosa
- ☐ **B** Wegener's granulomatosis
- ☐ **C** Systemic lupus erythematosus
- ☐ **D** Pulmonary eosinophilia
- ☐ **E** Churg-Strauss syndrome

2. How would you confirm the diagnosis?

- ☐ **A** Lung biopsy
- ☐ **B** Nasal biopsy
- ☐ **C** Renal angiogram
- ☐ **D** Anti-neutrophil cytoplasmic antibodies (ANCA)
- ☐ **E** Antibodies to double-stranded DNA

3. What is the most important prognostic factor?

☐ **A** Degree of renal involvement
☐ **B** Degree of arterial involvement
☐ **C** Degree of CNS involvement
☐ **D** Pattern of autoantibodies
☐ **E** CRP levels

66 (4 marks)

A 33-year-old Jamaican woman is referred for investigation of heartburn and dysphagia. Gastroscopy is normal and blood results show:

Hb	113 g/l
WCC	$6.1 \times 10^9/l$
MCV	81 fl
ESR	33 mm/h

Anti-nuclear antibodies	1:640, speckled pattern
Anti-centromere	1:10
Scl-70	1:160
Anti-nucleolus	1:160
Anti-dsDNA	1:10
Anti-ENA	1:10

1. What is the likely diagnosis?

☐ **A**   Sjögren's syndrome
☐ **B**   Limited cutaneous systemic sclerosis (CREST)
☐ **C**   Diffuse systemic sclerosis
☐ **D**   Systemic lupus erythematosus
☐ **E**   Mixed connective tissue disease (Sharp syndrome)

2. What is the next investigation?

☐ **A**   Dipstix urine testing
☐ **B**   CRP
☐ **C**   Chest X-ray
☐ **D**   Blood pressure measurement
☐ **E**   MR of the oesophagus

67 (2 marks)

A 67-year-old diabetic is referred from Casualty after admission with syncope.

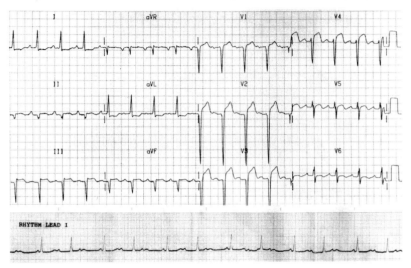

1. Which of the following is indicated?

☐ **A**   Warfarin
☐ **B**   24 h ECG
☐ **C**   Pacemaker insertion
☐ **D**   Thrombolysis
☐ **E**   Beta-blockers

68 (4 marks)

A 26-year-old West Indian woman presents with a flitting arthritis affecting predominantly both ankles and her knees and hands. She has an intermittent low-grade pyrexia and a dry cough. Investigations reveal:

Hb	124 g/l
WCC	12.1 × 10⁹/l
Plt	437 × 10⁹/l
ESR	88 mm/h
Na	140 mmol/l
K	4.2 mmol/l
Urea	14.2 mmol/l
Calcium	2.6 mmol/l
Albumin	37 g/l
ANA	1:10
ASO	1:40
Rheumatoid factor	1:20

1. What is your next investigation?

☐ **A**   Blood cultures
☐ **B**   Chest X-ray
☐ **C**   Throat swab
☐ **D**   Radio-isotope bone scan
☐ **E**   Serum ACE levels

2. What is the likely diagnosis?

☐ **A**   Systemic lupus erythematosus
☐ **B**   Infective endocarditis
☐ **C**   Non-Hodgkin's lymphoma
☐ **D**   Loefgren's syndrome
☐ **E**   Still's disease

69 (6 marks)

A 73-year-old man presents with increasing shortness of breath, worse at night, and pain around the left hip joint. The following results are obtained:

FBC	Normal
ESR	16 mm/h
U&Es	Normal
Calcium	2.35 mmol/l
Phosphate	1.2 mmol/l
Albumin	36 g/l
ALT	71 U/l
Gamma	GT 89 U/l
Bilirubin	18 μmol/l
Alkaline phosphatase	1190 U/l
Acid phosphatase	12 U/l (< 5 U/l)
Prostate-specific antigen	1.9 ng/ml (< 1 ng/ml)
Urinary hydroxyproline	730 mmol/24 h
	(70–300 mmol/24 h)

1. What is the likely underlying diagnosis?

- ☐ **A** Paget's disease
- ☐ **B** Osteomalacia
- ☐ **C** Multiple myeloma
- ☐ **D** Liver cirrhosis
- ☐ **E** Carcinoma of the prostate

2. What complication has occurred?

- ☐ **A** Stress fracture
- ☐ **B** Sarcomatous change
- ☐ **C** Hepatoma
- ☐ **D** Congestive cardiac failure
- ☐ **E** Metastatic disease

3. What investigation would you perform in the first instance?

- ☐ **A** Liver ultrasound and biopsy
- ☐ **B** Transrectal biopsy of the prostate
- ☐ **C** Vitamin D levels
- ☐ **D** Serum and urine protein electrophoresis
- ☐ **E** Pelvic X-ray

70 (3 marks)

A 33-year-old Indian salesman presents with a ten-day history of low-grade pyrexia and polyarthralgia. On examination the left knee is hot, with an effusion, and a pustular rash surrounds the joint. He has previously been well, except for an episode of non-specific urethritis 18 months previously.

Investigations show:

Biochemical profile	Normal
Glucose	6.4 mmol/l
CRP	43 mg/l
Autoantibody screen	Negative
Rheumatoid factor	Negative
Joint aspirate	15 ml turbid fluid
Protein	53 g/l
Glucose	2.8 mmol/l
Culture	Negative

1. What is the likely diagnosis?

- ☐ **A** Pustular psoriasis
- ☐ **B** Reiter's syndrome
- ☐ **C** Secondary syphilis
- ☐ **D** Gonococcal arthritis
- ☐ **E** Tuberculous arthritis

2. What is your next investigation?

- ☐ **A** Blood cultures
- ☐ **B** Joint aspirate and culture
- ☐ **C** VDRL test
- ☐ **D** Chest X-ray
- ☐ **E** Mid-stream urine sample

Paper 3 – Questions

1 (4 marks)

A thin 15-year-old girl is referred to the Cardiology Department for investigation of palpitations. She also complains of recurrent flank pain.

Arterial blood: (on air) gas analysis
pH   7.31
pO_2 14.0 kPa (105 mmHg)
pCO_2 4.0 kPa (30 mmHg)
Bicarbonate   15 mmol/l
Dipstix urinalysis Blood +, Protein –, Glucose –

ECG: Sinus rhythm 72/min, multifocal ventricular extrasystoles, QRS axis +75°, descending ST depression in antero-lateral leads, U-waves

1. What is the likely diagnosis?

☐ **A** Chronic liquorice intoxication
☐ **B** Renal tubular acidosis type I
☐ **C** Fanconi syndrome
☐ **D** Renal tubular acidosis type II
☐ **E** Anorexia nervosa

2. What is your next investigation?

☐ **A** Abdominal X-ray
☐ **B** 24-hour cardiac monitoring
☐ **C** Intravenous urogram
☐ **D** Echocardiogram
☐ **E** Urine spectroscopy

2 (6 marks)

A 54-year-old woman is referred by her GP with a six-month history of shortness of breath, malaise and weight gain. She was successfully treated for lymphoma in her twenties, but this was complicated by tuberculosis at the time. Two years previously she had a severe flu-like illness with pleuritic chest pain which resolved with symptomatic treatment only.

On examination she is overweight but otherwise well. Her jugular venous pressure is raised 6 cm above the sternal angle with systolic collapse. The cardiac apex cannot be palpated, the heart sounds are soft and no murmurs are heard. Pulse 76/min, regular; BP 110/55 mmHg. There is bilateral pitting oedema of the ankles. Examination of the abdomen reveals no abnormality.

Blood results show:

Hb	114 g/l
WCC	4.9 × 10⁹/l (normal differential)
Plt	219 × 10⁹/l
ESR	21 mm/h

Na	133 mmol/l
K	5.5 mmol/l
Creatinine	198 µmol/l
Total cholesterol	6.1 mmol/l
LDL	4.3 mmol/l (< 3.9 mmol/l)
Glucose	6.3 mmol/l

Chest X-ray: Large globular heart; lungs clear except for some apical calcification

1. **What is the cardiological diagnosis?**

- ☐ **A** Constrictive pericarditis
- ☐ **B** Myocarditis
- ☐ **C** Endomyocardial fibrosis
- ☐ **D** Pericardial effusion
- ☐ **E** Restrictive cardiomyopathy

2. **Which of the following is the *least* likely precipitating cause?**

- ☐ **A** Recurrent lymphoma
- ☐ **B** Gout
- ☐ **C** Hypothyroidism
- ☐ **D** Tuberculosis
- ☐ **E** Bornholm disease

3. What treatment would you recommend?

☐ **A** Digoxin
☐ **B** ACE inhibitors
☐ **C** Pericardial fenestration
☐ **D** Systemic steroids
☐ **E** Thyroxine

3 (10 marks)

A 56-year-old man is admitted for increasing shortness of breath and confusion. He was well until a week ago when his wife noticed increasing dyspnoea and some erratic behaviour.

In the past he has been investigated for two episodes of haematuria, but iv urography, cystoscopy and ultrasound one month previously had not detected any abnormality. He had hepatitis A at the age of 23 and rheumatic fever and endocarditis as a child.

On examination he is orientated to person but not to time and place. He is hyper-reflexic in the left arm and leg, with a slight increase in tone but no other focal signs. Pulse 120/min, irregular; JVP elevated 4 cm; soft pansystolic murmur at the apex radiating to the axilla. Auscultation of the chest reveals a mild wheeze and bilateral basal crackles. The spleen can be palpated 1 cm below the costal margin, the liver is not enlarged and there is no lymphadenopathy.

The following results are obtained:

Hb	128 g/l
WCC	9.3×10^9/l
Plt	476×10^9/l
CRP	21 mg/dl (< 10 mg/dl)
Na	139 mmol/l
K	4.6 mmol/l
Urea	10.1 mmol/l
Creatinine	172 µmol/l
Bilirubin	18 U/l
AST	34 U/l
Dipstix urinalysis	Blood + +, Protein +, Glucose –

ECG: Atrial fibrillation, 116/min, QRS axis +15°, 1-mm ST depression in the lateral leads

1. Which of the following sets of investigations is the most useful?

☐ **A**   White cell differential, chest X-ray, urine culture and microscopy
☐ **B**   ESR, abdominal ultrasound, cardiac enzymes
☐ **C**   Repeat IVU, hepatitis serology, left-sided cardiac catheter
☐ **D**   Echocardiogram, blood cultures, CT brain
☐ **E**   Creatinine clearance, CT kidneys, right-sided cardiac catheter

2. What management would you recommend?

- ☐ **A**   100% O$_2$ and oral sotalol
- ☐ **B**   iv antibiotics and iv furosemide (frusemide)
- ☐ **C**   iv fluids and iv digoxin
- ☐ **D**   iv diamorphine and renal dose dopamine
- ☐ **E**   Insertion of central line and iv amiodarone

3. What is the likely diagnosis?

- ☐ **A**   Endocarditis
- ☐ **B**   Renal cell carcinoma
- ☐ **C**   Pyelonephritis
- ☐ **D**   Transitional cell carcinoma
- ☐ **E**   Perinephric abscess

4. What complication has arisen?

- ☐ **A**   Cerebral metastasis
- ☐ **B**   Cerebral abscess
- ☐ **C**   Subarachnoid haemorrhage
- ☐ **D**   Subdural empyema
- ☐ **E**   Cerebral haemorrhage

4 (7 marks)

A 43-year-old woman is admitted after having collapsed at home. Over the preceding weeks she has complained of some tiredness, but has not required any time off work. There is no past history of note.

On examination she is drowsy with weakness of all four limbs. There is no neck stiffness or papilloedema. Auscultation reveals no murmurs, but a loud third heart sound. There is no clinical evidence of cardiac failure. She is admitted and makes a general improvement overnight. However, the nursing staff point out that her eyesight now seems extremely poor. There is no residual weakness, she is alert and orientated and does not complain of any visual disturbances. Fundoscopy, eye movements and pupillary light reflexes are normal. However, she is unable to count fingers.

Examinations reveal:

Hb	139 g/l
WCC	4.6×10^9/l (normal differential)
Plt	401×10^9/l
ESR	56 mm/h

Na	142 mmol/l
K	4.8 mmol/l
Creatinine	105 μmol/l
Albumin	40 g/l
Total protein	95 g/l
AST	28 U/l

ECG: Sinus rhythm 64/min, QRS axis $+60°$, no ischaemic changes
Chest X-ray: Normal heart and lungs

1. What is the cause for the acute presentation?

- ☐ **A** Vertebro-basilar embolus
- ☐ **B** Subarachnoid haemorrhage
- ☐ **C** Transient ischaemic attack
- ☐ **D** Amaurosis fugax
- ☐ **E** Encephalitis

2. What is the underlying cause?

- ☐ **A** Subacute bacterial endocarditis
- ☐ **B** Systemic lupus erythematosus
- ☐ **C** Atrial myxoma
- ☐ **D** Waldenström's macroglobolinaemia
- ☐ **E** Berry aneurysm

5 (5 marks)

This patient is admitted to Casualty severely breathless.

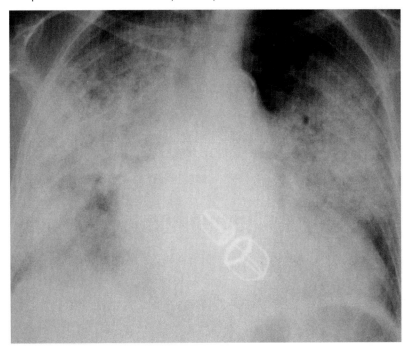

1. What is the diagnosis on chest X-ray?

- ☐ **A** Pneumonia
- ☐ **B** Tuberculosis
- ☐ **C** Adult respiratory distress syndrome
- ☐ **D** Cardiac failure
- ☐ **E** Pulmonary haemorrhage

2. Which of the following blood tests is most useful?

- ☐ **A** Full blood count
- ☐ **B** INR
- ☐ **C** Albumin
- ☐ **D** C-reactive protein
- ☐ **E** Urea and electrolytes

6 (2 marks)

The following readings are taken from a cardiac catheter of a 14-year-old cyanosed boy:

	Pressure [mmHg]
RA	Mean 6
RV	115/2
PA	22/12
LA	Mean 5
LV	110/0
Aorta	110/60

1. What is the likely diagnosis?

☐ **A**   Eisenmenger's complex
☐ **B**   Pulmonary stenosis
☐ **C**   Ebstein's anomaly
☐ **D**   Fallot's tetralogy
☐ **E**   Ventricular septal defect

7 (5 marks)

A 26-year-old woman is admitted to the Coronary Care Unit with suspected endocarditis. The following results are obtained from a right-sided cardiac catheter.

	Pressure [mmHg]	O$_2$ saturation
RA	Mean 3	71%
RV	28/1	72%
PA	28/15	81%
Pulmonary capillary wedge pressure	12	–

1. What is the diagnosis?

- ☐ **A** Atrial septal defect
- ☐ **B** Ventricular septal defect
- ☐ **C** Corrected transposition of the great arteries
- ☐ **D** Pulmonary stenosis
- ☐ **E** Patent ductus arteriosus

2. What definitive therapy would you recommend?

- ☐ **A** Balloon valvotomy
- ☐ **B** Surgical correction
- ☐ **C** Prostaglandin E1
- ☐ **D** Angiographic embolisation
- ☐ **E** Valve replacement

8 (5 marks)

This is an ECG of a 28-year-old man with intermittent palpitations.

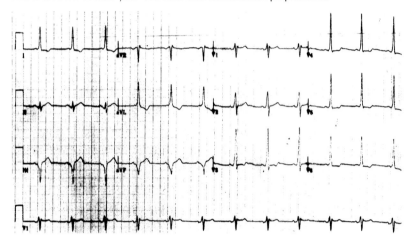

1. What is the diagnosis?

☐ **A**   Nodal rhythm
☐ **B**   Lown-Ganong-Levine syndrome
☐ **C**   Wolff-Parkinson-White type A
☐ **D**   Wolff-Parkinson-White type B
☐ **E**   Bi-fascicular block

2. What is the underlying cause?

☐ **A**   Sick sinus syndrome
☐ **B**   Septal ischaemia
☐ **C**   Central accessory bundle
☐ **D**   Right-sided accessory bundle
☐ **E**   Left-sided accessory bundle

9 (2 marks)

A 42-year-old woman has this blood film done as part of a medical assessment for life insurance.

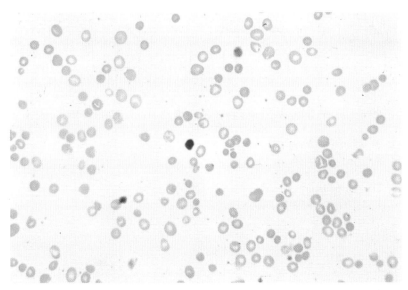

1. What does the blood film show?

- ☐ **A**   Iron deficiency anaemia
- ☐ **B**   Aplastic anaemia
- ☐ **C**   Hereditary spherocytosis
- ☐ **D**   Autoimmune haemolytic anaemia
- ☐ **E**   Folate deficiency

10 (2 marks)

A motorcyclist has collided with a bus and is brought into Casualty unconscious. Blood pressure and pulse are unrecordable. The following rhythm strip is obtained:

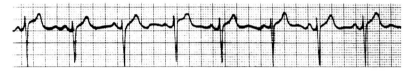

1. **Which of the following injuries is *unlikely* to account for the findings?**

- ☐ **A**   Serial rib fractures
- ☐ **B**   Aortic rupture
- ☐ **C**   Carotid dissection
- ☐ **D**   Air embolism
- ☐ **E**   Pericardial haemorrhage

11 (2 marks)

A 32-year-old woman is investigated for episodes of palpitations and anxiety.

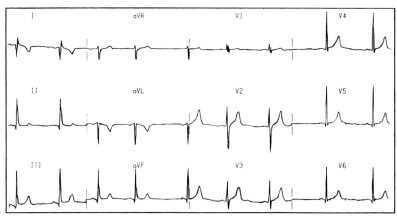

1. What abnormality does the ECG show?

☐ **A**   Jervell and Lange-Nielsen syndrome
☐ **B**   Limb lead reversal
☐ **C**   Right ventricular hypertrophy
☐ **D**   Acute right ventricular strain
☐ **E**   Dextrocardia

12 (5 marks)

An 11-year-old boy is referred for investigation of ataxia and exertional syncope. On examination there is a jerky pulse with an ejection systolic murmur. He also has clawing of the toes and fundoscopy shows temporal pallor of both discs.

Investigations show:

Chest X-ray: Normal
ECG: Left ventricular hypertrophy
Echocardiogram: Septal thickening and mild mitral regurgitation

1. What is the cardiac diagnosis?

☐ **A**   Mixed aortic valve disease
☐ **B**   Mixed mitral valve disease
☐ **C**   Supra-valvar aortic stenosis
☐ **D**   Hypertrophic obstructive cardiomyopathy
☐ **E**   Cardiac cushion defect

2. What is the underlying condition?

☐ **A**   Hereditary sensorimotor neuropathy
☐ **B**   Friedreich's ataxia
☐ **C**   Myotonic dystrophy
☐ **D**   Multiple sclerosis
☐ **E**   Poliomyelitis

13 (1 mark)

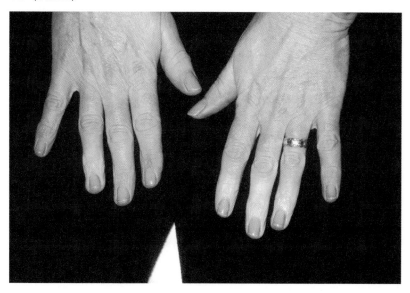

1. Which of the following should be avoided in this condition?

☐ **A**   Salbutamol
☐ **B**   Nifedipine
☐ **C**   Atenolol
☐ **D**   Aspirin
☐ **E**   Enalapril

14 (9 marks)

A 56-year-old butcher presents with an eight-month history of malaise, headaches, depression and backache. He has also found it difficult climbing the stairs at home and getting out of his car. He was previously healthy, smokes 25 cigarettes a day but does not drink alcohol. His only medication is diclofenac for back pain. On examination, he has a plethoric face, and multiple ecchymoses are present within the skin of his arms and abdomen. There is truncal obesity and striae are present over the abdomen.

There is some proximal muscle wasting, but no fasciculation and the reflexes are present.

Blood pressure is 190/105 mmHg and he has grade II hypertensive retinopathy. Investigations show:

Hb	159 g/l
WCC	7.8×10^9/l
Plt	238×10^9/l
Na	146 mmol/l
K	3.1 mmol/l
Creatinine	92 μmol/l

Oral glucose tolerance test					
Time [minutes]	0	30	60	90	120
Glucose [mmol/l]	6.9	8.5	11.2	9.8	8.9
Growth hormone [mU/l]	6.2 (2–8 mU/l)	4.8	4.5	3.9	2.8

1. What do these results imply?

- ☐ **A** Impaired glucose tolerance
- ☐ **B** Acromegaly
- ☐ **C** Manifest diabetes mellitus
- ☐ **D** Chronic liver disease
- ☐ **E** Pituitary dysfunction

A morning blood sample shows the following result:
9am cortisol   899 nmol/l (200–700 nmol/l)

After two days of 2 mg/day dexamethasone, the following result is obtained:
9am cortisol   801 nmol/l

Then after a further two days of 8 mg/day dexamethasone:
9am cortisol   769 nmol/l

2. **Which of the following two differential diagnoses are consistent with these results?**

☐ **A**   Pituitary adenoma and adrenal carcinoma
☐ **B**   Hyperthalamic dysfunction and pituitary adenoma
☐ **C**   Adrenal adenoma and ectopic ACTH secretion
☐ **D**   Factitious administration of cortisol and pituitary adenoma
☐ **E**   Bronchial carcinoma and Cushing's disease

3. **Which of the following tests is most likely to differentiate between the two?**

☐ **A**   Insulin stress test
☐ **B**   Renal ultrasound scan
☐ **C**   CRH test
☐ **D**   MR scan of the pituitary
☐ **E**   Serum ACTH levels

Following surgical treatment, the patient becomes hypotensive and oliguric. Examination of the abdomen reveals peritonism with absent bowel sounds. The following results are obtained:

Na	131 mmol/l
K	5.8 mmol/l
Urea	18.6 mmol/l
Creatinine	256 µmol/l

4. **What complication has developed?**

☐ **A**   Acute pituitary failure
☐ **B**   Acute tubular necrosis
☐ **C**   Acute adrenal failure
☐ **D**   Acute hydrocephalus
☐ **E**   Waterhouse-Friderichsen syndrome

15 (7 marks)

A 13-year-old girl is under investigation for tall stature, absent development of breasts and male distribution of pubic and body hair. She has never had a period and has recently developed hypertension. On examination, she is found to be on the 95th percentile for height and the 50th percentile for weight. No significant breast development is present, but there is hypertrophy of the clitoris and the labia majora. Her BP is 175/95 mmHg, pulse 88/min, regular, and examination of the chest and cardiovascular system is otherwise unremarkable. No focal neurology.

The following results are obtained:

FBC	Normal
Na	149 mmol/l
K	3.4 mmol/l
Urea	7.2 mmol/l
Creatinine	129 μmol/l
Albumin	42 g/l

Luteinising hormone	< 0.1 U/l (2.5–15 U/l)
FSH	< 0.1 U/l (0.3–3.0 U/l)
Testosterone	10.7 nmol/l (< 2.0 nmol/l)
9am cortisol	23 nmol/l (100–700 nmol/l)
Urinary 11-deoxycorticosterone	4.3 μg/24 h (0.1–0.4 μg/24h)
Plasma renin	16 pmol/l (85–410 pmol/l)

1. What is the diagnosis?

- ☐ **A** Congenital adrenal hyperplasia
- ☐ **B** Conn's syndrome
- ☐ **C** Phaeochromocytoma
- ☐ **D** Polycystic ovary syndrome
- ☐ **E** Craniopharyngioma

2. Why is the patient hypertensive?

- ☐ **A** Increased glucocorticoids
- ☐ **B** Increased growth hormone
- ☐ **C** Increased adrenaline (epinephrine)
- ☐ **D** Increased noradrenaline (norepinephrine)
- ☐ **E** Increased mineralocorticoids

3. Which of the following would be abnormally raised?

☐ **A**   Blood sugar
☐ **B**   Urinary sodium
☐ **C**   Thyroxine
☐ **D**   Parathormone
☐ **E**   ACTH

16 (5 marks)

A 56-year-old man presents with headaches and hypertension. The following results were obtained during an oral glucose tolerance test (75 g of oral glucose equivalent):

Time [minutes]	Plasma glucose [mmol/l]	Growth hormone [mU/l]
0	8.9	12
30	12.8	18
60	14.4	28
90	13.8	34
120	12.2	23

Prolactin: 1680 mU/l (75–350 mU/l)

1. What is the underlying diagnosis?

- ☐ **A**   Diabetes mellitus
- ☐ **B**   Prolactinoma
- ☐ **C**   Multiple endocrine neoplasia type I
- ☐ **D**   Multiple endocrine neoplasia type II
- ☐ **E**   Acromegaly

2. What complication has developed?

- ☐ **A**   Impaired glucose tolerance
- ☐ **B**   Malignant glucagonoma
- ☐ **C**   Pituitary failure
- ☐ **D**   Compression of the pituitary stalk
- ☐ **E**   Hyporthalamic failure

17 (2 marks)

This is the ECG of a 27-year-old woman with intermittent claudication. She is a life-long non-smoker and her lipid profile is normal.

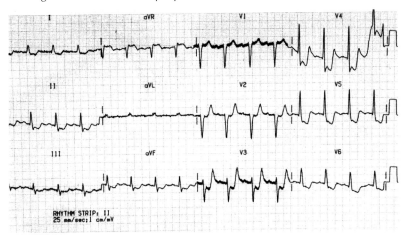

1. **Which of the following diagnoses is most likely?**

☐ **A**   Takayasu's disease
☐ **B**   Polyarteritis nodosa
☐ **C**   Pseudoxanthoma elasticum
☐ **D**   Thromboangiitis obliterans (Buerger's disease)
☐ **E**   Essential thrombocythaemia

18 (4 marks)

This is the abdomen of a 21-year-old man of short stature.

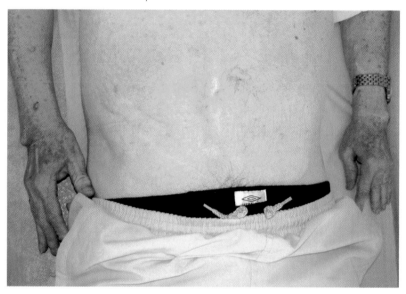

1. **What is the likely diagnosis?**

☐ **A** Inflammatory bowel disease
☐ **B** Rheumatoid arthritis
☐ **C** Whipple's disease
☐ **D** Psoriasis
☐ **E** Still's disease

2. **Which complication is _unlikely_ to have arisen?**

☐ **A** Hypertension
☐ **B** Upper lobe pulmonary fibrosis
☐ **C** Amyloidosis
☐ **D** Anaemia
☐ **E** Osteoporosis

19 (3 marks)

The following results were obtained during an insurance medical examination of a 48-year-old manager:

Na	138 mmol/l
K	4.1 mmol/l
Creatinine	92 µmol/l
Calcium	2.86 mmol/l
Phosphate	0.85 mmol/l
Alkaline phosphatase	99 U/l
Magnesium	1.3 mmol/l (0.7–1.0 mmol/l)
Parathormone	0.3 pmol/l (1.5–6.5 pmol/l)
Urinary calcium	0.9 mmol/24 h (2.5–6 mmol/24 h)

1. What is the diagnosis?

- ☐ **A** Milk-alkali syndrome
- ☐ **B** Sarcoidosis
- ☐ **C** Renal tubular acidosis type I
- ☐ **D** Familial hypocalciuric hypercalcaemia
- ☐ **E** Paget's disease

20 (5 marks)

A 50-year-old man presents with malaise and dizzy spells. These are his results after 250 µg tetracosactrin.

Cortisol at 0 minutes	128 nmol/l
Cortisol at 30 minutes	261 nmol/l
Cortisol at 60 minutes	301 nmol/l

1. What diagnosis is excluded by these results?

☐ **A**   Addison's disease
☐ **B**   Long-term steroid therapy
☐ **C**   Pituitary failure
☐ **D**   Cushing's syndrome
☐ **E**   Hypothalamic failure

Following the short Synacthen® test, the patient is given 1 mg of depot tetracosactrin im
Cortisol after 24 hours   612 nmol/l

2. What diagnosis is consistent with these results?

☐ **A**   Addison's disease
☐ **B**   Adrenal carcinoma
☐ **C**   Cushing's syndrome
☐ **D**   Nelson's syndrome
☐ **E**   Long-term steroid therapy

21 (5 marks)

A 26-year-old woman is under investigation for oligomenorrhoea and primary infertility. Blood results are as follows:

Na	134 mmol/l
K	4.1 mmol/l
Creatinine	94 µmol/l
Testosterone	2.7 nmol/l (0.8–1.6 nmol/l)
Follicle stimulating hormone	6 U/l (< 8 U/l in follicular phase)
Luteinising hormone	23 U/l (< 6 U/l in follicular phase)
7-hydroxyprogesterone	2.8 nmol/l (< 15 nmol/l)

1. **What diagnosis is the most likely?**

☐ A Testicular feminisation
☐ B Cushing's syndrome
☐ C Congenital adrenal hyperplasia
☐ D Polycystic ovary syndrome
☐ E Primary ovarian failure

2. **What investigation would be the most helpful?**

☐ A Urinary free cortisol
☐ B Urinary 17-corticosteroids
☐ C Ultrasound scan of the pelvis
☐ D Chromosomal analysis
☐ E Gonadotrophin-releasing hormone (GN-RH) test

22 (2 marks)

A 59-year-old retired accountant is referred by his General Practitioner for increasing unsteadiness and incontinence. A CT is performed.

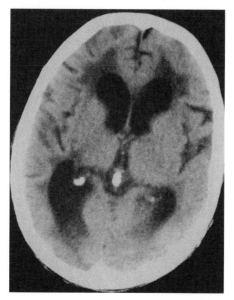

1. **What is the most likely diagnosis?**

☐ **A**   Chronic subdural haematoma
☐ **B**   Normal-pressure hydrocephalus
☐ **C**   Multi-infarct dementia
☐ **D**   Benign intracranial hypertension
☐ **E**   Subarachnoid haemorrhage

23 (8 marks)

A 36-year-old marathon runner presents to his GP with an itchy rash over both elbows. He has also noticed a slight decrease in his exercise tolerance, but otherwise feels well. On examination he is 180 cm tall, weighing 61 kg. Over the last few months he has noticed recurrent painful lesions in his mouth. The patient is taking oral retinoids for acne, but is on no other medication. Except for the rash, clinical examination is normal with no organomegaly and no lymphadenopathy. The patient experiences some symptomatic relief from topical steroids, but a blood sample taken returns the following results:

Hb	131 g/l
MCV	89 fl
WCC	7.2×10^9/l
Differential: 55% neutrophils, 31% lymphocytes, 6% eosinophils	
Plt	210×10^9/l
ESR	16 mm/h
Na	138 mmol/l
K	4.1 mmol/l
Urea	6.3 mmol/l
Albumin	30 g/l
Bilirubin	16 μmol/l
ALT	19 U/l

1. Which of the following tests is likely to be the most useful?

- ☐ **A** Endoscopy and small bowel biopsy
- ☐ **B** Skin biopsy
- ☐ **C** Stool microscopy and cultures
- ☐ **D** Small bowel aspirate and culture
- ☐ **E** Small bowel enema

2. What is the likely diagnosis?

- ☐ **A** Whipple's disease
- ☐ **B** *Cryptosporidium* infection
- ☐ **C** Tropical sprue
- ☐ **D** Small bowel lymphoma
- ☐ **E** Coeliac disease

With the appropriate treatment the patient becomes asymptomatic, but presents two years later with prolonged episodes of diarrhoea.

3. What is the likely precipitating cause?

☐ **A**   Malignant change
☐ **B**   Bacterial overgrowth
☐ **C**   Poor diet
☐ **D**   Pseudomembranous colitis
☐ **E**   Ileocaecal abscess

16 years later he is admitted as an emergency. The GP indicates that the patient has been asymptomatic up until the last six weeks when he started to lose weight and developed intermittent abdominal pain. On admission the patient is pale and has symptoms of small bowel obstruction.

4. What complication is likely to have developed?

☐ **A**   Adhesions
☐ **B**   Small bowel carcinoma
☐ **C**   Ileocaecal abscess
☐ **D**   Small bowel lymphoma
☐ **E**   Carcinoma of the colon

24 (10 marks)

A 19-year-old Asian man is admitted after two days of profound watery diarrhoea and colicky abdominal pain. He was previously perfectly well with normal developmental milestones. His elder brother, who returned from a trip to Bangladesh three weeks previously, has developed similar symptoms, although to a lesser degree.

On examination the patient is pyrexial at 38.6 °C, he looks profoundly ill and is badly dehydrated. The abdomen is tender but soft. The bowel sounds are hyperactive. Liver and spleen are not enlarged and the chest is clear. Examination of the CNS is unremarkable.

Hb	159 g/l
WCC	7.8×10^9/l (normal differential)
Plt	361×10^9/l
Na	134 mmol/l
K	3.8 mmol/l
Urea	15.2 mmol/l
Creatinine	101 µmol/l

On the ward the patient has an episode of explosive diarrhoea, and Dipstix testing shows a trace of blood.

1. What test is most likely to be diagnostic?

- ☐ **A** Anal swab and microscopy
- ☐ **B** Stool microscopy and culture
- ☐ **C** Colonoscopy and full-thickness biopsy
- ☐ **D** Serology for rotavirus
- ☐ **E** Small bowel aspirate and culture

After two days of aggressive resuscitation, the patient starts to recover, but on the third day after admission, develops tender erythematous lesions on both forearms. By this stage his brother has fully recovered and no other family member has become ill.

2. What complication is likely to have developed?

- ☐ **A** Erythema multiforme
- ☐ **B** Haemolytic uraemic syndrome
- ☐ **C** Henoch-Schönlein purpura
- ☐ **D** Bacterial endocarditis
- ☐ **E** Erythema nodosum

Over the following weeks the patient develops tender swellings of both wrists, the right shoulder and the left ankle. He also describes a very acute pain above his right buttock. He has sore eyes, a low-grade pyrexia and mild shortness of breath.

3. What further test is likely to be the most useful?

- ☐ **A** X-ray of both wrists and pelvis
- ☐ **B** Chest X-ray
- ☐ **C** Joint aspiration and culture
- ☐ **D** Blood culture
- ☐ **E** Rheumatoid factor

4. What condition is likely to have developed?

- ☐ **A** Reactive arthritis
- ☐ **B** Bacterial endocarditis
- ☐ **C** Reiter's syndrome
- ☐ **D** Septic arthritis
- ☐ **E** Autoimmune vasculitis

5. What is the treatment?

- ☐ **A** Non-steroidal anti-inflammatory drugs
- ☐ **B** Six weeks of appropriate antibiotics
- ☐ **C** Reducing course of oral steroids
- ☐ **D** Low-dose methotrexate
- ☐ **E** Intravenous immunoglobulins

25 (4 marks)

A 49-year-old woman complains of difficulty swallowing, recurrent episodes of sore eyes and generalised itch. She is not jaundiced, but she has periorbital xanthelasmata. The following results are obtained:

Hb	118 g/l
WCC	3.2 × 10⁹/l
Plt	281 × 10⁹/l
ESR	28 mm/h
Albumin	36 g/l
Total protein	88 g/l
3-day faecal fat excretion	42 g

1. Which of the following tests would be the most useful?

☐ **A**   Liver function tests
☐ **B**   Hepatitis serology
☐ **C**   Protein electrophoresis
☐ **D**   Antibodies to double-stranded DNA
☐ **E**   Anti-mitochondrial antibodies

2. What is the likely diagnosis?

☐ **A**   Chronic persistent hepatitis
☐ **B**   Chronic aggressive hepatitis
☐ **C**   Primary biliary cirrhosis
☐ **D**   Sclerosing cholangitis
☐ **E**   Mixed connective tissue syndrome

26 (4 marks)

A 63-year-old type 2 diabetic, well controlled on gliclazide, is admitted unconscious after being knocked off his bike. CT scan shows a small frontal lobe haematoma only and he is treated conservatively. He is managed on the neurosurgical ward with intravenous fluids and soluble insulin. His results on admission and on day 3 are as follows:

	On admission	Day 3
Na	134 mmol/l	125 mmol/l
K	4.5 mmol/l	3.6 mmol/l
Cl	118 mmol/l	92 mmol/l
Bicarbonate	28 mmol/l	25 mmol/l
Urea	9.4 mmol/l	5.2 mmol/l
Creatinine	151 μmol/l	64 mmol/l
Glucose	7.5 mmol/l	4.6 mmol/l

1. **Which two of the following are the most likely contributing factors?**

☐ **A** Central diabetes insipidus
☐ **B** Peripheral diabetes insipidus
☐ **C** Inappropriate ADH secretion
☐ **D** Renal ischaemia
☐ **E** Renal trauma
☐ **F** Small bowel ischaemia
☐ **G** Dilutional hyponatraemia
☐ **H** Acute adrenal failure
☐ **I** Rhabdomyolysis
☐ **J** Pontine myelinolysis

27 (4 marks)

A 63-year-old man is referred for an investigation of episodic bloating and diarrhoea. He was treated in his forties for presumed recurrent duodenal ulcers. The following results are obtained:

Hb   104 g/l
MCV   103 fl
WCC 6.2×10^9/l
Plt 217×10^9/l
Electrolytes   Normal

1. Suggest a diagnosis for the patient's symptoms.

☐ **A**   Dumping syndrome
☐ **B**   Pernicious anaemia
☐ **C**   Blind loop syndrome
☐ **D**   Malabsorption
☐ **E**   Hypothyroidism

An oral glucose tolerance test shows:

Time (minutes)	Plasma glucose [mmol/l]
0	4.5
30	10.1
60	6.3
120	4.8

2. Suggest a further investigation.

☐ **A**   ERCP
☐ **B**   Gastric biopsy
☐ **C**   Barium swallow
☐ **D**   Gastrin levels
☐ **E**   Radiocarbon (C14) breath test

28 (6 marks)

A 52-year-old patient with an 18-year history of recurrent peptic ulcer disease is investigated for a further relapse. He has not undergone any previous surgery. These are the results of his secretin test:

Baseline gastrin   380 pmol/l (20–100 pmol/l)
After injection of secretin (2 U/kg)   280 pmol/l

1. What is the most likely cause for these results?

- ☐ **A** Pernicious anaemia
- ☐ **B** Zollinger-Ellison syndrome
- ☐ **C** Gastric carcinoma
- ☐ **D** Proton pump inhibitor therapy
- ☐ **E** Erosive gastritis

2. Give two further differential diagnoses.

- ☐ **A** Gastric lymphoma
- ☐ **B** Chronic atrophic gastritis
- ☐ **C** Glucagonoma
- ☐ **D** *Helicobacter* gastritis
- ☐ **E** Gallstones
- ☐ **F** Chronic pancreatitis
- ☐ **G** Gastric leiomyoma
- ☐ **H** Linitis plastica
- ☐ **I** Small bowel carcinoma
- ☐ **J** Chronic pancreatitis

3. What is the next investigation?

- ☐ **A** Abdominal ultrasound
- ☐ **B** Schilling test
- ☐ **C** Abdominal CT scan
- ☐ **D** *Helicobacter* serology
- ☐ **E** Gastroscopy and biopsy

29 (6 marks)

A 69-year-old diabetic is admitted with right upper quadrant pain, and rigors. His bowel habit has been irregular for the last three years and he has had intermittent left iliac fossa pain. His investigations show:

Hb	98 g/l
MCV	82 fl
WCC	9.1×10^9/l
Differential: 85% neutrophils, 12% lymphocytes	
Plt	512×10^9/l
ESR	78 mm/h

Electrolytes	Normal
Bilirubin	22 μmol/l
ALT	56 U/l
Albumin	22 g/l
Total protein	71 g/l

1. What investigation is likely to be the most useful?

- ☐ **A** Blood cultures
- ☐ **B** Abdominal ultrasound
- ☐ **C** Barium enema
- ☐ **D** Radionuclide white cell scan
- ☐ **E** Chest X-ray

2. What is the likely underlying cause?

- ☐ **A** Streptococcal liver abscess
- ☐ **B** Mycobacterial empyema
- ☐ **C** Emphysematous cholecystitis
- ☐ **D** Enterococcal perinephric abscess
- ☐ **E** *Escherichia coli* psoas abscess

3. What treatment would you recommend?

- ☐ **A** Oral co-amoxiclav
- ☐ **B** iv erythromycin
- ☐ **C** Oral antituberculous triple therapy
- ☐ **D** iv benzylpenicillin plus gentamicin
- ☐ **E** Percutaneous drainage

30 (2 marks)

This is a 15-minute tomogram from an IVU performed on a patient with haematuria.

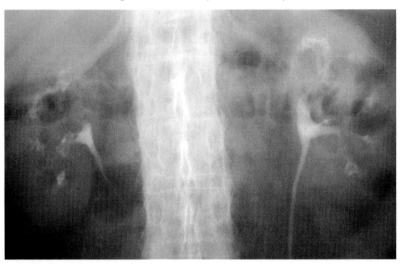

1. Which of the following is the most appropriate management?

☐ **A**   Radiotherapy
☐ **B**   Cystoscopy
☐ **C**   Change medication
☐ **D**   Urine culture
☐ **E**   Hyperhydration

31 (9 marks)

A 59-year-old publican presents with two episodes of haematemesis in the space of 24 hours. He has a seven-month history of mild dyspepsia but has not required any specific treatment. Two years previously he had developed a full-length thrombosis of his right leg, following a cholecystectomy. He was treated with warfarin for three months and had made a good recovery. On admission he is on no regular medication, but smokes 15 cigarettes per day and drinks two to three pints of beer daily.

On examination, he is pale, blood pressure 135/75 mmHg, pulse 92/min, regular, no murmurs. Chest is clear. Abdominal examination reveals a spleen palpable 3 cm below the left costal margin, but no associated hepatomegaly. He is not jaundiced and no spider naevi can be found. PR examination reveals melaena stools but no palpable mass.

Investigations show the following results:

Hb	112 g/l
MCV	66 fl
WCC	14.6 × 10⁹/l
Differential: 91% neutrophils, 6% lymphocytes, 2% monocytes	
Plt	917 × 10⁹/l
MCH	24 pg
MCHC	30 g/dl

Na	139 mmol/l
K	4.9 mmol/l
Urea	17.2 mmol/l
Creatinine	127 µmol/l
Albumin	37 g/l
AST	52 U/l
Gamma-GT	197 U/l
Uric acid	536 µmol/l (< 420 µmol/l)

Gastroscopy shows a normal oesophagus but a bleeding pre-pyloric ulcer which is successfully injected with alcohol. Biopsy from the margin shows no malignant cells.

1. What examination would you perform next?

- ☐ **A** Philadelphia chromosome
- ☐ **B** Leucocyte alkaline phosphatase (LAP)
- ☐ **C** Blood film
- ☐ **D** Repeat gastric biopsy
- ☐ **E** CT of the abdomen

2. What treatment would you recommend?

- ☐ **A** Aspirin
- ☐ **B** Intravenous heparin
- ☐ **C** Gastrectomy
- ☐ **D** Splenectomy
- ☐ **E** α-interferon

The following day the patient deteriorates and the following results are obtained:

Hb	109 g/l
WCC	13.6×10^9/l
Plt	871×10^9/l
Na	135 mmol/l
K	5.1 mmol/l
Urea	31 mmol/l
Creatinine	238 µmol/l
Dipstix urinalysis	Blood +++, Protein +, Bilirubin −

3. What complication has occurred?

- ☐ **A** Obstructing renal stone
- ☐ **B** Renal vein thrombosis
- ☐ **C** Cerebral haemorrhage
- ☐ **D** Recurrent GI haemorrhage
- ☐ **E** Acute hepatic failure

4. What is the underlying diagnosis?

- ☐ **A** Metastatic gastric carcinoma
- ☐ **B** Chronic myeloid leukaemia
- ☐ **C** Essential thrombocythaemia
- ☐ **D** Waldenström's macroglobulinaemia
- ☐ **E** Kaposi's sarcoma

32 (7 marks)

A 72-year-old farmer complains of progressive shortness of breath and increasing fatigue. He recently required a course of antibiotics from his GP for a chest infection. He complains of occasional indigestion and, on two occasions, has noticed some dark blood in his stools. There is no history of haematuria, haemoptysis or bruising. His health is otherwise good with a steady weight and good appetite. He is an ex-smoker and drinks approximately two units of alcohol per night. His only other complaint is of long-standing lower backache.

On examination he is pale, no lymphadenopathy, BP 140/80 mmHg, chest clear, abdominal examination unremarkable.

Investigations show:

Hb	86 g/l
MCV	70 fl
WCC	9.5×10^9/l
Plt	479×10^9/l
MCH	17.1 pg
MCHC	22.9 g/dl
Hct	38%

Blood film: Microcyctic, hypochromic, some rouleaux formation

Na	138 mmol/l
K	4.6 mmol/l
Urea	7.9 mmol/l
Creatinine	136 μmol/l
Calcium	2.15 mmol/l
Albumin	38 g/l
Total protein	95 g/l
Alkaline phosphatase	95 U/l
Serum electrophoresis	Narrow peak in the gamma region

Lumbar spine X-ray	Old wedge fracture of L1
Bone marrow biopsy	6% plasma cells
Barium enema	Normal

Mesenteric angiography: shows an abnormal vascular blush in the ascending colon

1. What is the likely cause for the anaemia?

- ☐ **A** Colon carcinoma
- ☐ **B** Colonic varices
- ☐ **C** Angiodysplasia
- ☐ **D** Meckel's diverticulum
- ☐ **E** Caecal lymphoma

2. **What therapy would you recommend?**

☐ **A**   Right hemicolectomy
☐ **B**   Resection of terminal ileum
☐ **C**   Chemotherapy
☐ **D**   Porto-caval shunt
☐ **E**   Endoscopic sclerotherapy

3. **How do you interpret the immune electrophoresis?**

☐ **A**   Reactive elevation
☐ **B**   Myeloma
☐ **C**   Waldenström's macroglobulinaemia
☐ **D**   Benign monoclonal gammopathy
☐ **E**   Lymphoma

33 (6 marks)

A 28-year-old Ghanaian woman attends the antenatal clinic with her first pregnancy. Her last menstrual period was normal, seven weeks previously.

The following results are obtained:

Hb	109 g/l
MCV	86 fl
WCC	$6.2 \times 10^9/l$
Plt	$238 \times 10^9/l$

Haemoglobin electrophoresis   HbA 61% (HbA$_2$ 5.5%); HbS 39%

Her partner is screened and the following results are found:

Hb	116 g/l
RCC	$5.9 \times 10^{12}/l$
MCV	65 fl
Haemoglobin electrophoresis	HbA 84% (HbA$_2$ 12%); HbF 16%

Of the following list, what are the likely diagnoses of:

1. **The mother?**
2. **The father?**

- ☐ **A**   α-thalassaemia minor
- ☐ **B**   Haemoglobin SC disease
- ☐ **C**   β-thalassaemia minor
- ☐ **D**   Haemoglobin C disease
- ☐ **E**   Sickle cell trait
- ☐ **F**   β-thalassaemia major
- ☐ **G**   Hereditary elliptocytosis
- ☐ **H**   Aplastic anaemia
- ☐ **I**   Dietary deficiency
- ☐ **J**   Hypersplenism

3. **What is the likelihood of the child inheriting a severe (i.e. requiring treatment) haemoglobinopathy?**

- ☐ **A**   No significant risk
- ☐ **B**   25%
- ☐ **C**   50%
- ☐ **D**   66%
- ☐ **E**   75%

34 (2 marks)

This is the hand of a 17-year-old patient with seizures, resistant to phenytoin.

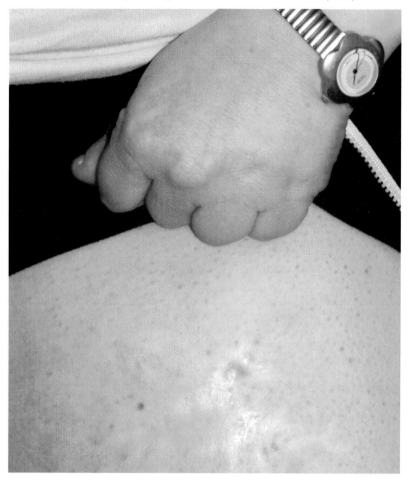

1. What is the most appropriate management?

- ☐ **A**   Change to sodium valproate
- ☐ **B**   Combination therapy
- ☐ **C**   MR scan of the brain
- ☐ **D**   Calcium substitution
- ☐ **E**   Family screening

35 (5 marks)

A 9-year-old boy is admitted with acute abdominal pain. On examination he is pale and of small stature.

A hand X-ray shows a skeletal maturity of approximately 4.5 years and dense bands across the metacarpal metaphyses.

Hb	101 g/l
MCV	81 fl
WCC	6.3×10^9/l
Plt	183×10^9/l
MCH	21 pg

Blood film: Dimorphic erythropoiesis, occasional ring sideroblast

1. What is the likely diagnosis?

- [ ] **A** Wilson's disease
- [ ] **B** Glue sniffing
- [ ] **C** Hereditary sideroblastic anaemia
- [ ] **D** Acute leukaemia
- [ ] **E** Lead poisoning

2. What simple tests may confirm the diagnosis?

- [ ] **A** Abdominal X-ray
- [ ] **B** Ham's test
- [ ] **C** Abdominal ultrasound
- [ ] **D** ESR
- [ ] **E** White cell differential

36 (4 marks)

A 54-year-old woman with long-standing active rheumatoid arthritis is referred for the investigation of anaemia. Her blood results show:

Hb   94 g/l
MCV   99 fl
WCC 6.2×10^9/l (76% neutrophils)
Plt 173×10^9/l
ESR   32 mm/h

1. **Which of the following is *unlikely* to be the cause for these results?**

☐ **A**   Methotrexate
☐ **B**   Sulfasalazine
☐ **C**   Gold
☐ **D**   Hypothyroidism
☐ **E**   Pernicious anaemia

2. **Which of the following tests would be the most helpful?**

☐ **A** B_{12} levels
☐ **B**   Folate levels
☐ **C**   Haptoglobin levels
☐ **D**   Blood film
☐ **E**   Gastroscopy and biopsy

37 (8 marks)

A 48-year-old woman with SLE is on haemodialysis for end-stage renal failure. She now complains of pain in her left hand and paraesthesia over the thenar eminence which is aggravated during haemodialysis. She has her second fistula at the radial aspect of her left forearm. This had required angioplasty three months previously but has been working satisfactorily since. Her lupus is well controlled on immunosuppressants, except for a mild polyarthropathy of the small joints.

On examination, there is wasting of the thenar eminence and a 3/5 weakness of abduction and opposition of the thumb. There is also reduction of sensation to pin prick and soft touch over the tips of thumb and index finger. The following results are obtained prior to dialysis:

Hb	108 g/l
WCC	6.3 × 10⁹/l
Plt	207 × 10⁹/l
Na	133 mmol/l
K	5.1 mmol/l
Urea	18.5 mmol/l
Creatinine	986 µmol/l
Calcium	2.05 mmol/l
Phosphate	1.5 mmol/l
Albumin	39 g/l
Total T4	69 nmol/l (75–150 nmol/l)
TSH	2.4 mU/l

Hand X-ray shows subperiosteal bone resorption of most phalanges, widespread arterial calcification and a well-defined lytic lesion expanding the left first metacarpal.

1. What two complications have arisen?

☐ **A** Hypothyroidism
☐ **B** Mononeuritis multiplex
☐ **C** Aneurysmal bone cyst
☐ **D** Osteomyelitis
☐ **E** Ischaemic neuritis
☐ **F** Carpal tunnel syndrome
☐ **G** Secondary hyperparathyroidism
☐ **H** Tertiary hyperparathyroidism
☐ **I** Pseudohypoparathyroidism
☐ **J** Syringomyelia

2. Suggest two further investigations.

☐ **A**   Anti-nuclear antibody levels
☐ **B**   Ultrasound scan of the neck
☐ **C**   Nerve conduction studies
☐ **D**   C-reactive protein
☐ **E**   Bone biopsy
☐ **F**   Parathormone levels
☐ **G**   Sural nerve biopsy
☐ **H**   MR scan of the hand
☐ **I**   Angiogram of the fistula
☐ **J**   Growth hormone levels

3. What two treatments would you recommend?

☐ **A**   Local steroid injection
☐ **B**   Median nerve decompression
☐ **C**   Azathioprine
☐ **D**   Increased dialysis frequency
☐ **E**   Parathyroidectomy
☐ **F**   Change of dialysate
☐ **G**   Increased calcium and vitamin D supplements
☐ **H**   Systemic steroids
☐ **I**   Peritoneal dialysis
☐ **J**   Pamidronate

38 **(2 marks)**

These are the pulmonary function tests of a 54-year-old housewife with increasing breathlessness.

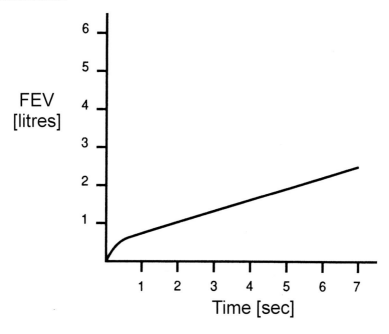

Which of the following values is best related to the severity of breathlessness?

☐ **A**   Peak expiratory flow rate (PEFR)
☐ **B**   Forced expiratory volume in the first second (FEV$_1$)
☐ **C**   Forced vital capacity (FVC)
☐ **D**   FEV$_1$/FVC ratio
☐ **E**   Pulmonary transfer factor

39 (9 marks)

A 73-year-old pensioner is referred to the Urology Department with a five-month history of frequency and a two-day history of acute lower left-sided back pain. Over the last year she has lost 1.5 kg in weight and complained of increased thirst. A random blood glucose was found to be 9 mmol/l and she has been started on gliclazide 40 mg by her GP. Her only other medication was bendroflumethiazide (bendrofluazide) 2.5 mg for mild hypertension.

Blood results on admission:

Hb	99 g/l
WCC	3.9 × 10⁹/l
Plt	109 × 10⁹/l
ESR	108 mm/h

Na	144 mmol/l
K	3.2 mmol/l
Urea	11.6 mmol/l
Creatinine	168 µmol/l
Corrected calcium	3.4 mmol/l

An abdominal X-ray showed some calcification projecting over the left kidney, but an IVU performed on the same day showed no evidence of renal obstruction.

1. **Suggest two non-invasive further investigations.**

- ☐ **A** Haemoglobin A,c
- ☐ **B** Radio-isotope bone scan
- ☐ **C** Serum electrophoresis
- ☐ **D** Renal biopsy
- ☐ **E** Urinary hydroxyproline
- ☐ **F** Dynamic CT of the kidneys
- ☐ **G** Skeletal survey
- ☐ **H** Chest X-ray
- ☐ **I** MAG-3 renogram
- ☐ **J** Creatinine clearance

2. **What is the likely diagnosis?**

- ☐ **A** Glucagonoma
- ☐ **B** Metastasised renal cell carcinoma
- ☐ **C** Waldenström's macroglobulinaemia
- ☐ **D** Metastasised phaeochromocytoma
- ☐ **E** Multiple myeloma

The patient's condition deteriorates over the following two days. She becomes very dyspnoeic and requires 35% oxygen. Repeat electrolytes show the following results:

Na	145 mmol/l
K	5.8 mmol/l
Urea	28.3 mmol/l
Creatinine	612 μmol/l

3. What complication has arisen?

- ☐ **A** Renal artery occlusion
- ☐ **B** Renal vein thrombosis
- ☐ **C** Renal papillary necrosis
- ☐ **D** Lactic acidosis
- ☐ **E** Acute tubular necrosis

4. What additional information is provided by this complication?

- ☐ **A** Microvascular disease
- ☐ **B** Secretion of active hormones
- ☐ **C** Presence of light chains
- ☐ **D** Bone metastases
- ☐ **E** Renal artery stenosis

40 (2 marks)

These are the arterial blood gases of a 69-year-old woman with chronic obstructive airways disease (COAD) (room air).

pH	7.21
pO_2	6.8 kPa
pCO_2	7.9 kPa
Bicarbonate	18 mmol/l
O_2 saturation	87%

1. What is the best way to describe these results?

- ☐ **A** Respiratory acidosis
- ☐ **B** Combined respiratory and metabolic acidosis
- ☐ **C** Combined respiratory acidosis and metabolic alkalosis
- ☐ **D** Venous sample
- ☐ **E** Laboratory error

41 (4 marks)

A 53-year-old woman with long-standing active rheumatoid arthritis presents with shortness of breath and tiredness. Blood samples show the following results:

Hb	78 g/l
WCC	1.9×10^9/l
Plt	57×10^9/l
ESR	57 mm/h
Na	141 mmol/l
K	3.2 mmol/l
Albumin	25 g/l
Urinary protein	2.8 g/24 h

Renal biopsy shows diffuse thickening of the glomerular basement membrane.

1. What is the likely mechanism for the abnormality in the blood count?

- ☐ **A**　Aplastic anaemia
- ☐ **B**　Haemolytic anaemia
- ☐ **C**　Anaemia of chronic disease
- ☐ **D**　Folate deficiency
- ☐ **E**　Sideroblastic anaemia

2. What is the cause for the renal abnormality?

- ☐ **A**　Small vessel vasculitis
- ☐ **B**　Immune complex deposition
- ☐ **C**　Analgesic nephropathy
- ☐ **D**　Drug-induced glomerulonephritis
- ☐ **E**　Papillary necrosis

42 (2 marks)

A 53-year-old builder complains of increasing breathlessness. This is a section of a helical CT scan through the lower thorax.

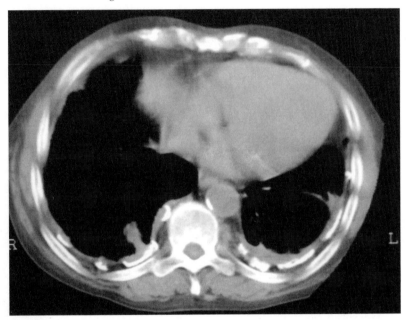

1. **Which of the following investigations is most useful?**

☐ **A** Bronchoscopy
☐ **B** Pulmonary function tests
☐ **C** Sputum microscopy
☐ **D** Pleural biopsy
☐ **E** Radio-isotope bone scan

43 (5 marks)

A 42-year-old man is referred to the clinic after an insurance medical revealed hypertension. The following results are obtained:

Na	145 mmol/l
K	Haemolysed
Bicarbonate	32 mmol/l
Creatinine	131 µmol/l
Urinary Na	48 mmol/l (< 40 mmol/l)

The following results are obtained after 25 mg oral captopril:

Time [min]	0	120
Aldosterone [80–400 pmol/l]	489	280
Renin [3–19 ng/l]	21	48

1. What is the diagnosis?

- ☐ **A** Essential hypertension
- ☐ **B** Conn's syndrome
- ☐ **C** Renal artery stenosis
- ☐ **D** Adrenocortical hyperplasia
- ☐ **E** Renin-secreting tumour

2. Which further investigation is the most appropriate?

- ☐ **A** CT scan of upper adenoma
- ☐ **B** Urinary electrolytes
- ☐ **C** Urinary cortisol
- ☐ **D** Isotope renogram
- ☐ **E** Synacthen® test

44 (5 marks)

A 68-year-old woman presents to the GP with low back pain (relieved by rest) and bilateral knee pain. She is given painkillers, but presents five weeks later to the Casualty Department with orthopnoea, bilateral leg oedema and clinical evidence of ascites. Immediate results show:

Na	143 mmol/l
K	5.6 mmol/l
Creatinine	199 µmol/l
Dipstix urinalysis	Glucose + +, Protein + + +, Blood +, Ketones –

1. What is the most likely diagnosis?

☐ **A** Renal vein thrombosis
☐ **B** Allergic interstitial nephritis
☐ **C** Renal papillary necrosis
☐ **D** Analgesic nephropathy
☐ **E** Acute tubular necrosis

2. What treatment would you suggest?

☐ **A** Oral steroids
☐ **B** Ciclosporin
☐ **C** Forced diuresis
☐ **D** Anticoagulation
☐ **E** Withdrawal of all medication

45 (7 marks)

A 23-year-old man presents to the A&E Department with a one-week history of increasing malaise and tiredness. In addition, he has experienced increasing difficulties in walking and in the last two days has had problems feeding himself, with liquid dribbling from the corners of his mouth.

On examination he has a mild ptosis of his left eye and is unable to whistle. Reduced tone is present in the legs and limb weakness is noted. Power is reduced to 3/5 for ankle extension and to 4/5 for knee and wrist extension. The ankle jerks are absent; knee and biceps jerks are present with reinforcement. There is reduced sensation to pinprick and soft touch to the level of both knees and the fingertips of the right hand. Fundoscopy reveals mild swelling of the right disc. Blood pressure 125/70 mmHg; pulse 96/min, regular. Respiratory rate 24/min; normal breath sounds on auscultation. Examination of the abdomen is unremarkable.

The following results are obtained:

Hb	146 g/l
WCC	6.2×10^9/l
Plt	193×10^9/l
ESR	13 mm/h
Biochemical profile	Normal
Glucose	5.8 mmol/l

The following CSF results are obtained at lumbar puncture:

Opening pressure	24 cmH$_2$O
Protein	2.3 g/l
Glucose	4.9 mmol/l
Microscopy	6 lymphocytes/mm^3, no polymorphs

Peroneal nerve conduction velocity	21 m/s (> 45 m/s)

1. What is the likely diagnosis?

- ☐ **A** Tetanus
- ☐ **B** Guillain-Barré syndrome
- ☐ **C** Botulism
- ☐ **D** Multiple sclerosis
- ☐ **E** Herpes simplex encephalitis

2. Which further investigation is indicated?

- ☐ **A**   Chest X-ray
- ☐ **B**   CT brain
- ☐ **C**   Pulmonary function tests
- ☐ **D**   *Clostridium* serology
- ☐ **E**   Visual-evoked potentials

3. What treatment has to be considered?

- ☐ **A**   im antitoxin
- ☐ **B**   Ventilation
- ☐ **C**   iv interferon
- ☐ **D**   Pyridostigmine
- ☐ **E**   iv penicillin

46 (3 marks)

A 38-year-old chemist is under investigation for hypertension. A MAG-3 renogram is performed which shows the following excretion curves:

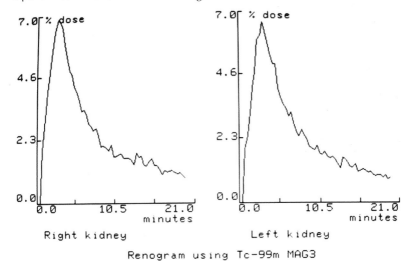

Renogram using Tc-99m MAG3

	RIGHT KIDNEY	LEFT KIDNEY
RELATIVE FUNCTION from 80 to 150 s	54 %	46 %

Na	143 mmol/l
K	3.1 mmol/l
Creatinine	72 µmol/l

1. **Which is the most appropriate treatment?**

☐ **A** Beta-blocker
☐ **B** Loop diuretic
☐ **C** ACE inhibitor
☐ **D** Renal artery stent
☐ **E** Surgery

47 (9 marks)

A 49-year-old bachelor is admitted to the Casualty Department with a one-day history of worsening diplopia, blurred vision and shortness of breath. This had been preceded by diarrhoea and vomiting. A keen gardener, he had previously been fit and well, keeping himself healthy with work on his allotment and buying organic produce from the local farm. In the past he had rheumatic fever at the age of eight and suffered a basal skull fracture three years previously falling out of a cherry tree. He is on no regular medication.

On examination the patient is extremely agitated. There is a mild convergent squint in both eyes with poor abduction; the pupils are of normal size but show a very sluggish response to light. He has difficulty swallowing his saliva and there is a moderate, global reduction in tone and power (3/5) and the reflexes are markedly depressed.

The chest is clear. A rumbling mid-systolic murmur is heard over the cardiac apex; BP 175/70 mmHg; pulse 92/min, regular.

Liver and spleen are not enlarged, but a smooth, firm mass is palpated in the lower abdomen arising from the pelvis. The patient is apyrexial but tachypnoeic at 28/min.

The following results are obtained:

Hb	142 g/l
WCC	6.1×10^9/l
Plt	329×10^9/l
Na	142 mmol/l
K	4.1 mmol/l
Creatinine	119 µmol/l
Albumin	39 g/l
Random glucose	5.9 mmol/l
C-reactive protein	7.9 mg/l (< 10 mg/l)

ECG: Sinus rhythm, complete left bundle branch block, axis $-45°$, 1-mm ST depression in V_5 and V_6

1. What is the likely diagnosis?

- ☐ **A** Botulism
- ☐ **B** Tetanus
- ☐ **C** Organophosphate poisoning
- ☐ **D** Rabies
- ☐ **E** Cerebral abscess

2. Which of the following investigations is the most important?

☐ **A**   CT of the brain
☐ **B**   Arterial blood gases
☐ **C**   Blood cultures
☐ **D**   Toxicology screen
☐ **E**   Viral serology

3. Which of the following should be administered?

☐ **A**   iv benzylpenicillin
☐ **B**   iv gentamicin
☐ **C**   Depolarising muscle relaxant
☐ **D**   Atropine
☐ **E**   Antitoxin

4. What further measures are indicated?

☐ **A**   Inspect patient for bite wounds and inform local council
☐ **B**   Stool cultures and referral of involved staff to Occupational Health
☐ **C**   Neurosurgical referral and screening of immediate relatives
☐ **D**   Admit to intensive care and inform Public Health
☐ **E**   Saliva samples and barrier nursing of the patient

48 (5 marks)

A 36-year-old woman presents with a right-sided facial weakness with inability to close the right eye. There is mild swelling of the right cheek. A lumbar puncture reveals:

Opening pressure	12 cmH$_2$O
Protein	0.8 g/l
Glucose	3.8 mmol/l
	(blood glucose 4.3 mmol/l)
Microscopy (/mm^3)	85 lymphocytes, 2 erythrocytes

1. Which of the following is the most likely diagnosis?

- ☐ **A** Bell's palsy
- ☐ **B** Cerebral sarcoid
- ☐ **C** Ramsay-Hunt syndrome
- ☐ **D** Right acoustic neuroma
- ☐ **E** Pleomorphic adenoma of the parotid

2. Which of the following investigations would you perform?

- ☐ **A** Chest X-ray
- ☐ **B** CT scan of the brain
- ☐ **C** Viral serology
- ☐ **D** Visual-evoked potentials
- ☐ **E** Ultrasound scan of the parotid

49 (6 marks)

An unemployed 42-year-old labourer presents with difficulties walking and palpitations. He has wasting of the facial muscles, bilateral ptosis and a distal muscle weakness. The sexual characteristics are underdeveloped. Visual acuity is 3/6 with glasses.

The following results are obtained:

Full blood count   Normal
Urea and electrolytes   Normal
Random glucose   7.8 mmol/L
Testosterone   6 nmol/l (12–30 nmol/l)
LH   27 µmol/l (2–10 µmol/l)

The following blood glucose levels are obtained after oral administration of 75g disaccharides:

0 minutes	7 mmol/l
60 minutes	9.5 mmol/l
120 minutes	10.1 mmol/l

ECG   PR   0.38 seconds
               QRS   0.13 seconds
               QT   0.4 seconds

1. What does the oral glucose tolerance test indicate?

- ☐ **A** Normal results
- ☐ **B** Chronic liver disease
- ☐ **C** Glucagonoma
- ☐ **D** Impaired glucose tolerance
- ☐ **E** Vomiting during the test

2. What do the sex hormone levels suggest?

- ☐ **A** Hypogonadotrophic hypogonadism
- ☐ **B** Hypergonadotropic hypogonadism
- ☐ **C** Thalamic dysfunction
- ☐ **D** Androgen resistance
- ☐ **E** Pituitary failure

3. **Which of the following is the most likely diagnosis?**

☐ **A**   Myotonic dystrophy
☐ **B**   Craniopharyngioma
☐ **C**   Kallmann's syndrome
☐ **D**   Friedreich's ataxia
☐ **E**   Hereditary sensorimotor neuropathy

50 (2 marks)

This is the chest X-ray of a 28-year-old African immigrant with exercise-induced dyspnoea.

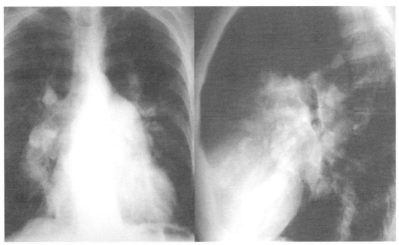

1. What is the likely diagnosis?

- ☐ **A**   Endomyocardial fibrosis
- ☐ **B**   Atrial septal defect
- ☐ **C**   Mitral stenosis
- ☐ **D**   Chagas' disease
- ☐ **E**   Ventricular septal defect

51 (4 marks)

A 22-year-old woman presents with bilateral foot drop, slowly worsening over the last five years.

The following neurophysiological results are obtained:

Radial nerve sensory action potential	< 3 microvolt (> 20 microvolt)
Sural nerve sensory action potential	< 1 microvolt (> 15 microvolt)
Median nerve motor conduction velocity	23 m/s (> 50 m/s)
Peroneal nerve motor conduction velocity	15 m/s (> 45 m/s)

1. What is the likely diagnosis?

- ☐ **A** Friedreich's ataxia
- ☐ **B** Subacute combined degeneration of the cord (SACD)
- ☐ **C** Multiple sclerosis
- ☐ **D** Hereditary sensorimotor neuropathy
- ☐ **E** Tabes dorsalis

2. What is fundoscopy likely to demonstrate?

- ☐ **A** Normal fundi
- ☐ **B** Roth spots
- ☐ **C** Angioid streaks
- ☐ **D** Papilloedema
- ☐ **E** Optic atrophy

52 (6 marks)

A 48-year-old farmer is admitted with an episode of haemoptysis. He has had no previous episodes, but has felt unwell with malaise and headaches for the preceding seven weeks. He has lost 3 kg in weight.

On examination he is pyrexial at 37.8 °C. Respiratory rate is 22/min, with right-sided basal crackles.

Examination of the cardiovascular system and abdomen is normal. There is mild proptosis of the left eye, which is tender to palpation. There is minimal diplopia on upward gaze.

Investigations show:

Hb	121 g/l
WCC	7.8×10^9/l

Differential: 58% neutrophils, 31% lymphocytes, 2% monocytes

Plt	468×10^9/l
MCV	84 fl
ESR	76 mm/h

Na	138 mmol/l
K	5.2 mmol/l
Urea	13.3 mmol/l
Creatinine	197 μmol/l
Dipstix urinalysis	Protein + +, Blood + +, Bilirubin –

Chest X-ray: Several ill-defined nodules present in both lungs

1. What is the likely diagnosis?

- ☐ **A** Wegener's granulomatosis
- ☐ **B** Polyarteritis nodosa
- ☐ **C** Non-Hodgkin's lymphoma
- ☐ **D** Goodpasture's syndrome
- ☐ **E** Extrinsic allergic alveolitis

2. Which of the following is likely to be *least* useful?

- ☐ **A** ENT referral
- ☐ **B** Renal biopsy
- ☐ **C** Lateral chest X-ray
- ☐ **D** Autoantibodies
- ☐ **E** Serum precipitins

3. What treatment would you recommend?

☐ **A**   iv methylprednisolone
☐ **B**   iv cyclophosphamide
☐ **C**   Radiotherapy
☐ **D**   Exposure prophylaxis
☐ **E**   Methotrexate

53 (7 marks)

A 64-year-old bachelor presents to the Accident & Emergency Department with severe epigastric pain and nausea and vomiting of three days' duration. This was preceded by several weeks of malaise and increasing difficulties getting out of his armchair. He smokes 15 cigarettes per day and has a chronic, dry cough.

On examination he is cachectic with increased skin turgor. The chest is clear. BP 110/70 mmHg with a postural drop of 15 mmHg. No organomegaly. There is bilateral gynaecomastia.

Blood results show:

Hb	108 g/l
WCC	5.6 × 10⁹/l (normal differential)
Plt	217 × 10⁹/l
MCV	76 fl
ESR	38 mm/h

Na	144 mmol/l
K	3.2 mmol/l
Urea	16.9 mmol/l
Creatinine	168 μmol/l
Bilirubin	21 U/l
Alkaline phosphatase	428 U/l
ALT	29 U/l
AST	35 U/l
Albumin	33 g/l
Total protein	59 g/l
Calcium	2.95 mmol/l

Radio-isotope bone scan	Generalised increased activity, no focal hot-spots
Bone marrow biopsy	Active erythropoiesis, normal granulopoiesis, 7% plasma cells

1. Which of the following investigations would be the most helpful?

☐ **A** Skeletal survey
☐ **B** Serum phosphate
☐ **C** Ultrasound of the liver
☐ **D** Urinary hydroxyproline
☐ **E** Hand X-ray

2. What is the underlying diagnosis?

☐ **A** Squamous cell carcinoma of the lung
☐ **B** Multiple myeloma
☐ **C** Sarcomatous change in Paget's disease
☐ **D** Small cell carcinoma of the lung
☐ **E** Metastasised carcinoma of the colon

3. What is your further management?

☐ **A** iv hydrocortisone and CT scan of the chest
☐ **B** iv diphosphonates and serum electrophoresis
☐ **C** iv saline and barium enema
☐ **D** Rectal ion-exchange resins and neck ultrasound
☐ **E** Forced diuresis and chest X-ray

54 (8 marks)

A 46-year-old woman is complaining of increasing difficulties driving her car and climbing stairs. She has developed a nasal quality to her speech and is repeatedly choking on drinks.

On examination she has proximal muscle weakness, but no obvious wasting or fasciculation. Palatal weakness is confirmed on examination. Reflexes are reduced but present and plantar response is flexor. Respiratory rate is 22/min and blood pressure is 115/65 mmHg.

The following results are obtained:

Na	138 mmol/l	Hb	139 g/l
K	4.2 mmol/l	WCC	6.8 x10⁹/l
Urea	4.5 mmol/l	Plt	192 x10⁹/l
Creatinine	72 µmol/l	ESR	13 mm/h
Albumin	38 g/l	CK	25 U/l

Chest X-ray shows a lobulated mass projecting over the aortic arch.

1. What is the diagnosis?

☐ **A**   Myasthenia gravis
☐ **B**   Non-Hodgkin's lymphoma
☐ **C**   Malignant teratodermoid
☐ **D**   Eaton-Lambert syndrome
☐ **E**   Motor neurone disease

2. Of the following, which are the two most appropriate tests?

☐ **A**   Tensilon® test
☐ **B**   High-resolution chest CT
☐ **C**   Bronchoscopy and biopsy
☐ **D**   Muscle biopsy
☐ **E**   Electromyography
☐ **F**   Acetylcholine receptor antibodies
☐ **G**   Arterial blood gases
☐ **H**   Nerve conduction studies
☐ **I**   Spirometry
☐ **J**   Spiral CT of the chest

3. What is the medical treatment?

- ☐ **A** Polychemotherapy
- ☐ **B** Radiotherapy
- ☐ **C** Gammaglobulins
- ☐ **D** Plasmapheresis
- ☐ **E** Pyridostigmine

4. Of the following name two drugs that must be used with great caution.

- ☐ **A** Triamcinolone
- ☐ **B** Digoxin
- ☐ **C** Midazolam
- ☐ **D** Fluoxetine
- ☐ **E** L-Dopa
- ☐ **F** Sulphonamides
- ☐ **G** Heparin
- ☐ **H** Curare derivatives
- ☐ **I** Amiodarone
- ☐ **J** Nitroglycerin

55 (6 marks)

A 69-year-old Haematology patient is admitted with pleuritic chest pain and a one-week history of increasing cough and shortness of breath. Her only current medication is α-interferon.

On examination the patient is tachypnoeic at rest. Temperature 37.9 °C (axilla); BP 115/70 mmHg; pulse 104/min, regular. Examinations of chest and cardiovascular system are normal. There is no lymphadenopathy.

The following results are obtained:

Hb 68 g/l
WCC 25.2 × 10⁹/l
Differential: 39% neutrophils, 15% promyelocytes, 23% myeloblasts, 12% lymphocytes, 8% monocytes, 2% eosinophils
Plt 107 × 10⁹/l
ESR 48 mm/h

U&Es Normal
Pulse oximetry 93% O₂ saturation on air
Chest X-ray: cavitating left upper lobe pneumonia

1. What do the blood results indicate?

- [ ] **A** Chronic myeloid leukaemia in blast crisis
- [ ] **B** Chronic myelomonocytic leukaemia
- [ ] **C** Acute myeloid leukaemia
- [ ] **D** Myelodysplasia
- [ ] **E** Leukaemoid reaction

2. Which of the following is the *least* likely cause for the respiratory symptoms?

- [ ] **A** Staphylococcal pneumonia
- [ ] **B** Tuberculosis
- [ ] **C** Cytomegalovirus
- [ ] **D** *Mycobacterium avium intracellulare*
- [ ] **E** *Klebsiella* pneumonia

3. What management would you recommend?

- [ ] **A** iv amphotericin B and bronchoscopy
- [ ] **B** Isolation and sputum examination
- [ ] **C** iv cotrimoxazole and chemotherapy
- [ ] **D** Intensive care and high-dose oxygen
- [ ] **E** iv ganciclovir and transfusion

56 (4 marks)

A 64-year-old publican presents with a three-week history of lethargy and coughing up bloodstained sputum. Chest X-ray shows an area of consolidation in the right mid-zone.

Blood results reveal:

FBC	Normal
Na	136 mmol/l
K	5.4 mmol/l
Urea	29 mmol/l
Creatinine	428 µmol/l

Arterial blood gases (air):

pH	7.29
pO_2	8.8 kPa (66 mmHg)
pCO_2	4.8 kPa (36 mmHg)
Bicarbonate	16 mmol/l

1. **Which of the following is the *least* likely diagnosis?**

□ **A** Bronchial carcinoma
□ **B** Polyarteritis nodosa
□ **C** Goodpasture's syndrome
□ **D** Allergic bronchopulmonary aspergillosis
□ **E** *Mycoplasma* pneumonia

2. **Which of the following investigations is *least* likely to be helpful?**

□ **A** Sputum microscopy and culture
□ **B** Lung biopsy
□ **C** CT of the thorax
□ **D** Renal biopsy
□ **E** Blood film

57 (4 marks)

A 23-year-old woman presents with acute onset of breathlessness. She is nine weeks pregnant and has always been well. Respiratory rate 28/min; pulse 92/min, regular; BP 155/70 mmHg.

FBC   Normal

Arterial blood gases (room air) reveal:

pH   7.55
pO_2 13.8 kPa (99 mmHg)
pCO_2 2.9 kPa (21 mmHg)
Bicarbonate   20 mmol/l

1. What would be your management?

- ☐ **A**   iv heparin
- ☐ **B**   Chest X-ray
- ☐ **C**   iv midazolam
- ☐ **D**   Re-breathing from a paper bag
- ☐ **E**   Administration of 40% O_2

2. What is the likely diagnosis?

- ☐ **A**   Hyperventilation
- ☐ **B**   Pulmonary embolus
- ☐ **C**   Pneumothorax
- ☐ **D**   Diaphragmatic splinting
- ☐ **E**   Pulmonary oedema

58 (2 marks)

This is the abdominal X-ray of a patient with bilateral loin pain.

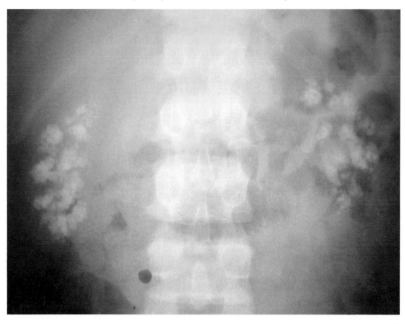

1. Which two of the following are the most useful investigations?

- [ ] **A**   Renal ultrasound scan
- [ ] **B**   Biochemical profile
- [ ] **C**   Intravenous urogram
- [ ] **D**   Radio-isotope renogram
- [ ] **E**   Renal biopsy
- [ ] **F**   Autoantibody screen
- [ ] **G**   Urinalysis
- [ ] **H**   Chest X-ray
- [ ] **I**   HbA$_1$c
- [ ] **J**   Urine culture for TB

59 (4 marks)

A 23-year-old man with progressive breathlessness shows the following results on lung function tests:

FEV_1	2.0 l
FVC	3.8 l
FEV_1/FVC	53%
TLC	6.1 l (predicted 4.5–5.9 l)
Transfer coefficient (KCO)	73%

1. What do the results suggest?

☐ **A**   Emphysema
☐ **B**   Small airway obstruction
☐ **C**   Bronchiectasis
☐ **D**   Fibrosis
☐ **E**   Haemorrhage

2. What is the likely diagnosis?

☐ **A**   Asthma
☐ **B**   Cystic fibrosis
☐ **C**   Rheumatoid arthritis
☐ **D** α_1-antitrypsin deficiency
☐ **E**   Hereditary haemorrhagic telangiectasia

60 (4 marks)

A 36-year-old patient with recurrent nose bleeds presents with haemoptysis and shortness of breath. The following results are obtained:

Hb	119 g/l
MCV	70 fl
ESR	28 mm/h

FEV$_1$/ FVC	85%
Transfer coefficient (KCO)	162%

Arterial blood gases (room air):

pH	7.49
pO$_2$	9.2 kPa (69 mmHg)
pCO2	3.6 kPa (27 mmHg)
Bicarbonate	23 mmol/l

Chest X-ray: Right basal consolidation

1. What has precipitated the acute presentation?

- ☐ **A** Pulmonary embolus
- ☐ **B** Pulmonary haemorrhage
- ☐ **C** Aspiration
- ☐ **D** Pneumothorax
- ☐ **E** Superinfection

2. What is the likely diagnosis?

- ☐ **A** Haemophilia
- ☐ **B** Idiopathic thrombocytopenic purpura
- ☐ **C** von Willebrand's disease
- ☐ **D** Hereditary haemorrhagic telangiectasia
- ☐ **E** Wegener's granulomatosis

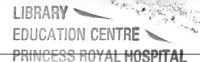

61 (4 marks)

A 57-year-old patient presents with dysphagia and breathlessness.

The following results are obtained:

Hb	106 g/l
WCC	5.6 × 10⁹/l (normal differential)
Plt	227 × 10⁹/l
MCV	73 fl
ESR	21 mm/h
CRP	4.5 mg/dl (< 10 mg/dl)
FEV₁	3.6 l (predicted 3.4–4.2 l)
FVC	4.0 l (predicted 4.8–5.4 l)
Transfer coefficient (KCO)	87%

Chest X-ray: Interstitial shadowing in both lower zones

1. Which of the following is the most appropriate investigation?

- ☐ **A** Barium swallow
- ☐ **B** Autoantibody screen
- ☐ **C** Transbronchial lung biopsy
- ☐ **D** Spiral CT of the thorax
- ☐ **E** Oesophageal manometry

2. Which of the following diagnoses is *unlikely*?

- ☐ **A** Achalasia
- ☐ **B** Systemic sclerosis
- ☐ **C** Tylosis
- ☐ **D** Whipple's disease
- ☐ **E** Hiatus hernia

62 (4 marks)

A retired teacher with chronic rheumatoid arthritis is admitted after an acute angina attack. She gives a three-month history of malaise and exercise-induced dyspnoea. Physical examination is unremarkable. Her blood results show:

Hb	64 g/l
WCC	39 × 10⁹/l
Differential	92% lymphocytes, 6% neutrophils, 1% eosinophils
Plt	118 x10⁹/l
MCV	92 fl

The blood film shows normochromic red cells with polychromasia and micro-spherocytes; 6% reticulocytes are seen and a large number of 'smudge' cells.

1. What two diagnoses can be inferred from these results?

☐ **A**   Myelodysplasia
☐ **B**   Iron deficiency anaemia
☐ **C**   Sézary syndrome
☐ **D**   Acute lymphocytic leukaemia
☐ **E**   Gold toxicity
☐ **F**   Sulfasalazine therapy
☐ **G**   Myelofibrosis
☐ **H**   Hypersplenism
☐ **I**   Chronic lymphocytic leukaemia
☐ **J**   Autoimmune haemolysis

63 (4 marks)

A 61-year-old woman presents with malaise, weight loss and copious amounts of frothy sputum, worst in the morning.

Investigations show:

Hb	102 g/l
MCV	73 fl
WCC	6.9 × 10⁹/l (normal differential)
Plt	191 × 10⁹/l
Pulse oximetry	94% saturation on air

Chest X-ray: Large area of consolidation in left upper lobe

1. What investigation would you recommend?

- ☐ **A** Sputum Gram stain and culture
- ☐ **B** Bronchoscopy and biopsy
- ☐ **C** Video fluoroscopy
- ☐ **D** Gastroscopy
- ☐ **E** High-resolution CT of the thorax

2. What is the likely diagnosis?

- ☐ **A** Tracheo-oesophageal fistula
- ☐ **B** Alveolar cell carcinoma
- ☐ **C** Bronchiectasis
- ☐ **D** Cardiac failure
- ☐ **E** Zenker's diverticulum

64 (9 marks)

A 34-year-old prostitute is referred from the Casualty Department with a left-sided weakness affecting the arm more than the leg. This had developed overnight, but had been preceded by two previous episodes of weakness in the left, non-dominant hand. Prior to this she had always been well and apart from the oral contraceptive pill was on no other medication. She does not drink alcohol, but smokes 10 cigarettes per day.

On examination there is a 3/5 weakness of the left arm and 4/5 weakness of the left leg, the plantar is up-going and non-sustained clonus is present at the left ankle. There is minor impairment of rapid alternating movements and a few beats of nystagmus are present in both eyes on extreme abduction. There is no meningism. On fundoscopy the discs appear normal but some silver-wiring is present on both sides.

BP 170/95 mmHg; pulse 88/min, regular; no heart murmurs on auscultation. The lungs are clear. Axillary temperature 38.3 °C. Examination of the gait reveals a right-sided limp and difficulties walking heel-to-toe.

The following results are obtained:

Hb	100 g/l
MCV	81 fl
WCC	3.9 × 10⁹/l
Plt	127 × 10⁹/l
MCH	27 pg

Na	130 mmol/l
K	4.9 mmol/l
Creatinine	168 µmol/l
Total protein	76 g/l
Albumin	31 g/l
Bilirubin	17 µmol/l
AST	39 U/l
CRP	8.5 mg/l (< 10 mg/l)
VDRL	Positive 1: 512
Dipstix urinalysis	Blood +, Protein + + +

1. What is the likely diagnosis?

- ☐ **A** Multiple sclerosis
- ☐ **B** Neurosyphilis
- ☐ **C** Systemic lupus erythematosus
- ☐ **D** HIV infection
- ☐ **E** Polyarteritis nodosa

2. Which of the following investigations is the most useful?

- ☐ **A**   Blood and urine cultures
- ☐ **B**   Lumbar puncture
- ☐ **C**   CT scan of the brain
- ☐ **D**   *Treponema pallidum* haemagglutination tests
- ☐ **E**   Renal biopsy

Over the following fortnight, the patient makes a slow recovery, but the limp is becoming worse. A plain radiograph shows no abnormality but a bone scan shows increased uptake of radioisotope over the right hip.

3. What is the likely pathology?

- ☐ **A**   Avascular necrosis
- ☐ **B**   Septic arthritis
- ☐ **C**   Neuropathic joint
- ☐ **D**   Reactive arthritis
- ☐ **E**   Stress fracture

While awaiting orthopaedic review, the patient develops bilateral ankle swelling and dyspnoea. The percussion note is stony dull at both lung bases.

4. What complication has developed?

- ☐ **A**   Myocarditis
- ☐ **B**   Nephrotic syndrome
- ☐ **C**   Pyelonephritis
- ☐ **D**   Pericarditis
- ☐ **E**   Aortic dissection

65 (9 marks)

A 13-year-old Chinese boy is referred with a three-week history of intermittent pyrexia and night sweats. He has also been complaining of pain in the right knee and left ankle and he has developed tender nodules over both shins.

His mother complains that, over the last week, he has started to drop things and has broken both teapots. The patient had a previously unremarkable childhood, had all routine vaccinations, but had caught chickenpox eight months previously and scarlet fever two months ago.

On examination he has tender, swollen wrists and elbows but the joints of the lower limbs appear to have settled. Mild erythema nodosum is present. The chest is clear and the abdomen is soft without organomegaly. Examination of the CNS is unremarkable without evidence of cerebellar signs, although some involuntary movements of the right hand are observed. BP 110/55 mmHg; pulse 88/min; no murmurs on auscultation.

The following results are obtained:

Hb	106 g/l
WCC	9.8×10^9/l (72% neutrophils)
Plt	428×10^9/l
CRP	28 mg/dl
Na	136 mmol/l
K	4.1 mmol/l
Urea	5.6 mmol/l
Creatinine	73 µmol/l
LFTs	Normal
Paul-Bunnell test	Negative
Rheumatoid factor	Negative
Chest X-ray	Normal
X-rays of hands and feet	No osteoporosis, no erosions

The patient is started on aspirin with a rapid symptomatic improvement.

1. **Suggest two further investigations.**

- ☐ **A** Serial blood cultures
- ☐ **B** Joint aspiration
- ☐ **C** Electrocardiogram
- ☐ **D** Chest X-ray
- ☐ **E** Echocardiogram
- ☐ **F** Electroencephalogram
- ☐ **G** ASO titres
- ☐ **H** Brain CT
- ☐ **I** Skin biopsy
- ☐ **J** Abdominal ultrasound

2. **What is the likely underlying diagnosis?**

- ☐ **A** Rheumatic fever
- ☐ **B** Subacute bacterial endocarditis
- ☐ **C** Lesch-Nyhan syndrome
- ☐ **D** Borreliosis
- ☐ **E** Systemic lupus erythematosus

3. **What is the cause for the neurological findings?**

- ☐ **A** Brain abscess
- ☐ **B** Cerebral vasculitis
- ☐ **C** Viral meningoencephalitis
- ☐ **D** Subdural empyema
- ☐ **E** Chorea minor (Sydenham's)

4. **What further management has to be considered?**

- ☐ **A** Chloroquine
- ☐ **B** Seven years of oral penicillin
- ☐ **C** Brain biopsy
- ☐ **D** Prolonged systemic steroids
- ☐ **E** Ventriculo-peritoneal shunt

66 (2 marks)

This is the barium swallow of a 71-year-old patient with increasing dysphagia.

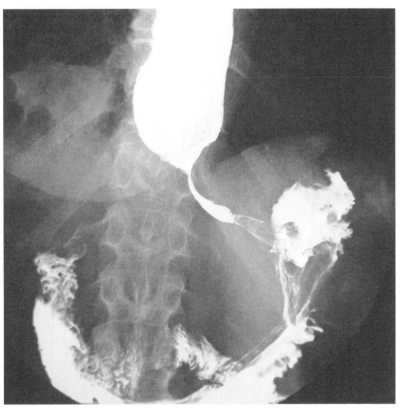

1. What is your next investigation?

- ☐ **A** Staging CT
- ☐ **B** Oesophageal manometry
- ☐ **C** Ultrasound abdomen
- ☐ **D** Full blood count
- ☐ **E** Gastroscopy

67 (4 marks)

A 36-year-old man on polychemotherapy for a relapse of stage IIIB Hodgkin's disease, presents with increasing shortness of breath. On examination there are bilateral basal crackles and pitting oedema of the lower legs. Palpation of the abdomen reveals hepatosplenomegaly.

Na	132 mmol/l
K	5.1 mmol/l
Urea	13.6 mmol/l
Creatinine	197 µmol/l
Albumin	28 g/l

Chest X-ray: Widened mediastinum, cardiomegaly, interstitial pulmonary oedema
Ultrasound abdomen: Hepatosplenomegaly, large kidneys without evidence of obstruction

1. What is the likely diagnosis?

- ☐ **A** Renal lymphoma
- ☐ **B** Membranous glomerulonephritis
- ☐ **C** Cytostatic-induced cardiomyopathy
- ☐ **D** Reactive amyloidosis
- ☐ **E** Renal vein thrombosis

2. What investigation would confirm this?

- ☐ **A** Echocardiogram
- ☐ **B** Renal biopsy
- ☐ **C** MAG-3 renogram
- ☐ **D** Intravenous urogram
- ☐ **E** Enhanced CT of the abdomen

68 (4 marks)

A 49-year-old woman presents with red eyes, a purpuric rash on both legs and polyarthralgia affecting the small joints of both hands.

A Schirmer test shows:

Left eye	2 mm/5 min (> 5 mm)
Right eye	3 mm/5 min (> 5 mm)

An autoantibody screen shows:

Rheumatoid factor	> 1:5000
Anti-nuclear antibodies	1:620
Anti-dsDNA	1:10
SS-A-(Ro) antibodies	1:320
SS-B-(La) antibodies	1:320

Hand X-ray: Normal bone density, no erosions

1. What is the likely diagnosis?

- ☐ **A** Rheumatoid arthritis
- ☐ **B** Mikulicz's syndrome
- ☐ **C** Heerfordt's syndrome
- ☐ **D** Systemic lupus erythematosus
- ☐ **E** Sjögren's syndrome

2. What therapy would you recommend?

- ☐ **A** Non-steroidal anti-inflammatory drugs
- ☐ **B** Oral steroids
- ☐ **C** Symptomatic therapy only
- ☐ **D** Plasmapheresis
- ☐ **E** Chloroquine

69 (4 marks)

A 38-year-old woman presents with fatigue and increasing pain in both arms. On examination there is a mild bilateral polyarthritis affecting the arms and knees.

Blood pressure measurements:

Right arm	105/65 mmHg
Left arm	140/80 mmHg

Investigations show:

Hb	104 g/l
MCV	82 fl
WCC	12.4×10^9/l
Plt	481×10^9/l
ESR	68 mm/h
Biochemical profile	Normal

1. What is the likely diagnosis?

☐ **A** Polymyalgia rheumatica
☐ **B** Coarctation
☐ **C** Polymyositis
☐ **D** Syphilitic aortitis
☐ **E** Takayasu's arteritis

2. What investigation is indicated?

☐ **A** Temporal artery biopsy
☐ **B** Muscle biopsy
☐ **C** Arch-aortogram
☐ **D** Contrast-enhanced CT of the thorax
☐ **E** MR scan of the aorta

70 (2 marks)

1. A 32-year-old student is admitted after taking a significant paracetamol overdose. With which of the following confounding factors should therapy be initiated, even below the treatment line?

☐ **A**   Aspirin
☐ **B**   Diazepam
☐ **C**   Furosemide (frusemide)
☐ **D**   Alcohol
☐ **E**   Beta-blockers

Paper 4 – Questions

1 (3 marks)

A 23-year-old patient with Down's syndrome is brought to Casualty in a confused state.

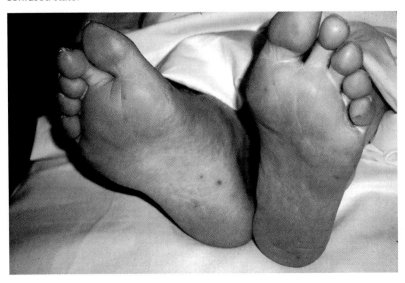

1. Which of the following investigations is the most appropriate?

☐ **A**   Ultrasound of the abdomen
☐ **B**   CT of the brain
☐ **C**   Urine microscopy
☐ **D**   Full blood count
☐ **E**   Echocardiogram

2 (7 marks)

A 28-year-old man, who was awaiting an appointment in the Cardiology Clinic for repeated syncope, is admitted as an emergency after collapsing in the gym. On arrival, he is unconscious without cardiac output. His brother indicates that there is a strong family history of cardiac disease, but he is on no current medication.

The monitor shows a broad-complex tachycardia of variable amplitude, no pulse is palpable, there is no respiratory effort and the pupils are small.

1. What is the correct management?

☐ **A**   Precordial thump, DC shocks, adrenaline (epinephrine) 1:1000 iv
☐ **B**   DC shocks, intubation and cardiac compressions
☐ **C**   1:5 CPR, iv fluids, chest aspiration
☐ **D**   DC shocks, 1:15 CPR, adrenaline (epinephrine) 1:10,000 iv
☐ **E**   External pacing, adenosine iv, carotid sinus massage

During resuscitation the arrhythmia terminates spontaneously and the patient slowly regains consciousness, remaining confused but obeying verbal commands.

The following results are obtained:

Na	142 mmol/l
K	5.9 mmol/l
Urea	6.2 mmol/l
Creatinine	141 µmol/l

Arterial blood gases:

pH	7.28
pO_2	19.7 kPa (148 mmHg)
pCO_2	7.7 kPa (58 mmHg)
Bicarbonate	13 mmol/l
O_2 sat.	100%

ECG: Sinus rhythm 168/min, axis +90°, PQ 0.1 s QRS 0.09 s, corrected QT 0.50 s, 1-mm ST elevation in V_4 to V_6

2. What is the likely underlying cause?

☐ **A**   Hyperkalaemia
☐ **B**   Wolff-Parkinson-White syndrome
☐ **C**   Romano-Ward syndrome
☐ **D**   Jervell and Lange-Nielsen syndrome
☐ **E**   Lown-Ganong-Levine syndrome

3. What was the nature of the arrhythmia?

☐ **A**   Ventricular tachycardia
☐ **B**   Junctional tachycardia
☐ **C**   Ventricular fibrillation
☐ **D**   Torsade-de-pointes tachycardia
☐ **E**   AV re-entrant tachycardia

3 (10 marks)

A tall 19-year-old woman presents to the Casualty Department with an acute episode of severe central chest and back pain. There is a family history of diabetes and ischaemic heart disease. The only past medical history includes a motorbike accident two years previously. She smokes 15 cigarettes per day and her only medication is the oral contraceptive pill.

On examination she looks unwell. Pulse 104/min, regular; BP 100/50 mmHg in the right arm, and 160/65 mmHg in the left arm. The jugular venous pressure is raised 4 cm with a normal waveform. The right carotid pulse is weak, the left is impalpable. The heart sounds are normal. A short diastolic murmur is audible at the left sternal edge and basal crackles are present at both bases.

Investigations reveal the following results:

Hb	142 g/l
WCC	6.3×10^9/l
Plt	229×10^9/l
ESR	17 mm/h
Na	141 mmol/l
K	4.3 mmol/l
Urea	5.2 mmol/l
Creatinine	78 µmol/l

Chest X-ray: Cardiothoracic ratio 61%, upper mediastinal widening, upper lobe blood diversion
ECG: Sinus rhythm 108/min, QRS axis +60°, 3-mm ST elevation in leads II, III and aVF

1. What is the diagnosis?

- ☐ **A** Aortic thrombosis
- ☐ **B** Aortic dissection
- ☐ **C** Rupture of aortic pseudo-aneurysm
- ☐ **D** Haemorrhagic pericarditis
- ☐ **E** Superior vena cava syndrome

2. What two complications have arisen?

- ☐ **A** Myocardial infarction
- ☐ **B** Pericardial effusion
- ☐ **C** Septal perforation
- ☐ **D** Rupture of papillary muscle
- ☐ **E** Left subclavian artery occlusion
- ☐ **F** Left ventricular rupture
- ☐ **G** Left common carotid occlusion
- ☐ **H** Autoimmune pericarditis
- ☐ **I** Mitral valve ring dilatation
- ☐ **J** Acute pulmonary oedema

3. Which of the following investigations is *not* indicated?

- ☐ **A** Hand X-ray
- ☐ **B** Contrast-enhanced CT of the thorax
- ☐ **C** Carotid Doppler
- ☐ **D** Echocardiogram
- ☐ **E** Aortic arch angiogram

4. What underlying cause has to be considered?

- ☐ **A** Previous trauma
- ☐ **B** Pseudoxanthoma elasticum
- ☐ **C** Buerger's disease
- ☐ **D** Polyarteritis nodosa
- ☐ **E** Marfan's syndrome

4 (8 marks)

A 15-year-old boy is admitted with headaches, palpitations and nausea. On examination he is pale, has mild photophobia, but is fully alert and orientated. Auscultation of heart and chest reveal no abnormalities. The abdomen is tender, bowel sounds are increased but no mass or organomegaly can be palpated. Pulse 100/min, regular; BP 195/110 mmHg; respiratory rate 18/min.

Preliminary investigations show:

Hb	153 g/l
WCC	4.9×10^9/l (normal differential)
Plt	271×10^9/l
ESR	8 mm/h
Na	142 mmol/l
K	3.6 mmol/l
Urea	8.9 mmol/l
Creatinine	109 µmol/l

1. Which of the following is the *least* likely diagnosis?

☐ **A** Cocaine abuse
☐ **B** Nephroblastoma (Wilms' tumour)
☐ **C** Renal artery stenosis
☐ **D** Conn's syndrome
☐ **E** Amphetamine overdose

The patient is resuscitated and further investigations show the following results:

Liver function tests   Normal
Dipstix urinalysis   Blood −, Protein +, Bilirubin −
ECG: QRS axis −15°, sinus rhythm 92/min, $S_{V2} + R_{V5} = 4.2$ mV, T inversion V_5 and V_6
Ultrasound abdomen: Normal liver, spleen and kidneys

2. Which of the following investigations would you recommend?

☐ **A** Renal angiogram
☐ **B** Urinary catecholamines
☐ **C** Chest X-ray
☐ **D** CT of the abdomen
☐ **E** Urinary 5-hydroxyindoleacetic acid

The patient is prepared for surgery.

3. What are two important preoperative measures?

☐ **A**   Estimation of creatinine clearance and octreotide administration
☐ **B**   Administration of beta-blockers and bronchodilators
☐ **C**   Salt-free diet and aspirin
☐ **D**   Administration of ACE inhibitors and diuretics
☐ **E**   iv rehydration and alpha-blockade

5 (2 marks)

This is the chest X-ray of a 49-year-old woman with a long-standing history of productive cough.

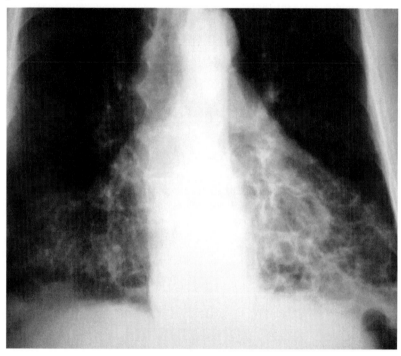

1. Which of the following is *not* a likely cause?

☐ **A**   Cystic fibrosis
☐ **B**   Measles
☐ **C**   Kartagener's syndrome
☐ **D**   Mumps
☐ **E**   Whooping cough

6 (5 marks)

A 6-year-old girl with short stature is under investigation for hypertension. Auscultation reveals a systolic murmur throughout the precordium with an early systolic click. Cardiac catheterisation reveals the following pressures:

	Pressure [mmHg]
RA	Mean 2
RV	25/0
PA	24/8
LA	Mean 5
LV	195/5
Ascending aorta	170/95
Descending aorta	120/60

1. What combination of lesions is present?

☐ **A** Aortic stenosis and aortic incompetence
☐ **B** Aortic stenosis and patent ductus arteriosus
☐ **C** Coarctation and pulmonary incompetence
☐ **D** Atrial septal defect and aortic stenosis
☐ **E** Coarctation and bicuspid aortic valve

2. What is your next investigation?

☐ **A** Growth hormone levels
☐ **B** Chromosomal analysis
☐ **C** Hand X-ray
☐ **D** Urinary 17-ketosteroids
☐ **E** Combined pituitary function tests

7 (2 marks)

This is a lesion on the scalp of a 69-year-old lady.

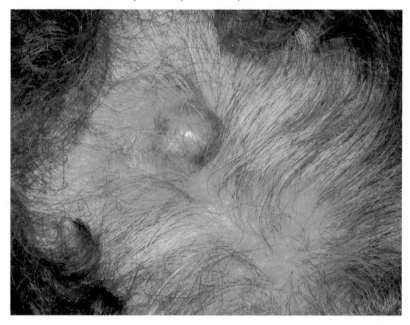

1. What is the likely diagnosis?

☐ **A**   Cholangiocarcinoma
☐ **B**   Basal cell carcinoma
☐ **C**   Infected dermoid cyst
☐ **D**   Seborrhoeic wart
☐ **E**   Haemangioma

8 (5 marks)

A 56-year-old man is under investigation for increasing shortness of breath on exercise. His chest X-ray shows cardiomegaly and pulmonary congestion. There is no history of chest pain.

The following results are obtained:

Hb	126 g/l
WCC	3.8×10^9/l
MCV	101 fl

Echocardiogram:

LV end-systolic volume	150 ml
LV end-diastolic volume	180 ml
Ejection fraction	17%
Moderate mitral regurgitation	

1. What is the likely diagnosis?

☐ **A** Dilating (congestive) cardiomyopathy
☐ **B** Restrictive cardiomyopathy
☐ **C** Hypertrophic obstructive cardiomyopathy (HOCM)
☐ **D** Mixed mitral valve disease
☐ **E** Aortic stenosis

2. What is the likely aetiology?

☐ **A** Viral infection
☐ **B** Rheumatic fever
☐ **C** Congenital defect
☐ **D** Endocardial fibrosis
☐ **E** Alcohol abuse

9 (4 marks)

The following are the readings from a cardiac catheter of a 42-year-old woman with worsening dyspnoea:

	Pressure [mmHg]	O$_2$ saturation
RA	Mean 12	66%
RV	58/10	65%
PA	56/28, Mean 39	64%
LA	Mean 15	95%
LV	120/2	93%
Aorta	120/75	94%

Cardiac output 3.0 l/min

1. What is the diagnosis?

- ☐ **A**   Hypertrophic obstructive cardiomyopathy
- ☐ **B**   Primary pulmonary hypertension
- ☐ **C**   Mixed aortic valve disease
- ☐ **D**   Mitral stenosis
- ☐ **E**   Ventricular septal defect

2. What complication has arisen?

- ☐ **A**   Shunt reversal
- ☐ **B**   Atrial thrombus
- ☐ **C**   Pulmonary hypertension
- ☐ **D**   Right ventricular dysfunction
- ☐ **E**   Left ventricular infarction

10 (3 marks)

A 71-year-old retired policeman is referred by the GP after three blood pressure readings of 175/95 mmHg. He is a non-smoker, there is no significant past medical history and clinical examination of the cardiovascular system is unremarkable except for mild bilateral ankle oedema.

1. Which of the following is the most appropriate treatment?

- ☐ **A**   Amlodipine
- ☐ **B**   Bendroflumethiazide (bendrofluazide)
- ☐ **C**   Beta-blocker
- ☐ **D**   Doxazosin
- ☐ **E**   Enalapril

11 (5 marks)

A 62-year-old smoker is admitted with severe epigastric pain. Pulse 44/min regular; BP 155/65 mmHg.

Creatinine kinase	350 U/l
AST	75 U/l
ESR	28 mm/h

The following rhythm strip is obtained:

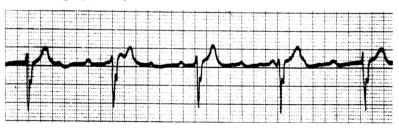

1. What is the abnormality?

- ☐ **A**   Left bundle branch block
- ☐ **B**   Sinus bradycardia
- ☐ **C**   Nodal rhythm
- ☐ **D**   Second-degree atrioventricular block
- ☐ **E**   Complete heart block

2. Which of the following should be considered?

- ☐ **A**   Thrombolysis
- ☐ **B**   Transient pacemaker
- ☐ **C**   External pacemaker
- ☐ **D**   iv atropine
- ☐ **E**   iv heparin

12 (2 marks)

This patient is referred to the Outpatient Department for assessment of malaise and weight gain.

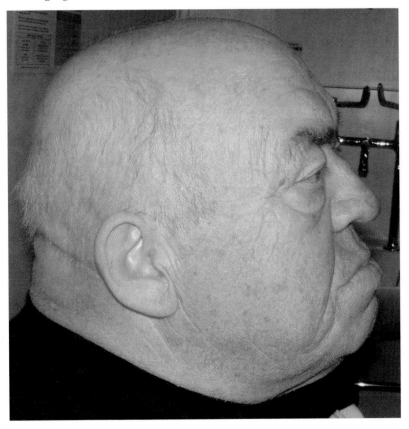

1. **Which of the following is *not* indicated?**

□ **A** Lateral skull X-ray
□ **B** Oral glucose tolerance test
□ **C** Random T4 levels
□ **D** Ophthalmology assessment
□ **E** MR scan

13 (2 marks)

The following are the results of a left-sided cardiac catheter of a 21-year-old patient with increasing breathlessness.

	Pressure [mmHg]	O$_2$ saturation
LA	Mean 8	98%
LV	155/10	90%
Aorta	150/70	91%

1. What is the correct diagnosis?

- ☐ **A**   Atrial septal defect
- ☐ **B**   Ventricular septal defect
- ☐ **C**   Tetralogy of Fallot
- ☐ **D**   Ebstein's anomaly
- ☐ **E**   Eisenmenger's complex

14 (3 marks)

This 38-year-old teacher is referred with increasing shortness of breath.

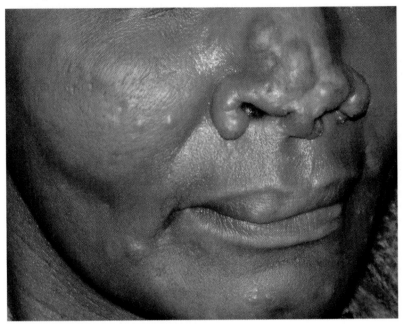

The following results are obtained on spirometry:

FVC	2.8 l (predicted 3.6 l)
FEV_1	2.4 l (predicted 3.0 l)

1. What is the likely diagnosis?

☐ **A**   Tuberculosis
☐ **B**   Tropical pulmonary eosinophilia
☐ **C**   Sarcoidosis
☐ **D**   Leprosy
☐ **E**   Rheumatoid arthritis

15 (8 marks)

A 69-year-old woman presents with weight loss, polyuria and polydipsia. She complains of upper abdominal and back pain and has lost 3 kg in weight. She is a lifelong non-smoker, drinks one glass of sherry a night and her only medication is bendroflumethiazide (bendrofluazide) 2.5 mg for hypertension. On examination, she is pale, pulse 72/min regular, BP 155/90 mmHg. Her apex beat is displaced into the anterior axillary line and there are fine crackles at both lung bases. She is tender in the epigastrium, but there is no palpable enlargement of liver or spleen and no lymph nodes can be felt.

Blood results:

Hb	121 g/l
WCC	3.2 × 10⁹/l
Plt	105 × 10⁹/l
ESR	28 mm/h

Hb   121 g/l
WCC 3.2×10^9/l
Plt 105×10^9/l
ESR   28 mm/h

The blood film shows a small number of nucleated red cells and myeloblasts.

Na   138 mmol/l
K   3.3 mmol/l
Urea   9.8 mmol/l
Calcium   3.7 mmol/l
Phosphate   1.4 mmol/l (0.75–1.5 mmol/l)
Bilirubin   18 μmol/l
Alkaline phosphatase   180 U/l (20–120 U/l)
Albumin   38 g/l
Total protein   62 g/l

The patient is given 40 mg hydrocortisone tds for 10 days.

Calcium   3.1 mmol/l

1. What further investigation would you recommend?

☐ **A**   Abdominal X-ray
☐ **B**   Parathormone levels
☐ **C**   Radio-isotope bone scan
☐ **D**   Ultrasound scan of the neck
☐ **E**   Immune electrophoresis

2. What is the likely diagnosis?

- ☐ **A** Primary hyperparathyroidism
- ☐ **B** Sarcoidosis
- ☐ **C** Ectopic PTH secretion
- ☐ **D** Metastatic carcinoma
- ☐ **E** Myeloma

3. How do you interpret the blood film?

- ☐ **A** Leucoerythroblastic film due to marrow invasion
- ☐ **B** Myelofibrosis
- ☐ **C** Myelodysplasia
- ☐ **D** Aplastic anaemia
- ☐ **E** Rebound phenomenon

4. What initial management do you suggest?

- ☐ **A** iv saline
- ☐ **B** High-dose systemic steroids
- ☐ **C** Chlorambucil
- ☐ **D** Parathyroid injection with alcohol
- ☐ **E** Radiotherapy of primary tumour

16 (7 marks)

A 6-year-old boy presents with a generalised seizure to his GP and is referred to the endocrine clinic for investigation of hypocalcaemia. There is a weak family history of 'bone problems' which his paternal grandfather was diagnosed with at the age of 12.

On examination, the patient is on the 25th percentile for height and shows swelling of most large joints and the costo-sternal junction. Trousseau's and Chvostek's signs are positive. Mental development is normal for his age. No soft tissue calcifications are seen. He has always been on an healthy diet, has no prolonged episodes of diarrhoea and takes no regular medication.

Blood results show:

Hb	146 g/l
WCC	4.2 × 10⁹/l
Plt	173 × 10⁹/l
ESR	6 mm/h

Na	139 mmol/l
K	4.1 mmol/l
Calcium	1.8 mmol/l
Phosphate	0.45 mmol/l (0.75–1.5 mmol/l)
Creatinine	55 µmol/l
Bilirubin	12 µmol/l
Alkaline phosphatase	761 U/l
Parathormone	273 pmol/l (10–90 pmol/l)

X-rays of his hands show widened growth plates with cupped and frayed metaphyses.

1. What is the most likely diagnosis?

☐ **A**   Rickets
☐ **B**   Hypoparathyroidism
☐ **C**   Multiple endocrine neoplasia type 2
☐ **D**   Pseudohypoparathyroidism
☐ **E**   Hereditary vitamin D-dependent rickets

2. Which of the following would be the most useful investigation?

☐ **A**   Small bowel biopsy
☐ **B**   Neck ultrasound
☐ **C**   Vitamin D levels
☐ **D**   Renal biopsy
☐ **E**   Radio-isotope parathyroid scan

3. What is the most likely inheritance based on the information given?

☐ **A**   Autosomal dominant
☐ **B**   Autosomal recessive
☐ **C**   X-linked dominant
☐ **D**   X-linked recessive
☐ **E**   Sporadic

17 (4 marks)

A 23-year-old man is under investigation for significantly taller stature than his parents. He is 1.93 m tall with an armspan of 1.97 m. Pubis-to-heel distance is 99 cm, pubis-to-vertex 95 cm. The metacarpal index estimated on a hand X-ray indicates arachnodactyly.

Blood results show:

Testosterone	4.6 nmol/l (10–30 nmol/l)
Luteinising hormone	28 U/l (< 6 U/l)
Follicle stimulating hormone	43 U/l (< 6 U/l)

Buccal smear: Barr bodies present

1. What is the diagnosis?

- ☐ **A** Turner's syndrome
- ☐ **B** Klinefelter's syndrome
- ☐ **C** Noonan's syndrome
- ☐ **D** Marfan's syndrome
- ☐ **E** Testicular feminisation

2. What management is appropriate?

- ☐ **A** Family screening
- ☐ **B** Testicular biopsy
- ☐ **C** MR scan of the pituitary
- ☐ **D** Combined pituitary function test
- ☐ **E** Testosterone replacement

18 (2 marks)

This is the brain scan of a 62-year-old patient admitted unconscious to Casualty.

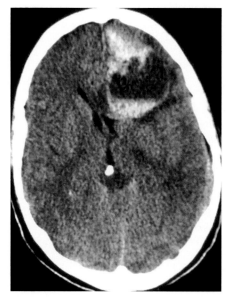

1. Which of the following is *not* indicated?

☐ **A**   Clotting screen
☐ **B**   Abdominal ultrasound scan
☐ **C**   Neurosurgical referral
☐ **D**   Oral nimodipine
☐ **E**   Blood cultures

19 (5 marks)

A 49-year-old man is under investigation for hypertension. He has a two-month history of malaise and weight loss. The following blood results are obtained:

Na	144 mmol/l
K	4.2 mmol/l
Urea	11.8 mmol/l
Calcium	2.9 mmol/l
Phosphate	0.4 mmol/l

A radio-isotope bone scan shows no evidence of metastases. 24-hour blood pressure monitoring shows hypertension between 170/95 and 195/105 mmHg.

1. Which two of the following investigations would be the most useful?

☐ **A** Blood sugar
☐ **B** Full blood count
☐ **C** Bone marrow biopsy
☐ **D** Sputum microscopy and culture
☐ **E** Barium swallow
☐ **F** Neck ultrasound
☐ **G** Parathormone levels
☐ **H** Chest X-ray
☐ **I** ENT referral
☐ **J** Skeletal survey

2. What is the likely diagnosis?

☐ **A** Conn's syndrome
☐ **B** Multiple endocrine neoplasia type I
☐ **C** Extra-adrenal phaeochromocytoma
☐ **D** Small cell carcinoma of the lung
☐ **E** Multiple endocrine neoplasia type 2

20 (2 marks)

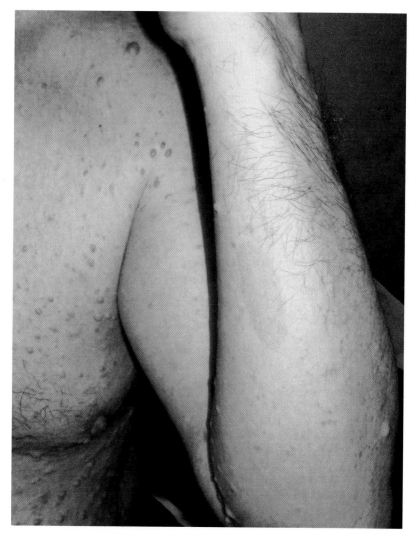

1. Which of the following is *not* a recognised feature of the syndrome shown?

☐ **A**   Phaeochromocytoma
☐ **B**   Scoliosis
☐ **C**   Autosomal dominant transmission
☐ **D**   Renal cell carcinoma
☐ **E**   Renal artery stenosis

21 (5 marks)

A 15-year-old boy is under investigation for the following blood results:

Na	136 mmol/l
K	3.2 mmol/l
Urea	6.1 mmol/l
Creatinine	62 μmol/l
Bicarbonate	21 mmol/l
Calcium	2.1 mmol/l
Albumin	41 g/l
Urine pH	6.9

After oral administration of 100 mg/kg ammonium chloride, the following results are obtained:

Time [min]	0	120
Serum bicarbonate [mmol/l]	23	15
Urine pH	6.1	5.8

1. What is the most likely diagnosis?

☐ **A** Lactic acidosis
☐ **B** Renal tubular acidosis type I
☐ **C** Renal tubular acidosis type II
☐ **D** Cystinuria
☐ **E** Alport's syndrome

2. What investigation would be the most useful?

☐ **A** Plain abdominal radiograph
☐ **B** Urinary calcium excretion
☐ **C** Urinary protein electrophoresis
☐ **D** Renal biopsy
☐ **E** Renal ultrasound scan

22 (5 marks)

A 15-year-old boy is sent to the endocrine clinic for investigation of short stature and obesity. He has underdeveloped genitals, but normal intellectual development. The following blood results are obtained:

Na	140 mmol/l
K	5.0 mmol/l
Urea	8.5 mmol/l
Creatinine	112 μmol/l
Glucose	6.5 mmol/l
Testosterone	2.5 nmol/l
	(pre-puberty 1–4 nmol/l,
	post-puberty 12–30 nmol/l)
Urine osmolality	242 mOsmol/kg

After administration of 100 μg gonadotrophin-releasing hormone (GN-RH), the following results are obtained:

Time [mins]	0	30	60	120
LH [U/l]	1.5 (1–10)	1.8	3.2 (10–50)	17.3
FSH [U/l]	0.3 (1–5)	0.8	1.2 (1–7)	7.4

1. What does the GN-RH test indicate?

☐ **A** Hypogonadotrophic hypogonadism
☐ **B** Hypergonadotrophic hypogonadism
☐ **C** Pituitary failure
☐ **D** Testicular failure
☐ **E** Androgen resistance

2. What is the likely underlying diagnosis?

☐ **A** Noonan's syndrome
☐ **B** Kallmann's syndrome
☐ **C** Craniopharyngioma
☐ **D** Klinefelter's syndrome
☐ **E** Constitutional delay

23 (2 marks)

This is the flow-volume loop of a 59-year-old miner.

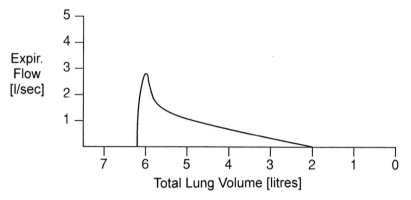

1. **What is the diagnosis?**

☐ **A** Asthma
☐ **B** Pulmonary fibrosis
☐ **C** Emphysema
☐ **D** Tracheal carcinoma
☐ **E** Pleural encasement

24 (8 marks)

A 63-year-old woman with an 18-year history of relapsing ulcerative colitis is admitted with increasing malaise and jaundice. She has lost 2 kg in weight over the last two months and was started on 30 mg prednisolone by her GP for worsening diarrhoea three weeks ago. On examination, she looks unwell, there is scleral icterus and she is mildly dehydrated. Scratch marks are present over her arms and legs, there is no adenopathy, but a tender liver is palpable under the costal margin. The chest is clear and the examination of the CNS is unremarkable.

Hb	102 g/l
WCC	4.2 × 10⁹/l
Plt	168 × 10⁹/l
ESR	39 mm/h
Na	131 mmol/l
K	3.9 mmol/l
Urea	4.2 mmol/l
Bilirubin	98 μmol/l
ALT	42 U/l
AST	51 U/l
Albumin	32 g/l

1. What is the likely cause for her jaundice?

- ☐ **A** Drug side-effect
- ☐ **B** Primary biliary cirrhosis
- ☐ **C** Primary sclerosing cholangitis
- ☐ **D** Autoimmune hepatitis
- ☐ **E** Viral hepatitis

2. What test is the most appropriate?

- ☐ **A** MR-cholangiogram (MRCP)
- ☐ **B** Autoantibody screen
- ☐ **C** Liver biopsy
- ☐ **D** Hepatitis serology
- ☐ **E** Abdominal ultrasound

The patient has a biliary drain inserted and a percutaneous cholangiogram shows irregular intrahepatic bile ducts, with a long, smooth stricture in the common hepatic duct and normal common bile duct.

3. What other differential diagnosis has to be considered?

- ☐ **A**   Lymphoma
- ☐ **B**   Metastasised carcinoma of the colon
- ☐ **C**   Mirizzi's syndrome
- ☐ **D**   Cholangiocarcinoma
- ☐ **E**   Carcinoma of the pancreas

4. What test would be most useful at this stage?

- ☐ **A**   Barium enema
- ☐ **B**   Colonoscopy
- ☐ **C**   Anti-mitochondrial antibodies
- ☐ **D**   Liver colloid scan
- ☐ **E**   CT of the abdomen

25 (12 marks)

A 48-year-old stonemason is referred to the clinic for investigation of a six-month history of malaise and weight gain. He is a non-smoking bachelor without a significant past medical history and is on no current medication. He admits to drinking half a bottle of spirits a day. On examination he has a sallow complexion, is slightly overweight, with normal conjunctivae and mucous membranes. The liver edge is palpable 3 cm under the costal margin. The spleen is not enlarged and there is no adenopathy. Examination of the chest and cardiovascular system is unremarkable. Examination of the legs shows mildly swollen and tender knees and reduction of light touch below the ankles.

Full blood count	Normal
ESR	8 mm/h
Na	139 mmol/l
K	4.1 mmol/l
Creatinine	108 μmol/l
ALT	98 U/l
Bilirubin	28 μmol/l

X-rays of the knees show advanced degenerative changes.

1. Suggest two further investigations.

☐ **A** Creatinine clearance
☐ **B** Ceruloplasmin
☐ **C** Blood glucose
☐ **D** Smooth muscle antibodies
☐ **E** 9am cortisol
☐ **F** Serum ferritin
☐ **G** ERCP
☐ **H** D-dimer levels
☐ **I** Alpha-fetoprotein
☐ **J** Vitamin B_{12} levels

2. What is the likely underlying diagnosis?

☐ **A** Chronic active hepatitis
☐ **B** Haemochromatosis
☐ **C** Systemic lupus erythematosus
☐ **D** Nelson's syndrome
☐ **E** Wilson's disease

3. How is it confirmed?

- ☐ **A** Liver biopsy
- ☐ **B** Synacthen® test
- ☐ **C** 24 h urine collection
- ☐ **D** Liver colloid scan
- ☐ **E** Autoantibodies screen

4. How is it acquired?

- ☐ **A** Autosomal recessive inheritance
- ☐ **B** Autosomal dominant inheritance
- ☐ **C** Viral infection
- ☐ **D** Ischaemic degeneration
- ☐ **E** Prion disease

Nine years later the patient is readmitted with a weight loss of 3 kg over the space of four months. The liver can no longer be palpated, but there is a smooth mass in the left upper quadrant.

Hb	187 g/l
PCV	66%
WCC	5.3×10^9/l
Plt	128×10^9/l
ESR	1 mm/h
Normal U&Es	

5. What two important complications have to be excluded?

- ☐ **A** Non-Hodgkin's lymphoma
- ☐ **B** Portal hypertension
- ☐ **C** Myelofibrosis
- ☐ **D** Chronic myeloid leukaemia
- ☐ **E** Polycythaemia rubra vera
- ☐ **F** Felty's syndrome
- ☐ **G** Hepatocellular carcinoma
- ☐ **H** Acute myeloid leukaemia
- ☐ **I** Hodgkin's lymphoma
- ☐ **J** Multiple myeloma

26 (4 marks)

A 42-year-old vagrant is admitted to the A&E Department with the following results:

Hb	109 g/l
MCV	101 g/l
WCC	4.8×10^9/l
Plt	197×10^9/l
Blood film	Rouleaux formation, reticulocytes 5%
Na	108 mmol/l
K	5.6 mmol/l
Urea	2.8 mmol/l
Total cholesterol	9.6 mmol/l
Bilirubin	48 μmol/l
Direct bilirubin	16 μmol/l (normal <5 μmol/l)

1. What is the diagnosis?

- ☐ **A**   Acute alcoholic hepatitis
- ☐ **B**   Zieve's syndrome
- ☐ **C**   Rhabdomyolysis
- ☐ **D**   Scurvy
- ☐ **E**   Methanol intoxication

2. What is the cause for the hyponatraemia?

- ☐ **A**   Inappropriate ADH secretion
- ☐ **B**   Hyperaldosteronism
- ☐ **C**   Water intoxication
- ☐ **D**   Central diabetes insipidus
- ☐ **E**   Spurious hyponatraemia

27 (2 marks)

A 53-year-old farmer's wife is referred with increasing shortness of breath. She smokes 10 cigarettes per day and has one son with asthma. On examination the chest is clear. An outpatient chest X-ray is reported as normal.

1. Which of the following is the most appropriate next investigation?

- ☐ **A** Peak expiratory flow rate (PEFR)
- ☐ **B** Serum precipitins
- ☐ **C** Spirometry and reversibility
- ☐ **D** High-resolution chest CT
- ☐ **E** Sputum microscopy

28 (3 marks)

A 54-year-old man presents with a three-month history of polyarthralgia and mild pyrexia up to 37.8 °C. Over the last month he has developed a diarrhoea which intermittently he has found difficult to flush down the toilet. The following results are obtained:

Hb	114 g/l
MCV	98 fl
WCC	5.6 × 10⁹/l (normal differential)
Plt	322 × 10⁹/l
Total protein	60 g/l
Globulin	35 g/l

A small bowel biopsy shows infiltration with PAS-positive macrophages.

1. What is the likely diagnosis?

- ☐ **A** Non-Hodgkin's lymphoma
- ☐ **B** Small bowel tuberculosis
- ☐ **C** Whipple's disease
- ☐ **D** Polyarteritis nodosa
- ☐ **E** Familial Mediterranean fever

2. How could the diagnosis be confirmed?

- ☐ **A** Lymph node biopsy
- ☐ **B** Stool culture
- ☐ **C** Joint aspiration for microscopy and culture
- ☐ **D** Polymerase chain reaction from duodenal biopsy
- ☐ **E** Autoantibody screen

29 (5 marks)

A 56-year-old farmer is admitted with a sudden onset of right upper quadrant pain and mild jaundice. He has previously been well, but is now wheezy with a respiratory rate of 28/min and a temperature of 38.7 °C. He has a blood pressure of 100/45 mmHg, pulse rate of 112/min and a tender lobulated mass is palpable in the right flank.

Hb	141 g/l
MCV	88 fl
WCC	7.9×10^9/l
Differential: 64% neutrophils, 25% lymphocytes, 8% eosinophils	
Electrolytes	Normal
Dipstix urinalysis	Blood −, Protein −, Bilirubin + +

Six hours later the patient has a generalised seizure.

1. What is the likely diagnosis?

- ☐ **A** Adult polycystic disease
- ☐ **B** Tuberose sclerosis
- ☐ **C** Liver abscesses
- ☐ **D** Wegener's granulomatosis
- ☐ **E** Hydatid disease

2. What is the next investigation?

- ☐ **A** CT of the abdomen
- ☐ **B** Chest X-ray
- ☐ **C** EEG
- ☐ **D** Blood cultures
- ☐ **E** CT of the brain

30 (6 marks)

A 17-year-old girl is investigated for a Parkinsonian syndrome. This has presented insidiously over the space of two years with a low frequency tremor, stiffness of the upper limbs and dysarthria. The following are the results of a glucose tolerance test after 75 g oral disaccharides:

Time [min]	Glucose [mmol/l]
0	4.6
30	12.8
60	10.9
90	6.5
120	3.2

1. What abnormality is shown?

- ☐ **A** Impaired glucose tolerance
- ☐ **B** Dumping syndrome
- ☐ **C** Lag storage
- ☐ **D** Malabsorption
- ☐ **E** Hyperinsulinaemia

2. What is the likely diagnosis?

- ☐ **A** Complicated diabetes mellitus
- ☐ **B** Glucagonoma
- ☐ **C** Haemochromatosis
- ☐ **D** Insulinoma
- ☐ **E** Wilson's disease

3. How would you confirm it?

- ☐ **A** Liver biopsy
- ☐ **B** Gastroscopy
- ☐ **C** Barium meal
- ☐ **D** Ceruloplasmin levels
- ☐ **E** Autoantibody screen

31 (3 marks)

A 66-year-old type 2 diabetic of Asian origin presents for a routine follow-up. His medication consists of aspirin 75 mg and gliclazide 80 mg. Blood pressure is 155/85 mmHg in both arms. The following results are obtained:

Na	134 mmol/l
K	4.1 mmol/l
Urea	8.6 mmol/l
Creatine	158 μmol/l
Total cholesterol	5.2 mmol/l
HbA$_1$c	8.6%
Dipstix urinalysis	Blood −, Protein +, Ketones +

1. **What is the best treatment to prevent progression of microvascular renal disease?**

- ☐ **A** Insulin
- ☐ **B** Beta-blocker
- ☐ **C** Introduction of statin
- ☐ **D** ACE inhibitor
- ☐ **E** Metformin

32 (10 marks)

A 29-year-old female accountant presents with a swollen right leg. One year previously she had been on warfarin for a suspected pulmonary embolism but she had refused a VQ lung scan as she thought she was pregnant at the time. She is otherwise well and on no regular medication except simple analgesics for tension headaches.

The following results are obtained:

Hb	106 g/l
MCV	103 fl
WCC	$6.1 \times 10^9/l$ (63% neutrophils)
RCC	$2.9 \times 10^{12}/l$ (7% reticulocytes)
Plt	$172 \times 10^9/l$
PT	15 s (control 12–14 s)
APTT	78 s (control 32 s)
APTT after 1:1 addition of normal plasma	72 s
Bleeding time	6 min (5–8 min)
Na	136 mmol/l
K	5.1 mmol/l
Creatinine	151 µmol/l
Direct Coombs' test	Positive

1. What do the clotting results suggest?

- ☐ **A** Platelet defect
- ☐ **B** Defect in the extrinsic clotting pathway
- ☐ **C** Defect in the intrinsic clotting pathway
- ☐ **D** Anti-phospholipid antibodies
- ☐ **E** Red cell defect

2. What is the cause for the anaemia?

- ☐ **A** Chronic disease
- ☐ **B** Autoimmune haemolytic anaemia
- ☐ **C** Sideroblastic anaemia
- ☐ **D** Vitamin B$_{12}$ deficiency
- ☐ **E** Hypersplenism

3. What is the next investigation?

☐ **A**   Haemoglobin electrophoresis
☐ **B**   Indirect Coombs' test
☐ **C**   Ultrasound of the abdomen
☐ **D**   Red cell sequestration studies
☐ **E**   Autoantibody screen

Ten months later, the patient presents to the eye hospital complaining of a 'dark cloud' in the top right corner of her right eye. Fundoscopy shows a focal haemorrhage in the right retina; the remainder of the retina and the left fundus are normal. Her blood pressure is found to be 155/100 mmHg and a trace of protein is found in the urine.

4. What is the likely cause for the visual problem?

☐ **A**   Retinal vein branch occlusion
☐ **B**   Retinal artery branch occlusion
☐ **C**   Hypertensive haemorrhage
☐ **D**   Retinal detachment
☐ **E**   Amaurosis fugax

5. What treatment would you recommend?

☐ **A**   Heparin
☐ **B**   Aspirin
☐ **C**   Warfarin
☐ **D**   Fresh frozen plasma
☐ **E**   Laser treatment

33 (4 marks)

A 26-year-old woman has become profoundly unwell two hours after a Caesarean section for delivery of monozygotic twins.

Investigations show:

Hb	93 g/l
MCV	96 fl
WCC	8.6×10^9/l (87% neutrophils)
Plt	51×10^9/l
Blood film: Reticulocytosis, red cell fragmentation	
PT	21 s (control 12–14 s)
APTT	42 s (control 34 s)
Thrombin time	29 s (control 16 s)

1. Which one of the following sets of tests would you perform?

- ☐ **A**   D-dimer levels and antithrombin levels
- ☐ **B**   Thrombin time with protamine and chest X-ray
- ☐ **C**   Fibrin degradation products (FDP) and blood cultures
- ☐ **D**   Abdominal ultrasound scan and bleeding time
- ☐ **E**   Biochemical profile and arterial blood gases

2. What is the most likely underlying cause?

- ☐ **A**   Pelvic sepsis
- ☐ **B**   Amniotic fluid embolus
- ☐ **C**   Ligation of the iliac artery
- ☐ **D**   Perforation of the colon
- ☐ **E**   Pyelonephritis

34 (5 marks)

A 76-year-old man is referred by his GP for episodes of acrocyanosis when washing his hands.

The fingers develop a purple discoloration directly after exposure to cold water. No blanching phase is observed.

Blood samples obtained in the evening show the following results:

Na	138 mmol/l
K	3.9 mmol/l
Urea	6.3 mmol/l
Creatinine	121 µmol/l
Albumin	39 g/l
Total protein	83 g/l

The full blood count sample is kept in the fridge overnight and the following day the pathology staff request a new sample as it has haemolysed.

1. Which of the following investigations is likely to be most helpful?

- [ ] **A** White cell differential
- [ ] **B** Blood film
- [ ] **C** Immune electrophoresis
- [ ] **D** Rheumatoid factor
- [ ] **E** Bone marrow biopsy

2. What is the likely diagnosis?

- [ ] **A** Chronic lymphocytic leukaemia
- [ ] **B** Paroxysmal nocturnal haemoglobinuria
- [ ] **C** Cold haemagglutinin disease
- [ ] **D** Hereditary spherocytosis
- [ ] **E** Mixed connective tissue disease

35 (2 marks)

This is the chest X-ray of a 68-year-old pensioner complaining of malaise and weight loss.

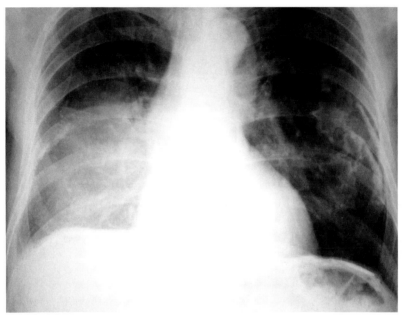

1. Which of the following examination is the *least* helpful?

- ☐ **A** CT of the thorax
- ☐ **B** Bronchoscopy
- ☐ **C** Pulmonary function tests
- ☐ **D** Lateral chest X-ray
- ☐ **E** Arterial blood gases

36 (1 mark)

The following blood results are returned for a man on outpatient follow-up for recurrent episodes of ventricular tachycardia. His current medication is aspirin and amiodarone.

Na	131 mmol/l
K	7.1 mmol/l
Urea	19.2 mmol/l
Glucose	1.1 mmol/l

1. What would you expect to see in the blood film?

- [ ] **A** Normal appearance
- [ ] **B** Haemolysis
- [ ] **C** Basophilic stippling
- [ ] **D** Heinz bodies
- [ ] **E** Howell-Jolly bodies

37 (9 marks)

A 17-year-old man is referred by the GP for investigation of haematuria. Examination of the abdomen is unremarkable. BP 165/95 mmHg; pulse 72/min, regular. Despite mydriatic eye-drops, the fundi cannot be adequately assessed. In addition, a mild hearing deficit is identified and tuning-fork tests show the following results: Weber lateralises to the right; Rinne demonstrates air conduction is better than bone conduction in both ears.

Blood results in clinic are as follows:

Hb	162 g/l
WCC	$5.1 \times 10^9/l$
Plt	$265 \times 10^9/l$
Na	138 mmol/l
K	4.8 mmol/l
Creatinine	286 µmol/l
Dipstix urinalysis	Protein +, Blood + +

1. How do you interpret the hearing tests?

☐ **A** Right sensorineural deficit
☐ **B** Left sensorineural deficit
☐ **C** Right middle ear conductive deficit
☐ **D** Left middle ear conductive deficit
☐ **E** Artefactual

2. What is the likely reason for the failed fundoscopy?

☐ **A** Myopia
☐ **B** Cataract
☐ **C** Anisocoria
☐ **D** Retinal detachment
☐ **E** Lenticonus

3. What is the unifying diagnosis?

☐ **A** Congenital rubella
☐ **B** IgA nephritis
☐ **C** Complicated type 1 diabetes
☐ **D** Alport's syndrome
☐ **E** Systemic lupus erythematosus

4. What is the prognosis for the kidneys and their function?

- ☐ **A** Spontaneous recovery
- ☐ **B** Development of hypernephroma
- ☐ **C** Progressive renal failure
- ☐ **D** Full recovery with treatment
- ☐ **E** Renal papillary necrosis

38 (8 marks)

A 28-year-old male presents to the A&E Department with acute, right-sided flank pain.

There were no previous episodes. Brought up as a single adopted child he has always been well and never been to see his GP. He admits, however, to a one-year history of intravenous substance abuse. On examination, there are needle marks at both elbows with thrombosis of the cephalic veins. No palpable AV fistula. BP 165/100 mmHg; pulse 80/min, regular; no heart murmurs. He is breathless at rest with normal auscultation.

The liver is enlarged and a mass is palpable in the left upper quadrant.

The following results are obtained:

Hb	149 g/l
WCC	3.1×10^9/l (84% granulocytes)
Plt	238×10^9/l
ESR	6 mm/h

Na	139 mmol/l
K	4.6 mmol/l
Urea	14.1 mmol/l
Creatinine	289 µmol/l

Urine microscopy: Multiple red blood cells, several hyaline casts

IVU shows poor excretion through the left kidney; the right side shows compression of the collecting system with splaying and elongation of the calyces.

1. What is the likely cause for the presentation?

- ☐ **A** Passage of renal stone
- ☐ **B** Acute tubular necrosis
- ☐ **C** Haemorrhage into a cyst
- ☐ **D** Malignant transformation
- ☐ **E** Pyelonephritis

2. What is the likely diagnosis?

- ☐ **A** Adult polycystic kidney disease
- ☐ **B** Infantile polycystic kidney disease
- ☐ **C** Horseshoe kidney
- ☐ **D** Multicystic dysplastic kidney
- ☐ **E** Tuberose sclerosis

Pulse oximetry reveals an oxygen saturation of 95% on room air and chest X-ray shows bilateral diffuse mid-zone shadowing. On moderate exercise, the patient desaturates to 85%.

3. What diagnosis has to be considered?

☐ **A** Interstitial pulmonary oedema
☐ **B** Sarcoidosis
☐ **C** Pulmonary haemorrhage
☐ **D** *Pneumocystis carinii* pneumonia
☐ **E** Eosinophilic pneumonia

With treatment, the patient makes a good recovery but is lost to follow-up. Eight months later he is brought back to the A&E Department after having been found collapsed on a park bench. On examination, he has a Glasgow Coma Scale score of 5 with flexion to pain stimulus. Unenhanced CT of the brain is reported as normal.

A lumbar puncture reveals the following results:

Opening pressure	14 cmH$_2$O
Xanthochromia	++
Protein	0.28 g/l (0.2–0.4 g/l)
Glucose	59% of blood glucose
Microscopy	4 red cells/µl (< 5 per µl)

4. What is the likely explanation for these results?

☐ **A** Traumatic tap
☐ **B** Haemorrhagic stroke
☐ **C** Herpes encephalitis
☐ **D** Cerebral toxoplasmosis
☐ **E** Subarachnoid haemorrhage

39 (2 marks)

A 33-year-old woman is referred to the medical team from the delivery suite with worsening shortness of breath. She is being treated by her GP for fibromyalgia. Previous medical history includes surgery for cataracts. Her baby was born at term but suffered a respiratory arrest immediately after delivery. Blood results show:

Hb	93 g/l
WCC	10.1 × 10⁹/l (62% neutrophils)
Plts	129 × 10⁹/l
ESR	38 mm/h
CRP	<1 mg/l
Na	141 mmol/l
K	4.9 mmol/l
Urea	10.2 mmol/l
Creatinine	98 µmol/l

Chest X-ray shows bilateral peri-hilar consolidation.

1. What is the likely diagnosis?

- ☐ **A** Acute adrenal failure
- ☐ **B** Myasthenia gravis
- ☐ **C** Systemic lupus erythematosus
- ☐ **D** Hypothyroidism
- ☐ **E** Myotonic dystrophy

2. What is the cause for her acute symptoms?

- ☐ **A** Cardiomyopathy
- ☐ **B** Pulmonary embolus
- ☐ **C** Amniotic fluid embolus
- ☐ **D** Aspiration pneumonia
- ☐ **E** Pericardial effusion

40 (4 marks)

A 47-year-old man with familial hypercholesterolaemia is admitted to Coronary Care with 2-mm ST elevation in leads, II, III and AVF. A right-sided cardiac catheter gives the following results:

	Pressure [mmHg]
SVC	Mean 10
RA	Mean 10
RV	19/8
PA	18/5
Pulmonary Wedge Pressure	3
Radial Artery	95/50

1. What is the likely explanation for these results?

- ☐ **A** Atrial fibrillation
- ☐ **B** Complete heart block
- ☐ **C** Right ventricular infarction
- ☐ **D** Cardiac tamponade
- ☐ **E** Septal perforation

Two hours later the patient is found to be in a nodal bradycardia.

2. What does this indicate?

- ☐ **A** Thrombosis of right coronary artery
- ☐ **B** Thrombosis of circumflex artery
- ☐ **C** Re-perfusion injury
- ☐ **D** Lateral extension of infarct
- ☐ **E** Apical extension of infarct

41 (4 marks)

A 48-year-old unemployed electrician is admitted to Casualty after being found unconscious at a building site. His vital signs are stable and the following results are obtained:

Na	132 mmol/l
K	6.9 mmol/l
Urea	13.2 mmol/l
Creatinine	921 µmol/l
ALT	53 U/l
AST	348 U/l
Dipstix urinalysis	Blood + + +, Protein +, Ketones –

1. What do these results suggest?

- ☐ **A** Rhabdomyolosis
- ☐ **B** Acute tubular necrosis
- ☐ **C** Renal haemorrhage
- ☐ **D** Aortic dissection
- ☐ **E** Renal infarction

2. What is the likely precipitating cause?

- ☐ **A** Blunt abdominal trauma
- ☐ **B** Alcohol excess
- ☐ **C** Hypothermia
- ☐ **D** Benzene intoxication
- ☐ **E** Electric shock

42 (5 marks)

A 23-year-old Turkish woman presents with malaise, weight loss and polyuria. The following results are obtained:

Na	127 mmol/l
K	4.1 mmol/l
Urea	8.1 mmol/l
Creatinine	117 μmol/l

Urine microscopy:	
Red cells	8/μl (< 5/μl)
White cells	95/μl (< 10/μl)
Multiple hyaline casts	

Urinary Na excretion	410 mmol/24 h
	(40–220 mmol/24 h)
MSU × 3	No growth

1. What is the cause for the electrolyte imbalance?

☐ **A**   Pyelonephritis
☐ **B**   Acute tubular necrosis
☐ **C**   Salt-wasting nephropathy
☐ **D**   Nephrogenic diabetes insipidus
☐ **E**   Inappropriate ADH secretion

2. What is the likely underlying cause?

☐ **A**   Gonorrhoea
☐ **B**   Vesico-ureteric reflux
☐ **C**   *Chlamydia* infection
☐ **D**   Fanconi syndrome
☐ **E**   Renal tuberculosis

43 (2 marks)

This is the MR renal angiogram of a 52-year-old HGV driver with hypertension. Full blood count and biochemical profile are normal.

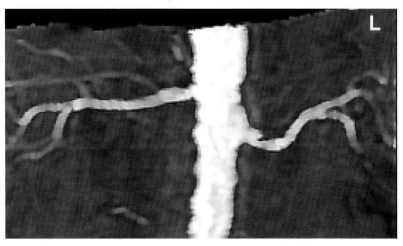

1. **Which of the following investigations is the most useful?**

- ☐ **A** Intravenous urogram
- ☐ **B** Glomerular filtration rate (GFR)
- ☐ **C** Selective renal arteriogram
- ☐ **D** Renal vein sampling
- ☐ **E** Isotope renogram

44 (4 marks)

A 43-year-old salesman presents, after two years in the Far East, with a macular erythematous rash, lymphadenopathy and painless buccal ulcers. On examination, he has a low-grade pyrexia with evidence of meningism. He is admitted as an emergency and given intravenous penicillin.

1. **What investigation is likely to be diagnostic?**

☐ **A**   Blood culture
☐ **B**   Lumbar puncture
☐ **C**   Oral swab and dark-field microscopy
☐ **D**   *Treponema pallidum* haemagglutination test (TPHA)
☐ **E**   Viral serology

The following day, the patient becomes extremely unwell with fever, polymyalgia and hypotension.

2. **What complication has occurred?**

☐ **A**   Waterhouse-Friderichsen syndrome
☐ **B**   Jarisch-Herxheimer reaction
☐ **C**   Anaphylactic reaction to penicillin
☐ **D**   Stevens-Johnson syndrome
☐ **E**   Septicaemia

45 (7 marks)

A four-year-old boy is referred from the GP with shortness of breath on exercise and unwillingness to play with his friends. This has come on over the previous six months after initially normal developmental milestones. When called into the examination room, he needs support from his mother to get up from the floor.

Examination shows a normal mental development. He is short of breath at rest; examination of chest and cardiovascular system are otherwise unremarkable. He has very well developed calves, but a symmetrical moderate weakness of the pelvic and shoulder girdle are present.

Investigations show:

Hb	138 g/l
WCC	5.2 × 10⁹/l
Plt	327 × 10⁹/l
ESR	8 mm/h
Na	134 mmol/l
K	4.9 mmol/l
Urea	4.1 mmol/l
Albumin	38 g/l
Chest X-ray	Mild cardiomegaly

An ECG shows first-degree heart block with occasional monotopic ventricular extrasystoles.

Electromyography shows polyphasic action potentials of short duration and low amplitude.

1. What is the likely diagnosis?

- ☐ **A** Guillain-Barré syndrome
- ☐ **B** Duchenne muscular dystrophy
- ☐ **C** Facio-scapulo-humeral dystrophy
- ☐ **D** Organophosphate poisoning
- ☐ **E** Becker's muscular dystrophy

2. What is your next investigation?

- ☐ **A** Echocardiogram
- ☐ **B** Liver function tests
- ☐ **C** Muscle biopsy
- ☐ **D** Autoantibody screen
- ☐ **E** Creatinine phosphokinase levels

3. What is the likely prognosis?

☐ **A** Death before age 10
☐ **B** Death as a teenager
☐ **C** Wheelchair-bound in middle age
☐ **D** End-stage cardiac failure in the third decade
☐ **E** Respirator dependency by the age of 30

46 (9 marks)

A 29-year-old woman is referred to the Neurology Department with recent onset of walking difficulties and dull backache. She seems to relate this to an accident three weeks previously where she was knocked off her bike. She had suffered blunt trauma to her thoracic spine, but X-rays performed in the A&E Department did not demonstrate a fracture. She is otherwise well and takes no regular medication.

Examination of the upper limbs is normal. In the left leg the reflexes are brisk and several beats of clonus can be elicited at the ankle. Pinprick sensation is normal but sensation to deep pain is reduced. Power deficit of 4/5 is present in the extension of the knee.

The only deficit noticeable in the right leg is a mild reduction in pinprick sensation over the anterior tibia and thigh to the groin with some hyperaesthesia along the right costal margins.

1. What do these findings suggest?

☐ **A**   Left-sided disc prolapse
☐ **B**   Right-sided thoracic tumour
☐ **C**   Right-sided disc prolapse
☐ **D**   Thoracic syrinx
☐ **E**   Left-sided thoracic tumour

It is also noted that the patient has a mild convergent squint in the left eye and on formal examination there is a deficit in abduction and elevation of gaze on the left, as well as a mild mydriasis. There is no proptosis and the eyes are not injected.

2. Which of the following processes is most likely to cause this deficit?

☐ **A**   Mononeuritis multiplex
☐ **B**   Extradural haemorrhage
☐ **C**   Superior orbital fissure meningioma
☐ **D**   Cerebellopontine angle tumour
☐ **E**   Cavernous sinus thrombosis

On further testing of the cranial nerves, a hearing deficit is detected. Testing with a tuning fork reveals the following results:

Weber: lateralising to the left
Rinne: positive in both ears (air conduction better than bone conduction)

3. What is indicated by these results?

- ☐ **A** Right sensorineural deficit
- ☐ **B** Left sensorineural deficit
- ☐ **C** Left conduction deficit
- ☐ **D** Right conduction deficit
- ☐ **E** Otosclerosis

4. Which of the following diagnoses has to be considered?

- ☐ **A** Multiple sclerosis
- ☐ **B** Basal skull fracture
- ☐ **C** Benign intracranial hypertension
- ☐ **D** Neurofibromatosis type II
- ☐ **E** Von Hippel-Lindau syndrome

47 (3 marks)

This patient has diplopia on right lateral gaze.

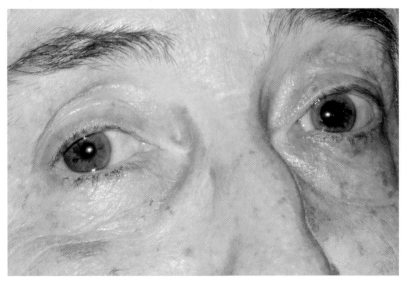

1. What is the diagnosis?

- ☐ **A** Right abducens nerve palsy
- ☐ **B** Left trochlear nerve palsy
- ☐ **C** Holmes-Adie pupil
- ☐ **D** Left oculomotor palsy
- ☐ **E** Right Horner's syndrome

2. Which of the following is the most appropriate investigation?

- ☐ **A** C-reactive protein
- ☐ **B** Lateral skull X-ray
- ☐ **C** HbA_{1c}
- ☐ **D** Chest X-ray
- ☐ **E** Visual-evoked potentials

48 (2 marks)

A 49-year-old patient with lupus nephritis is admitted after a short episode of crushing central chest pain. He has severe chronic renal impairment and is listed for dialysis. His results on admission are:

Hb	88 g/l
WCC	5.2×10^9/l
Plt	186×10^9/l
MCV	81 fl
ESR	28 mm/h
Na	133 mmol/l
K	5.8 mmol/l
Creatinine	688 µmol/l

1. What is the best treatment for the anaemia?

- ☐ **A** Oral iron supplements
- ☐ **B** Blood transfusion
- ☐ **C** Erythropoietin
- ☐ **D** iv hydrocortisone
- ☐ **E** iv iron

49 (6 marks)

A woman in her thirties is admitted from a nightclub having collapsed. She has extensive telangiectasia around her right eye.

An un-enhanced CT of the brain shows atrophy of the right parietal lobe with meningeal calcification.

The following day a lumbar puncture is performed, during which the patient has a fit.

CSF shows: Bloodstaining +, Xanthochromia + +
Pressure   17 cmH$_2$O
Protein   0.5 g/l
Glucose   4.2 mmol/l
Microscopy (/mm^3)   360 erythrocytes, 7 lymphocytes

1. What do the results imply?

- ☐ **A** Traumatic tap
- ☐ **B** Haemorrhagic stroke
- ☐ **C** Subarachnoid haemorrhage
- ☐ **D** Meningioma
- ☐ **E** Cerebral metastases

2. What is the underlying condition?

- ☐ **A** Von Hippel-Lindau syndrome
- ☐ **B** Renal cell carcinoma
- ☐ **C** Sturge-Weber syndrome
- ☐ **D** Adult polycystic kidney disease
- ☐ **E** Hereditary haemorrhagic telangiectasia

3. What is the most sensible investigation?

- ☐ **A** CT of the brain after iv contrast
- ☐ **B** Ultrasound of the abdomen
- ☐ **C** Cerebral angiogram
- ☐ **D** Radio-labelled red cell scan
- ☐ **E** MR scan of the brain

50 (3 marks)

A 17-year-old girl presents with a six-month history of headaches, worst in the morning. Clinical examination, including the cranial nerves and visual acuity, is normal. Fundoscopy shows no papilloedema. Her body mass index is 27 and her only medication is the oral contraceptive pill and vitamin supplements. Lumbar puncture shows:

Opening pressure	29 cmH$_2$O
Protein	0.4 g/l
Glucose	5.1 mmol/l
Microscopy	3 lymphocytes/mm^3, no red blood cells

1. **Which of the following investigations is the most appropriate?**

   ☐ **A** CT scan of the brain
   ☐ **B** Cytospin
   ☐ **C** Carotid angiography
   ☐ **D** MR scan of the brain
   ☐ **E** 24-hour blood pressure profile

2. **What is the likely diagnosis?**

   ☐ **A** Migraine
   ☐ **B** Leukaemic meningitis
   ☐ **C** Cushing's disease
   ☐ **D** Phaeochromocytoma
   ☐ **E** Benign intracranial hypertension

51 (6 marks)

A middle-aged vagrant woman is admitted to the ward after having fallen down the stairs in the local train station.

A CT scan shows a small right chronic subdural haematoma. Three days later she becomes confused with worsening ataxia and horizontal nystagmus in both eyes.

The following results are obtained:

Hb	137 g/l
MCV	102 fl
WCC	9.8×10^9/l (normal differential)
Prothrombin time	16.9 s

A lumbar puncture shows normal results.

1. What is the likely diagnosis?

- ☐ **A**   Subarachnoid haemorrhage
- ☐ **B**   Extradural haematoma
- ☐ **C**   Hepatic encephalopathy
- ☐ **D**   Central pontine myelinolysis
- ☐ **E**   Wernicke's syndrome

2. What treatment is indicated?

- ☐ **A**   iv nimodipine
- ☐ **B**   Surgical decompression
- ☐ **C**   iv thiamine
- ☐ **D**   Oral lactulose
- ☐ **E**   iv glucose

3. What other measures should be considered?

- ☐ **A**   Fresh frozen plasma
- ☐ **B**   Oral chlordiazepoxide
- ☐ **C**   im vitamin B_{12}
- ☐ **D**   iv hypertonic saline
- ☐ **E**   im vitamin K

52 (3 marks)

This is the unenhanced CT scan of a 48-year-old patient with a Glasgow Coma Scale score of 6/15.

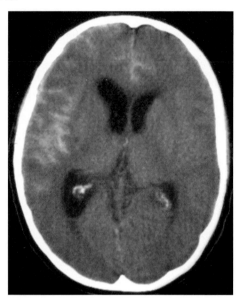

1. **Which of the following is indicated?**

☐ **A** Oral nimodipine
☐ **B** Lumbar puncture
☐ **C** iv cephalosporin
☐ **D** Neurosurgical referral
☐ **E** iv aciclovir

53 (7 marks)

A 41-year-old Cuban teacher presents with tiredness and three episodes of night sweats. She has lost 2.5 kg in weight over the last three months. She describes an irritating dryness in her throat and dry cough, which has plagued her for the best part of six weeks. Recently she complains of increasing dizzy spells and has fainted on two occasions. In addition, she has recently developed intermittent painful knees and wrists. She had a termination of pregnancy six months earlier and her symptoms seem to have followed on from this. There is no past medical history of note, and her only medication is temazepam for insomnia.

On examination she looks well with no anaemia or jaundice and no evidence of finger clubbing. BP 95/45 mmHg; pulse 56/min, regular; no heart murmurs. One or two lymph nodes are palpated in the axillae; no organomegaly is present in the abdomen. Normal neurological examination.

The following blood results are obtained:

Hb	113 g/l
WCC	6.2×10^9/l (normal differential)
Plt	193×10^9/l
ESR	59 mm/h
Na	141 mmol/l
K	4.4 mmol/l
Urea	9.2 mmol/l
Creatinine	112 μmol/l
Albumin	33 g/l
Calcium	2.85 mmol/l
Phosphate	1.3 mmol/l
FEV_1	1.7 l (predicted 2.4–3.7 l)
FVC	2.2 l (predicted 4.0–5.2 l)
TLC	4.8 l (predicted 5.7–7.6 l)

Chest X-ray: Mediastinal widening, clear lungs, normal heart
ECG: Axis –40°, PR 0.25 s, QRS 0.14 s, right bundle branch block, no evidence of ischaemia

1. **Suggest two further investigations.**

☐ **A**   Pathergy test
☐ **B**   Parathormone levels
☐ **C**   Blood cultures
☐ **D**   High-resolution CT scan
☐ **E**   Kveim test
☐ **F**   Lymph node biopsy
☐ **G**   24 h ECG
☐ **H**   Serum ACE levels
☐ **I**   Silver stain of sputum
☐ **J**   Bronchoscopy

2. **What is the likely diagnosis?**

☐ **A**   Non-Hodgkin's lymphoma
☐ **B**   Sarcoidosis
☐ **C**   Cryptogenic fibrosing alveolitis
☐ **D**   Langerhans cell histiocytosis
☐ **E**   Behçet's disease

3. **What two therapeutic measures have to be considered?**

☐ **A**   Erythromycin
☐ **B**   Forced diuresis
☐ **C**   Methotrexate
☐ **D**   Systemic steroids
☐ **E**   Cardiac pacing
☐ **F**   Amiodarone
☐ **G**   Rifampicin
☐ **H**   Cardiac transplant
☐ **I**   iv immunoglobulins
☐ **J**   Heart-lung transplant

54 (8 marks)

A 48-year-old switchboard operator is under long-term follow-up for seropositive nodular rheumatoid arthritis. She is referred by her GP as an urgency, with a ten-day history of intermittent diplopia.

Her arthritis had flared up eight months previously and she had been successfully started on indometacin 50 mg bd and D-penicillamine 500 mg daily. Blood results at that time were normal. She is also on thyroxine 200 µg following radioiodine ablation for thyrotoxicosis. On examination there is only mild synovial swelling in the small joints of the hands. Moderate ulnar deviation is present in the MCP joints. Neurological examination reveals mild weakness of the upper limbs, more pronounced after exercise, but there is no evidence of wasting or fasciculation. Reflexes are present with reinforcement. Cranial nerves are unremarkable. Some fine end-inspiratory crackles are heard at the lung bases which do not clear with coughing. BP 150/85 mmHg; pulse 76/min, regular; respiratory rate 22/min.

Blood results:

Hb	118 g/l
WCC	5.6×10^9/l
Plt	102×10^9/l
MCV	79 fl
ESR	16 mm/h
Na	141 mmol/l
K	3.9 mmol/l
Creatinine	168 µmol/l
Albumin	29 g/l

1. **Which one of the following pairs of investigations would be the most useful?**

☐ **A** Chest X-ray and 24 h creatinine clearance
☐ **B** Rheumatoid factor and bone marrow biopsy
☐ **C** Urinary protein and acetylcholine receptor antibodies
☐ **D** Renal biopsy and autoantibody screen
☐ **E** High-resolution CT chest and histone antibodies

2. **What is the likely underlying cause for the neurology?**

☐ **A** Recurrence of thyrotoxicosis
☐ **B** Myasthenia gravis
☐ **C** Drug-induced lupus
☐ **D** Drug-induced myasthenia
☐ **E** Mononeuritis multiplex

3. What therapeutic measure would you recommend?

- ☐ **A**   Reduce thyroxine
- ☐ **B**   Stop indometacin
- ☐ **C**   Stop penicillamine
- ☐ **D**   Introduce steroids
- ☐ **E**   Start pyridostigmine

4. What is the most likely cause for the respiratory signs?

- ☐ **A**   Rheumatoid lung
- ☐ **B**   Chronic aspiration
- ☐ **C**   Drug-induced fibrosis
- ☐ **D**   Cryptogenic fibrosing alveolitis
- ☐ **E**   Invasive aspergillosis

55 (5 marks)

A 41-year-old flight attendant is referred with intermittent cough and haemoptysis. She also describes intermittent episodes of wheeze, dyspnoea and palpitations. She has otherwise been well with the occasional episode of diarrhoea which she has put down to the frequent travelling. Her symptoms had been investigated 18 months earlier, but a blood test and a chest X-ray had shown normal results. She is on no regular medication and has had all the required vaccines.

On examination she looks well and clinical examination is normal except for a dull percussion note at the left lung base associated with some reduced breath sounds.

Investigations show:

Hb	141 g/l
WCC	$6.5 \times 10^9/l$ (normal differential)
Plt	$241 \times 10^9/l$
ESR	12 mm/h
Prothrombin time	14 s (control 12–14s)
U&Es	Normal

Chest X-ray: Partial collapse of left lower lobe, no adenopathy

Arterial blood gases (on air):

pH	7.38
pO_2	12.7 kPa (95 mmHg)
pCO_2	5.5 kPa (41 mmHg)
O_2 sat.	99%

1. What two examinations would you recommend?

- ☐ **A** Lateral chest X-ray
- ☐ **B** High-resolution CT
- ☐ **C** Thoracoscopy
- ☐ **D** Ventilation–perfusion scan
- ☐ **E** Ultrasound of liver
- ☐ **F** Gallium scintigraphy
- ☐ **G** Bronchoscopy
- ☐ **H** Positron emission tomography
- ☐ **I** Contrast of the enhanced CT-thorax
- ☐ **J** Bone marrow biopsy

2. What is the likely diagnosis?

- ☐ **A** Bronchial carcinoid
- ☐ **B** Langerhans cell histiocytosis
- ☐ **C** Allergic bronchopulmonary aspergillosis
- ☐ **D** Churg-Strauss syndrome
- ☐ **E** Small cell carcinoma of lung

56 (2 marks)

A 26-year-old hairdresser presents with a four-month history of weight loss and palpitations. Results show:

Hb	129 g/l
WCC	6.8 × 10⁹/l (38% lymphocytes)
Plts	208 × 10⁹/l
ESR	12 mm/h
T4	199 nmol/l
T3	12.8 pmol/l
Serum TSH	< 0.1 mU/l

1. What is the most likely diagnosis?

- ☐ **A** Viral thyroiditis
- ☐ **B** Multiple endocrine neoplasia
- ☐ **C** Thyrotoxicosis
- ☐ **D** Riedel's fibrosing thyroiditis
- ☐ **E** Autoimmune thyroiditis (Hashimoto's)

57 (2 marks)

A 43-year-old non-smoking veterinarian presents with an unproductive cough, worse at night.

Investigations show:

FEV$_1$	2.4 l (predicted 3.0–4.5)
FVC	3.8 l (predicted 3.9–5.9)
FEV$_1$/FVC	63%
PEFR	520 l/min
	(predicted 560–620 l/min)

Methacholine provocation test:

20% fall in FEV$_1$ is provoked by concentration of 1 mg/ml (normal > 4 mg/ml)

1. What diagnosis is suggested by these results?

- ☐ **A**   Tracheomalacia
- ☐ **B**   Occupational asthma
- ☐ **C**   Relapsing polychondritis
- ☐ **D**   Hyper-reactive bronchial system
- ☐ **E**   Thyroid enlargement

58 (5 marks)

A 36-year-old bank manager presents with a seven-day history of malaise, headaches and increasing cough.

Investigations show:

Hb	92 g/l
RCC	2.6×10^{12}/l
Reticulocytes	4.6%
WCC	9.8×10^9/l
Differential: 41% granulocytes, 52% lymphocytes, 4% monocytes	
Plt	381×10^9/l

Dipstix urinalysis	Blood + + +, Protein +, Glucose –

Chest X-ray: Bilateral patchy basal consolidation

1. What is the likely diagnosis?

- ☐ **A**   Glucose-6-phosphate dehydrogenase deficiency
- ☐ **B**   Haemolytic uraemic syndrome
- ☐ **C**   *Mycoplasma* pneumonia
- ☐ **D**   Paroxysmal nocturnal haemoglobinuria
- ☐ **E**   Sickle cell disease

2. Which of the following tests will be positive for haemolysis?

- ☐ **A**   Direct Coombs' test
- ☐ **B**   Indirect Coombs' test
- ☐ **C**   Ham's test (acidic resistance)
- ☐ **D**   Osmotic resistance
- ☐ **E**   Heat resistance at 40 °C

59 (2 marks)

A 21-year-old nurse is admitted for investigation of breathlessness and diplopia. Except for an episode of prolonged diarrhoea three months previously, she has always been well. The following results are obtained:

FEV$_1$ 2.1 l (predicted 3.8–4.2)
FVC   2.5 l (predicted 4.2–5.0)

Arterial gases (room air):

pH   7.30
pO$_2$ 9.8 kPa (73.5 mmHg)
pCO$_2$ 6.1 kPa (46 mmHg)

1. Which of the following is the most likely diagnosis?

☐ **A**   Phrenic nerve palsy
☐ **B**   Guillain-Barré syndrome
☐ **C**   Myasthenia gravis
☐ **D**   Multiple sclerosis
☐ **E**   Organophosphate poisoning

60 (2 marks)

A 41-year-old patient with polycystic disease is due to undergo a renal transplant the following day. His results are:

Na	137 mmol/l
K	5.6 mmol/l
Creatinine	726 μmol/l

1. What immediate treatment is indicated?

- ☐ **A** Subcutaneous insulin
- ☐ **B** Calcium
- ☐ **C** Haemodialysis
- ☐ **D** iv dextrose and insulin
- ☐ **E** None

61 (4 marks)

A 43-year-old woman with seropositive rheumatoid arthritis is prescribed indometacin for increasing pain in her right hip. Two months later she returns complaining of breathlessness.

Lung function tests in clinic show:

FEV$_1$	3.0 l (predicted 2.8–3.3 l)
FVC	3.8 l (predicted 3.4–4.3 l)
FEV$_1$/FVC	79%
PEFR	510 l/min
	(predicted 490–580 l/min)
O$_2$ sat.	98% on air

1. Which of the following investigations is *least* likely to be helpful?

- ☐ **A**   Full blood count
- ☐ **B**   Chest X-ray
- ☐ **C**   Arterial blood gases
- ☐ **D**   Biochemical profile
- ☐ **E**   Erythrocyte sedimentation rate

2. Which of the following is *least* likely to have produced her symptoms?

- ☐ **A**   Renal failure
- ☐ **B**   Bronchospasm
- ☐ **C**   Anaemia
- ☐ **D**   Pulmonary fibrosis
- ☐ **E**   Fluid retention

62 (5 marks)

A 73-year-old man is admitted to hospital with an infective exacerbation of chronic airflow limitation. Investigations show:

Arterial blood gases (on air):

pH	7.31
pO_2	6.5 kPa (49 mmHg)
pCO_2	7.1 kPa (53 mmHg)
Bicarbonate	27 mmol/l

He is treated with nebulisers but after an initial improvement where he deteriorates over the following two hours.

Repeat arterial gases show:

pH	7.23
pO_2	9.8 kPa (74 mmHg)
pCO_2	9.3 kPa (70 mmHg)
Bicarbonate	28 mmol/l

A portable chest X-ray shows extensive right mid-zone consolidation.

1. What is the likely cause for the deterioration?

- ☐ **A** Aspiration
- ☐ **B** Septicaemia
- ☐ **C** Adult respiratory distress syndrome (ARDS)
- ☐ **D** CO_2 narcosis
- ☐ **E** O_2 administration

2. What management would you recommend?

- ☐ **A** iv antibiotics
- ☐ **B** Insertion of a nasogastric tube
- ☐ **C** Intubation
- ☐ **D** iv doxapram
- ☐ **E** High-dose O_2 administration

63 (4 marks)

A 47-year-old line manager in a cheese factory presents with worsening chronic breathlessness. Examination reveals a few inspiratory crackles but no other abnormality.

The following results are obtained:

FBC	Normal
PEFR	550 l/min
	(predicted 590–650 l/min)
FEV$_1$/FVC	78%
O$_2$ sat.	95% on air
Transfer coefficient (KCO)	88%

1. What is the likely diagnosis?

- ☐ **A** Emphysema
- ☐ **B** Occupational asthma
- ☐ **C** Extrinsic allergic alveolitis
- ☐ **D** Chronic bronchitis
- ☐ **E** Allergic bronchopulmonary aspergillosis

2. What is his chest X-ray likely to show?

- ☐ **A** Apical fibrosis
- ☐ **B** Basal fibrosis
- ☐ **C** Bullae
- ☐ **D** Pleural thickening
- ☐ **E** Bronchiectasis

64 (2 marks)

This is the chest X-ray of a patient with slowly worsening dyspneoa.

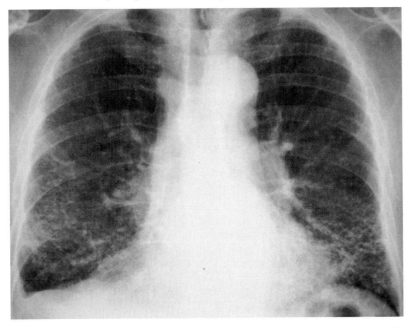

1. Which of the following is *not* a likely differential diagnosis?

☐ **A** Rheumatoid arthritis
☐ **B** Coal dust inhalation
☐ **C** Amiodarone toxicity
☐ **D** Systemic sclerosis
☐ **E** Asbestosis

65 (7 marks)

A 16-year-old girl under investigation for polyuria presents with acute dyspnoea. She had a previous episode six months earlier which had resolved spontaneously. On examination she looks well but distressed. Respiratory rate 28/min. Percussion note in the left upper thorax is hyper-resonant and the breath sounds are reduced. Examination of the abdomen is unremarkable. There is an ejection systolic murmur heard over the aorta; blood pressure 105/65 mmHg; pulse 104/min, regular.

An urgent chest X-ray shows a large, left-sided pneumothorax with early mediastinal shift. In addition there are bilateral interstitial abnormalities with some nodules and multiple cysts.

1. Which of the following diagnoses is *least* likely?

- ☐ **A**   Tuberose sclerosis
- ☐ **B**   Neurofibromatosis
- ☐ **C**   Eosinophilic granuloma
- ☐ **D**   Sarcoidosis
- ☐ **E**   Lymphangio-leiomyomatosis

A small chest drain is inserted in the X-ray Department and the patient makes a rapid recovery.

Investigations show the following results:

Na	141 mmol/l
K	4.0 mmol/l
Urea	11.0 mmol/l
Creatinine	129 μmol/l
Glucose	4.0 mmol/l
Liver function tests	Normal

Arterial blood gases after drainage of pneumothorax (room air):

pH	7.39
pO_2	9.2 kPa (69 mmHg)
pCO_2	4.3 kPa (29 mmHg)
Bicarbonate	21 mmol/l

2. Which of the following investigations are indicated?

- ☐ **A**   Sputum microscopy and lung function tests
- ☐ **B**   CT of the thorax and renal biopsy
- ☐ **C**   Lung biopsy and early morning urine sampling
- ☐ **D**   Kveim test and MR of the brain
- ☐ **E**   Skull X-ray and urine osmolality

3. What complication has probably arisen?

- ☐ **A** Thalamic dysfunction
- ☐ **B** Nephrogenic diabetes insipidus
- ☐ **C** Central diabetes insipidus
- ☐ **D** Bronchiectasis
- ☐ **E** Renal tubular acidosis type II

66 (5 marks)

A 43-year-old lady with long-standing, severe psoriasis is started on methotrexate 30 mg/week. After ten days her left knee becomes swollen, hot and painful overnight. The following results are obtained:

Hb	122 g/l
WCC	$4.2 \times 10^9/l$
Plt	$95 \times 10^9/l$
ESR	36 mm/h
U&Es	Normal

Knee X-ray: Small amount of calcification within the articular cartilage, no bone destruction

1. What is the likely diagnosis?

- ☐ **A** Calcium pyrophosphate deposition
- ☐ **B** Septic arthritis
- ☐ **C** Acute gout
- ☐ **D** Joint haemorrhage
- ☐ **E** Psoriatic arthritis

2. What investigation is likely to be diagnostic?

- ☐ **A** Joint aspirate and culture
- ☐ **B** MR scan
- ☐ **C** Clotting screen
- ☐ **D** Joint aspiration and polarised light microscopy
- ☐ **E** Complement levels

3. What therapy would you suggest?

- ☐ **A** Allopurinol
- ☐ **B** Diclofenac
- ☐ **C** Fresh frozen plasma
- ☐ **D** Co-amoxiclav
- ☐ **E** Methotrexate 60mg/week

67 (4 marks)

A 17-year-old boy is being investigated for a swinging pyrexia and recurrent painful swelling of both knees. Over the last three weeks he has developed a sore red eye and now presents to the A&E Department with acute visual deterioration over the preceding 24 hours. Blood samples reveal:

Hb	92 g/l
MCV	78 fl
WCC	19×10^9/l (94% neutrophils)
Plt	612×10^9/l
ESR	98 mm/h

Biochemical profile	Normal

Rheumatoid factor	1:10
Anti-nuclear antibodies (ANA)	1:160
Extractable nuclear antigen (ENA)	1:1
HLA-B27	Negative

Chest X-ray: Small right pleural effusion

1. What is the likely diagnosis?

- ☐ A Behçet's disease
- ☐ B Reiter's syndrome
- ☐ C Familial Mediterranean fever
- ☐ D Lyme disease
- ☐ E Still's disease

2. What is the appropriate management?

- ☐ A Paediatric referral
- ☐ B iv antibiotics
- ☐ C Rheumatology referral
- ☐ D Blood cultures
- ☐ E Ophthalmology referral

68 (2 marks)

A 29-year-old woman is under investigation for abdominal pain and weight loss. After a barium follow-through she is admitted with trismus and acute torticollis.

1. Which of the following treatments is indicated?

☐ **A**   Chlorpromazine
☐ **B**   Benzhexol
☐ **C**   Midazolam
☐ **D**   Paper bag re-breathing
☐ **E**   Haloperidol

69 (4 marks)

A 28-year-old woman is admitted with acute onset of shortness of breath, lower chest and epigastric pain. She is noticed to have peau d'orange on her neck. BP 95/65 mmHg; pulse 100/min; no murmurs. The pedal pulses are absent.

ECG shows sinus tachycardia with left bundle branch block.

FBC	Normal
ESR	28 mm/h
Na	136 mmol/l
K	4.1 mmol/l
Urea	8.5 mmol/l
Creatinine	123 µmol/l
Creatinine kinase	210 U/l
LDH	290 U/l
AST	38 U/l
Amylase	128 U/l

1. What is the underlying condition?

☐ **A**   Kawasaki disease
☐ **B**   Pseudoxanthoma elasticum
☐ **C**   Buerger's disease
☐ **D**   Ehlers-Danlos syndrome
☐ **E**   Systemic sclerosis

2. What is the cause for her symptoms?

☐ **A**   Aortic dissection
☐ **B**   Bacterial endocarditis
☐ **C**   Acute myocardial infarction
☐ **D**   Rhabdomyolysis
☐ **E**   Oesophageal dysmotility

70 (3 marks)

This is the mouth of a 28-year-old patient admitted with acute, severe dyspnoea.

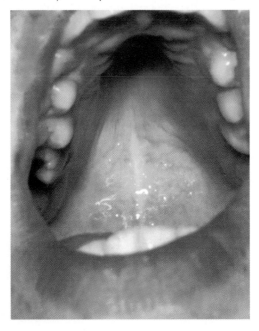

1. **Which of the following is the *least* likely precipitating cause for the patient's symptoms?**

- [ ] **A** Acute renal failure
- [ ] **B** Pneumothorax
- [ ] **C** Pulmonary oedema
- [ ] **D** Pericordial effusion
- [ ] **E** Rupture of chordae tendineae

Paper 1 - Answers

1 Answers (4 marks)

1. **C**   Ventricular septal defect
2. **B**   Shunt reversal

The patient has marked clubbing with deep peripheral cyanosis. The most likely cause for this is a congenital heart defect which has led to the development of secondary pulmonary hypertension and shunt reversal (Eisenmenger complex). The main symptoms in cystic fibrosis and bronchiectasis would be cough and recurrent chest infections.

2 Answers (9 marks)

1. **A**   Mitral stenosis
2. **E**   Mesenteric infarction
3. **D**   Lactic acidosis
4. **B**   Mesenteric angiogram

The patient has numerous features of **mitral stenosis**. Acute presentation with abdominal pain may indicate a posterior MI, but the patient also has a high anion gap acidosis ($[Na^+ + K^+] - [Cl^- + HCO_3^-] = 32$ mmol/l). **Mesenteric infarction** causes a rise in lactate. A surgical opinion needs to be sought urgently. Plain abdominal films may be normal. An ultrasound scan may show a swollen loop of atonic bowel and some free fluid. CT may be diagnostic, the investigation of choice is angiography.

3 Answers (8 marks)

1. **D**   Perforated ventricular septum
2. **E**   Transthoracic echocardiogram
3. **B**   Cardiac surgery

The presence of a significant **post-infarction VSD** is indicated by a high arterial pulmonary pressure, but the normal wedge pressure and a high O_2 saturation indicate a left-to-right shunt. Other acute complications of MI include rupture of papillary muscle and ventricular rupture; late complications include post-infarction pericarditis (Dressler's syndrome) and LV aneurysm.

4 Answers (5 marks)

1. **D** Autoimmune pericarditis
2. **C** Indometacin

Post-cardiotomy syndrome occurs up to one year following cardiac surgery. It is an acute febrile illness with pericarditis and/or pleuritis. Pleural and pericardial effusions are frequently found. The disease, similar to Dressler's syndrome (pericarditis two to four weeks after MI), is usually self-limiting but may require treatment with non-steroidal anti-inflammatories or, if these fail, steroids. Pericarditic pain is typically worse lying down and relieved by sitting forward. Typical ECG changes of pericarditis may be subtle or absent in the autoimmune form.

5 Answer (2 marks)

1. **E** Subdural haematoma

There are bilateral crescentic hypodense (darker than brain) collections extending from the frontal, over the temporal, to the parietal areas. The ventricles are normal in size and calcification is seen in the pineal gland and the choroid plexus. Fresh blood on CT-settings for brain is white. As it gets broken down it turns darker to the same shade of grey as the brain itself, over a period of 2–3 weeks, and becomes 'watery' (black) after 4–5 weeks.

6 Answers (4 marks)

1. **B** Significant ischaemia
2. **E** Coronary angiography

There is an ST-segment depression of >1 mm in leads II, III, AVF and V_{3-6} at 0.8 seconds after the 'J' point. This is a strongly **positive exercise test** and suggests multi-vessel disease because of involvement of anterior and inferior leads. This requires further investigation and treatment.

7 Answers (4 marks)

1. **C** Renal tubular acidosis (RTA) type I (distal)
2. **B** Primary biliary cirrhosis

The patient has a hypokalaemic acidosis and this constellation is highly suggestive of **renal tubular acidosis**. The age and the presence of renal calculi suggests RTA type I (distal tubular acidification defect). This may be inherited by any of the traits or may be secondary to a variety of diseases (for full list see Kumar and Clark's *Clinical Medicine*). Hypergammaglobulinaemia is excluded by the normal globulin fractions; Wilson's disease is unlikely to cause this degree of liver damage at this age.

8 **Answers (4 marks)**

1. **C** Second-degree heart block
2. **A** Observation only

The patient has a **Second-degree AV block** heart block with **Wenckebach periodicity** (Mobitz 1). The PR interval increases until one QRS complex is dropped. This has a better prognosis than a Mobitz 2 block with a fixed conduction deficit. Asymptomatic patients do not require treatment.

9 **Answer (2 marks)**

1. **C** Barium swallow

The patient has significant Barrett's oesophagus as indicated by the change from pale oesophageal to red gastric mucosa. Biopsy to exclude metaplasia, treatment of reflux disease and at least bi-annual repeat endoscopy is required.

10 **Answers (6 marks)**

1. **B** Ventricular fibrillation
2. **C** DC shock 200 J
3. **D** Myocardial infarction

The initial rhythm is disorganised without a definite pattern coarse ventricular fibrillation and the second ECG shows an acute postero-inferior MI, in combination this indicates. Management of cardiac arrest is an infrequent, but recurring theme of the exam. Detailed knowledge of the latest guidelines will be expected by the examiners, in particular in the clinical part of the exam.

11 **Answers (5 marks)**

1. **D** Ostium secundum atrial septal defect
2. **A** Ventilation–perfusion lung scan

There is a step-up of saturation in the right atrium, indicating a left-to-right shunt. However, of the four options given for a defect at this level, the ECG changes indicate an **ASD**. By far the commoner form is an ostium secundum defect which is also likely to present later on in life. Paradoxical emboli to the systemic circulation can be found despite the predominant left-to-right shunt. Injection of embolising particles (microalbumin aggregates) in a lung perfusion scan is therefore contraindicated as they usually end up in the brain or in the kidneys.

12 Answers (5 marks)

1. **C**   Toxic cardiomyopathy
2. **B**   Venesection

The patient has **haemochromatosis**. The cardinal features are diabetes, liver disease and skin pigmentation (beware the well-looking patient!). Myocardial deposition of iron leads to a dilating cardiomyopathy. Initial therapy is with iron removal by bloodletting.

13 Answer (2 marks)

1. **D**   Lymphoma

There is air within the right ureter, most likely due to a entero–vesical fistula. Lymphoma will cause adenopathy and may involve the bowel, particularly the terminal ileum, but it is extremely unlikely to cause fistula formation between organs.

14 Answers (9 marks)

1. **B**   Secondary hyperthyroidism
2. **C**   MR scan of the pituitary
3. **D**   Carbimazole
4. **C**   Trans-sphenoidal hypophysectomy

A raised TSH in the presence of a raised T4 indicates failure of the feedback to the pituitary and the presence of either a secondary (pituitary) hyperthyroidism or ectopic TSH production (trophoblastic disease). The latter is unlikely as the patient is on oral contraceptives. In primary (thyroid) hyperthyroidism TSH and TRH would be suppressed; in tertiary (hypothalamic) hyperthyroidism the TRH would be high, stimulating TSH and T4 secretion.

Increased secretion of TSH by the pituitary is usually due to an adenoma but may occur as 'simple' hypersecretion.

Pituitary adenomata, if very small, may even be missed by MRI scanning, but may be differentiated from TSH hypersecretion by failure of TSH to suppress with bromocriptine and with increase TRH. Conservative treatment (bromocriptine, octreotide) may be successful, but surgery will often be required.

Treatment of the end-organ thyroid with carbimazole, surgery or radioiodine will only produce a transient response as the continuing stimulation with TSH will facilitate regrowth of any residual thyroid tissue. Patients on thyrostatics need to be monitored for agranulocytosis.

15 Answers (10 marks)

1. B 240

The serum osmolality is calculated as follows: (Na + K) × 2 + urea + glucose.

2. E Syndrome of inappropriate ADH secretion (SIADH)

The patient has extremely low osmolality of the serum with an inappropriately high osmolality of the urine. Causes for **inappropriate ADH secretion** include any intracranial pathology (tumour, hydrocephalus, infection), intrathoracic pathology (tumour, empyema, infection, in particular *Legionella*), a number of drugs (in particular, drugs beginning with 'c', i.e. chlorpropamide, chlorothiazide, cytotoxics and carbamazepine) as well as lymphoma and acute intermittent porphyria.

3. D Fluid restriction and iv diazepam

The treatment for SIADH is fluid restriction. The patient, however, is in status epilepticus and requires appropriate treatment.

4. B Central pontine myelinolysis
5. B MR scan of the brain

Rapid correction of the electrolyte disturbance is contraindicated. The change in blood results suggests that the patient has been given (hypertonic) saline intravenously with a disastrous result. The posterior fossa and the brainstem are poorly demonstrated on CT but will be clearly shown on MR scanning.

16 Answer (2 marks)

1. C Pseudohypoparathyroidism type I

Parathormone increases the urinary phosphate excretion. This is mediated within the cell by the second messenger c-AMP. After infusion of intravenous PTH, urinary excretion of c-AMP and phosphate should increase by a factor of 10–15. In hypoparathyroidism, there is not enough end-ogenous parathormone. In **pseudohypoparathyroidism**, there is end-organ resistance within the kidney to PTH. In type I, there is a complete receptor defect and neither c-AMP nor phosphate excretion is increased. In type II, the cell receptor is intact and c-AMP rises, with a consequent increase in urinary excretion, but phosphate levels do not change.

Pseudohypoparathyroidism is associated with somatic features (short stature, moon face, short 4th and 5th metacarpals and intellectual impairment). In addition, ectopic soft tissue calcification is found more commonly in type I than in type II. In pseudo-pseudohypoparathyroidism, the skeletal abnormalities are found, but the biochemistry is normal.

17 Answer (2 marks)

1.   A   Ischaemic heart disease

The flexor aspects of the elbows show the 'plucked chicken skin' appearance of pseudoxanthoma elasticum. This familial condition is more than a cosmetic problem as abnormality of the elastic fibres in the arterial wall lead to peripheral vascular disease and ischaemic heart disease at an early age. Breaks in Bruch's membrane of the retina produce the angioid streaks seen on fundoscopy.

18 Answers (4 marks)

1.   C   T3 thyrotoxicosis
2.   A   Increased thyroxine-binding globulin (TBG)

T3 thyrotoxicosis is characterised by a normal free T4 concentration, but an elevated free T3 concentration (which is the investigation of choice). As in 'normal' hyperthyroidism, TSH levels are suppressed and fail to increase after administration of TRH.

T3 thyrotoxicosis is seen more frequently in patients with thyroid adenoma/multinodular goitre than in Graves' disease. As expected, this patient has a mild increase in hepatic synthesis of TBG due to the oestrogens contained in the contraceptive pill.

19 Answers (6 marks)

1.   A   Subacute thyroiditis
2.   C   Fine-needle aspiration and systemic steroids
3.   D   Hypothyroidism

The patient has evidence of active thyroiditis, but the white cells are not elevated, indicating **subacute thyroiditis (de Quervain's)**. This is characterised by raised ESR and raised T3 and T4 levels due to liberation of the hormones from the inflamed gland, which suppresses TSH. Prognosis is very good and most patients do not require treatment and, despite initial hyperthyroid status, return to normal function. However, hypothyroidism may ensue and, if severe, the patient may be treated with steroids.

Acute bacterial thyroiditis, of course, requires antibiotics and aspiration of any collections. Chronic lymphocytic thyroiditis (Hashimoto's) occurs in middle-aged women and is associated with thyroid autoantibodies. There is insidious onset of hypothyroidism which, potentially, leads to firm fibrosis of the gland (Riedel's goitre). Fine-needle aspiration is a safe procedure when done under ultrasound control.

20 Answers (5 marks)

1. **C** Polyglandular failure (Schmidt's syndrome)
2. **A** Autoantibody screen

The serum electrolytes and the low morning cortisol indicate adrenocortical insufficiency. In addition, the patient has features of hypothyroidism. The normal growth hormone and high TSH are against panhypopituitarism. **Polyglandular failure** is also associated with diabetes mellitus, pernicious anaemia, gonadal failure and hypoparathyroidism. Hyperthyroidism may be seen if the auto-antibodies are of a stimulating kind. In the majority of patients, antibodies to the affected glandular tissue are found.

21 Answers (8 marks)

1. **A** Normal vitamin B_{12} metabolism

Both phases of the test are normal. The Dicopac® test combines the two phases of the Schilling test in one injection, the B_{12} and the B_{12}/intrinsic factor compound being labelled with different radioactive markers. Either phase of the test is abnormal if urinary excretion is less than 8%. Correction with intrinsic factor indicates pernicious anaemia.

2. **B** *Candida* oesophagitis

The described appearances are typical of candidiasis. Herpes simplex is the main differential diagnosis. However, this is less common and less likely to be so extensive. CMV typically causes giant ulcers.

3. **C** HIV infection

4. **E** Secondary lymphoma

Usually non-Hodgkin's lymphoma. It can affect any site including small bowel and brain.

The features of watery diarrhoea, normal Dicopac® test and a **sub**mucosal process exclude Crohn's disease. Lymphoma, TB and possibly **y**ersiniosis, remain differential diagnoses. **AIDS-defining diseases** include Kaposi's sarcoma (can occur anywhere in the body), oesophageal *Candida*, Pneumocystiscarinii pneumonia, cerebral toxoplasmosis, CMV retinitis, recurrent *Salmonella* septicaemia, disseminated mycobacterial disease, non-Hodgkin's lymphoma, primary cerebral lymphoma and disseminated histoplasmosis (AIDS-defining means any of the above with evidence of HIV infection).

22 Answers (8 marks)

1. **C** Faecal porphyrins
   D Abdominal ultrasound
2. **C** Acute intermittent porphyria
3. **C** Stop fluoxetine
   D Sun avoidance

A combination of a low serum osmolality [(Na + K) × 2 + urea + glucose = 269 mmol/l] and a high urine osmolality indicates inappropriate ADH secretion. Causes for this include any intracranial pathology (tumour/abscess/increased pressure), intrathoracic pathology (infection, in particular *Legionella*, empyema, tumour), drugs (promazine, carbamazepine, chlopropramide), lymphoma and acute porphyrias.

A triad of recurrent episodes of peritonism, neuropsychiatric disturbances and hyponatraemia is typical of **acute intermittent porphyria**. Urine turns orange/brown on standing and there is a familial incidence (autosomal dominant). It is precipitated by a number of drugs, in particular alcohol, oral contraceptives, antidepressants, barbiturates, benzodiazepines and a number of antibiotics (for full list, see *BNF*). If the syndrome is combined with a photosensitive rash, this indicates the much rarer variegate porphyria, which is more common in white South Africans.

23 Answers (5 marks)

1. **C** Acquired hypogammaglobinaemia
2. **D** Chronic *Giardia* infection

There is isolated reduction of all the immunoglobulins. The age of the patient is against Hodgkin's disease; normal clinical examination and normal full blood count make non-Hodgkin's lymphoma unlikely and exclude yellow nail syndrome. Recurrent infections are the main manifestations of **acquired hypogammaglobulinaemia**. Causes for diarrhoea are bacterial overgrowth and chronic infections, in particular *Giardia*. An inflammatory colitis may occur.

24 Answer (2 marks)

1. **B** Aortic dissection

There is a renal transplant scar, a haemodialysis fistula and hirsutism indicating ciclosporin therapy. The main risks are hypertensive haemorrhage, electrolyte imbalance and immune suppression.

25 Answers (6 marks)

1. **B** Autoimmune chronic active hepatitis (CAH)
2. **C** Hepatitis serology
3. **A** Azathioprine

Autoimmune CAH in women typically presents with malaise, tender hepatomegaly, secondary amenorrhoea and elevated LFTs. Without immune suppressant therapy, prognosis is bad; with therapy ten-year survival rate is usually higher than 90%. Non-specific manifestations of chronic liver disease are found. The disease may be complicated by development of hepatocellular carcinoma.

26 Answers (6 marks)

1. **E** Budd-Chiari syndrome
2. **A** Prolonged severe illness in the neonatal period
3. **C** Fundal varices

Budd-Chiari syndrome or hepatic vein thrombosis is seen in the context of thrombophilia, red cell anomalies and severe illnesses associated with chronic sepsis and dehydration. It results in post-hepatic portal hypertension with consecutive liver damage. The caudate lobe (liver segment one) is usually spared as this has separate portal and arterial supply as well as venous drainage. It results in compensatory hypertrophy of this lobe. The ascites seen in this context is frequently an exudate rather than a transudate but the normal glucose essentially rules out infection. Fundal varices will not be treated by sclerotherapy of the oesophagus alone. Umbilical vein catheters cause portal vein thrombosis.

27 Answers (5 marks)

1. **D** Insulinoma
2. **D** CT pancreas

On one occasion the patient shows morning hypoglycaemia, on another morning hyperglycaemia, the latter likely to be due to a rebound phenomenon (Somogyi effect) or the patient having eaten to combat the hypoglycaemia in the early hours. The raised C-peptide after a fast indicates there is inappropriate insulin secretion. Factitious insulin administration would not result in elevation of the C-peptide, which is produced by cleavage from endogenous pro-insulin. Most insulinoma tumours are benign but are, however, frequently seen as part of multiple endocrine neoplasia type I (pancreatic tumours, parathyroid hyperplasia and medullary carcinoma of the thyroid).

28 Answer (1 mark)

1. C Pneumatosis coli

Pneumatosis intestinalis is most commonly found in the lower colon and may be idiopathic (15%) or secondary to obstructive airways disease or, rarely, inflammation, infection or ischaemia. It may cause recurrent asymptomatic pneumoperitoneum.

29 Answers (9 marks)

1. B Erythrocyte sedimentation rate
2. E Prothrombin time
3. C Venesection
4. D Myelofibrosis

A middle-aged patient with an increase in all cell lines and splenomegaly. The combination of polycythaemia and iron depletion indicates **polycythaemia rubra vera**.

This is a myeloprofilerative disorder with a peak incidence in the sixth decade, commoner in men than in women. Endogenous erythropoietin is reduced, distinguishing it from secondary polycythaemia, causes for which include chronic airways disease, EPO-secreting tumours (hepatoma, hypernephroma and cerebellar haemangioblastoma) and pseudopolycythaemia (stress polycythaemia, Gaissböck syndrome). Leucocyte alkaline phosphatase (LAP) is elevated in contrast to CML. Although platelets may be increased, platelet function is often reduced, with a tendency for bruising and an increased bleeding time. The increased cell turnover may precipitate gout.

Therapy in the first instance is with venesection in order to keep the haematocrit below 45%. Second-line treatment includes 5-hydroxyurea, but with an increased risk of secondary leukaemia.

Complications: embolism (stroke and PE accounting for up to 40% of deaths), haemorrhage, myelofibrosis and acute leukaemia. The latter occurs in under 2% when treated with venesection and in up to 10–15% under myelosuppressive chemotherapy.

As a late feature, the patient develops a leucoerythroblastic blood film with left shift of all cell lines, indicating extramedullary erythropoiesis.

30 Answers (7 marks)

1. **A** Thrombin time
2. **D** Antithrombin III (AT III) deficiency
3. **D** Heparin side-effect

A young patient presents with features of thrombophilia. Despite full heparinisation, the patient develops a further thrombosis. The resistance to heparin therapy is characteristic of **antithrombin III deficiency.**

Antithrombin III is an inhibitor of clotting factors, mainly directed against the activity of thrombin, Factor Xa and Factor IXa and other clotting factors. It is the mediator of the effect of heparin, in the presence of which it is an effective inhibitor of thrombin and Factor Xa. There is a spectrum of congenital AT III-deficiencies which vary in the levels of AT III as well as its activity. The commonest form is transmitted as an autosomal dominant trait. The main differential diagnoses are protein C deficiency and protein S deficiency.

An important side-effect of heparin is the induction of thrombocytopenia and the *BNF* (Edition 45) recommends monitoring of platelet levels for patients on heparin for longer than five days.

31 Answers (6 marks)

1. **C** Bone marrow biopsy
2. **B** Hodgkin's disease
3. **D** iv antibiotics

A young patient with no obvious precipitating cause for a profound pancytopenia. The most important and probably most likely cause is an **acute leukaemia with an aleukaemic blood film** (no blasts). The patient has evidence of sepsis in the presence of absolute granulocytopenia and requires immediate covering with broad-spectrum antibiotics.

Hodgkin's disease presents with lymphadenopathy, usually in the mediastinum. Severe bone marrow infiltration would be evidenced by a leucoerythroblastic blood film.

32 Answer (1 mark)

1. **D** Brachial plexus

There is wasting of the thenar eminence as well as the palmar interossei muscles, indicating a lower motor neurone lesion affecting the median as well as the ulnar nerve.

33 Answers (4 marks)

1. **A** Dietary deficiency
2. **B** Vitamin B$_{12}$ levels

A macrocytic anaemia with mild reduction in white cell count and platelets in an Asian woman is most likely to be **nutritional**. Strict Hindu diet is free of animal produce. Other causes to be considered would be toxic, including alcohol and myelodysplasia, but these are much less likely. Pernicious anaemia is essentially excluded by the low gastrin.

First-line investigations should confirm B$_{12}$ deficiency before any more invasive procedures are performed.

34 Answers (4 marks)

1. **C** Hodgkin's disease
2. **A** Radiotherapy

Hodgkin's disease has two age peaks, in the third and seventh decades, and is more common in men. Presentation is with fever, weight loss, malaise, lymphadenopathy and/or hepatomegaly. Staging depends on the number of lymph stations and extralymphatic organs involved.

As far as can be said, the patient has no adenopathy and no evidence of hepatosplenomegaly. The commonest presentation is with mediastinal adenopathy (stage one). The treatment for stage one is radiotherapy, the prognosis is excellent.

Alcohol-induced nodal pain is a rare but typical manifestation, as is an undulating fever (Pel-Ebstein fever).

35 Answers (6 marks)

1. **B** Discontinue any medication
2. **A** Glucose-6-phosphate-dehydrogenase (G-6-PD) deficiency
3. **E** X-linked recessive

G-6-PD deficiency (favism) is the second most common inherited condition worldwide after diabetes mellitus. Haemolytic crises are precipitated by ingestion of white beans (fava beans), most antimalarial drugs (Kenya!), antibiotics (sulphonamides, nitrofurantoin, chloramphenicol), vitamin K, aspirin and many others. Blood count and blood film are normal between attacks. During a crisis there is evidence of haemolysis (bite cells, Heinz bodies and reticulocytosis).

Diagnosis is by direct measurement of the enzyme levels. In a crisis any precipitating cause has to be removed; blood transfusions may be required in severe cases. Splenectomy is not indicated.

36 Answer (1 mark)

1. **A** Amiodarone

The commonest cause of gingival hyperplasia is ciclosporin treatment. Other causes include phenytoin, calcium antagonists and AML-M5.

37 Answers (9 marks)

1. **E** Hypernephroma
2. **D** Hyperreninaemia
3. **B** Renal vein thrombosis
4. **C** Vascular occlusion due to polycythaemia

An elderly patient has haematuria with back pain, polycythaemia and a painful varicocele. These features suggest a **left renal tumour** with increased production of erythropoietin and a possible occlusion of the left renal vein causing the varicocele. The raised Na, despite therapy with diuretics, suggests that the tumour is also producing renin (parathormone-related protein may also cause hypercalcaemia). An increasing number of renal cell carcinomas are now diagnosed incidentally on ultrasound. The main symptom is haematuria, the classical combination with low-grade pyrexia and flank pain becoming more rare. These are very vascular tumours and, if inoperable, may be successfully embolised. The metastases (cannonball to the lung and lytic to the bone) are also very vascular and single chest metastases may be resected.

A normal brain scan excludes a haemorrhagic stroke, but not arterial occlusion. The affected side does not correspond to the carotid plaque.

38 Answers (5 marks)

1. **E** IgA nephropathy
2. **C** Renal biopsy

IgA nephritis (Berger's disease) is a condition usually found in young men. It frequently follows a non-specific upper respiratory tract infection without interval. There is mesangial deposition of IgA and C3 with evidence of focal proliferative glomerulonephritis on microscopy. HLA-DR4 is positive in 50%. It may present without an obvious precipitating factor; prognosis is usually good but up to 10% develop chronic renal failure.

The main differential diagnosis here is towards poststreptococcal GN. However, there is typically an interval of two to three weeks between the upper respiratory tract infection, and the main symptom is proteinuria, although haematuria can be seen. C3 is normal or high in IgA nephritis, but low in post-streptococcal GN. In addition, the history indicates that there was no response to the therapy with penicillin and macrolide antibiotics, making a viral infection more likely.

There is no history of purpura or arthralgia to suggest Henoch-Schönlein purpura.

39 Answers (3 marks)

1. C Lactic acidosis type A

The patient has a **raised anion gap** $[Na^+ + K^+] - [Cl^- + HCO_3^-] = 29$ mmol/l. Normal range 10–18 mmol/l. In the context given, this is most likely to be due to shock and tissue hypoxia, indicating type A, rather than a toxic cause, such as biguanide therapy or salicylate overdose.

For the purpose of the exam, if the chloride is given (particularly if double figures only), this should immediately prompt for a calculation of the anion gap.

40 Answer (2 marks)

1. D Adult polycystic kidney disease

The kidneys are enlarged by multiple cysts which contain subtle areas of calcification. In addition multiple cysts are seen throughout both lobes of the liver. Note: A lack of accessible parents (adoption, fostering, orphan) should alert you to the possibility of a significant family history.

41 Answers (4 marks)

1. B Urate stones
2. D Bicarbonate supplements

Uric acid stones are not uncommon in patients with ileostomies. The increased loss of fluid and bicarbonate through the stoma results in the production of concentrated acidic urine, which causes precipitation of uric acid. Alkalinisation of urine will prevent stone formation.

Urate and **X**anthine stones are 'radio**lux**ent'.

42 Answers (4 marks)

1. D Lesch-Nyhan syndrome
2. B X-linked recessive enzyme defect

Lesch-Nyhan syndrome is characterised by a reduction (< 1%) in activity of hypoxanthine-guanine-phosphoribosyl transferase which leads to a chronic increase in uric acid, with all the symptoms of hyperuricaemia and progressive renal failure. This is associated with a variety of neurological symptoms, classically with a tendency to self-mutilation. The patient is too young for 'simple' gout. Gout arthropathy causes well defined (punched out) deep erosions along the shaft of the phalanges, adjacent to, but not necessarily involving, the articular surface. Involvement is usually unilateral but can be bilateral but asymmetrical. Calcified tophi indicate a chronic form.

43 Answers (4 marks)

1. **D** Cervical swab
2. **A** Gonorrhoea

In a small proportion of men and up to 30% of women, **gonorrhoea** can remain asymptomatic. Complications include ascending salpingitis and pelvic inflammatory disease, prostatitis, reactive arthritis (especially monarthritis of knee), septicaemia, endocarditis, and perihepatitis (Fitz-Hugh–Curtis syndrome). The Gram-negative diplococci require special media for culture, but can be identified on Gram stains. A co-existent venereal disease, i.e. syphilis, has to be considered.

44 Answer (2 marks)

1. **E** Hereditary sensorimotor neuropathy

There is predominantly distal muscle wasting with pes cavus and clawed toes. In addition trophic skin changes are seen around the ankles, suggesting a co-existing sensory deficit. Patients with Friedreich's ataxia have a shorter life expectancy and syringomyelia usually causes an upper motor neurone deficit of the legs.

45 Answers (7 marks)

1. **C** Carotid Doppler
2. **E** Chronic subdural haematoma
3. **A** Neurosurgical referral

An anticoagulated elderly patient has a mixture of neurological symptoms of subacute onset. The intermittent and fluctuating nature points towards a space-occupying lesion rather than an ischaemic process. A left-sided carotid problem would also localise to the other side. The most likely diagnosis is **subdural haematoma**. These may occur spontaneously without a history of trauma or anticoagulation. The two most important investigations are a prothrombin time/INR and a CT brain scan.

On a CT scan with brain settings, freshly clotted blood appears white. This turns to the same 'greyness' (isodense) as brain substance after two to three weeks and appears as dark as water (CSF in ventricles) after approximately one month. The sequence is dependent on haemoglobin concentration, clotting factors, including warfarin, and recurrent haemorrhage.

Clinical symptoms may be insidious, with confusion, ataxia or incontinence. If symptomatic, neurosurgical decompression should be considered.

Hyponatraemia should alert you to the possibility of inappropriate ADH secretion which may be caused by essentially any pathology within the head (tumour, haemorrhage, raised intracranial pressure, infection); any pathology within the chest (tumour, infection, particularly *Legionella*, empyema), drugs, acute porphyria and lymphoma.

46 Answers (7 marks)

1. **B** Blood film
2. **A** Subacute combined degeneration of the cord (SACD)
3. **C** Folate replacement

SACD is a consequence of protracted vitamin B_{12} deficiency, usually caused by pernicious anaemia. Classically there is evidence of upper motor neurone as well as lower motor neurone defects in the legs, as well as a mixed sensory deficit with emphasis on the posterior columns (hence 'combined' degeneration). The longest nerves are affected earliest in a peripheral neuropathy and the arc of the spinal reflex is lost distally in the ankle while upper motor neurone signs still dominate more proximally (plantar reflexes are not a spinal reflex).

There is no evidence of liver damage to suggest alcohol abuse as the underlying cause. The pancytopenia supports a diagnosis of pernicious anaemia. A blood film would show macrocytosis and hypersegmented neutrophils.

As B_{12} and folate deficiencies often co-exist, the replacement with folate may acutely exacerbate the B_{12} deficiency as the blood cells begin to regenerate. The peripheral neuropathy usually responds well to B_{12} replacement, whereas cord and brain damage may persist.

Reduction in amplitude of the motor neurone potentials with preserved conduction velocity indicate an axonal disease process.

47 Answers (4 marks)

1. **D** Tuberculous meningitis
2. **D** Communicating hydrocephalus

The combination of mild CSF lymphocytosis, increased protein and reduced glucose suggests **TB meningitis**. This affects the basal aspects of the brain and may involve cranial nerves at this site. The high protein reduces CSF re-absorption and causes communicating hydrocephalus (communicating as no CSF spaces are obstructed). This may cause brainstem descent with false localising signs.

Cysticercosis causes focal mass lesions causing seizures or focal signs.

48 Answer (2 marks)

1. **C** Multiple sclerosis

The MR scan shows multiple hyperintense areas affecting the white matter, the corpus callosum and the cerebellum. In conjunction with the normal CT these are very typical for demyelinating plaques.

49 Answers (5 marks)

1. **E** Acute intermittent porphyria
2. **D** Chlorpromazine

Acute psychosis, abdominal pain, peripheral polyneuropathy and hyponatraemia represent the full house of acute intermittent porphyria. Variegated porphyria has identical features plus photosensitivity.

The *BNF* contains a list of drugs unsafe in porphyria.

50 Answers (5 marks)

1. **C** Thyroid function tests
2. **E** Hypothyroidism and pernicious anaemia

The patient has extensive features of profound hypothyroidism with acute confusion/delusion (**myxoedema madness**). Alcohol abuse is the most likely differential diagnosis, but the normal liver function tests are strongly against this.

Hypothyroidism is associated with pernicious anaemia, but may cause a macrocytic anaemia on its own, although normochromic normocytic anaemia is more common.

Hyperlipidaemia may result in spurious hyponatraemia.

51 Answers (4 marks)

1. **B** Syringobulbia
2. **D** MR scan of the cervical spine

The patient has low motor neurone signs in the upper limbs and upper motor neurone signs in the lower limbs, indicating a lesion in the cervical cord. In addition, there is dissociate sensory loss (light touch is predominantly conducted in the posterior columns), typical features of a syrinx. However, the lower motor neurone lesion of the 12th cranial nerve indicates that it extends up into the brainstem in keeping with **syringobulbia**.

52 Answer (2 marks)

1. **A** Basal cell carcinoma

The ulcer with a surrounding 'pearly' edge is typical of a basal cell carcinoma (rodent ulcer).

53 Answers (9 marks)

1. **D** Compensated respiratory alkalosis
2. **C** High-resolution CT scan
3. **E** Asbestosis
4. **C** Pleural encasement

The wife of a plumber 'contracting' **asbestos-related lung disease** is an old classic of the exam. This is a well-documented occurrence from washing the husband's clothes (!).

The initial lung function tests show a restrictive defect with hyperventilation and mild compensatory reduction in bicarbonate. In combination with the clinical findings this indicates **asbestosis** (= asbestos-induced pulmonary fibrosis). Investigation of choice is a thin-section CT. (HRCT).

The spectrum of asbestos-related lung disease includes calcified pleural plaques, pleural thickening/encasement, recurrent *benign* pleural effusions, adenocarcinoma (particularly in smokers) and pleural/ peritoneal mesothelioma.

The latency of complications is 10–30 years and the expected peak incidence of asbestosis and mesothelioma is around 2010.

The subsequent deterioration of the lung function with exaggeration of the restrictive defect in the presence of a relatively normal transfer coefficient indicate an extrapulmonary restriction.

54 Answers (8 marks)

1. **D** Aspergilloma
2. **C** CT scan
3. **A** Emphysema
4. **D** Surgery

Aspergillus fumigatus is a fungus which causes three distinct clinical pictures:
- Allergic bronchial pulmonary aspergillosis (ABPA) – a hypersensitivity reaction typically occurring in young male patients presenting with asthma. Mucoid plugs are expectorated and the patient develops *proximal* bronchiectasis.
- Invasive aspergillosis – in immunocompromised patients, the fungus can become invasive and causes cavitating pneumonia, usually in the apices.
- Aspergilloma – a fungus ball develops in a pre-existing cavity, usually following TB. It can remain asymptomatic for a long time, but haemoptysis is the usual complication. Surgical excision is the treatment of choice; direct intra-cavity injection of antibiotics is a second-line treatment option.

55 Answers (5 marks)

1. **A**   Acute epiglottitis
2. **A**   Urgent ENT referral and intubation

Acute infective epiglottitis is a respiratory emergency caused by infection with *Haemophilus influenzae*. This may lead to acute upper airway obstruction, although this is much rarer in adults than in children. Instrumentation of the mouth should only be performed by experts as this may provoke airway closure. Treatment is with iv antibiotics (amoxicillin resistance is now common), humidification of room air and early intubation/tracheostomy to safeguard the airways.

Laryngitis (croup) is caused by viral infection; the commonest is parainfluenza virus.

56 Answer (2 marks)

1. **E**   Gilbert's syndrome

The patient has asymptomatic jaundice, diagnosed incidentally in adulthood. The absence of bilirubin excretion in the urine indicates an unconjugated hyperbilirubinaemia. This could be confirmed with a nicotinic acid test or a three-day fast.

57 Answers (4 marks)

1. **B**   Sleep apnoea
2. **E**   Hypothyroidism

Sleep apnoea typically occurs in obese patients, more commonly in men. Hypoventilation and desaturation occur during REM sleep. Loud snoring and morning headaches are typical findings and daytime blood gases are normal. Underlying diseases such as neuromuscular disorders, hypothyroidism (macrocytosis and hypercholesterolaemia), acromegaly, alcohol and sedative drugs need to be excluded.

58 Answers (4 marks)

1. **E**   High anion gap acidosis
2. **C**   Salicylate overdose

In **salicylic acid poisoning** there is initially a respiratory alkalosis due to direct stimulation of the respiratory centre. Trying to compensate, the body reduces the bicarbonate buffer. In addition to the acidic effect of the salicylate itself, there is uncoupling of oxidative phosphorylation of carbohydrates. Increased fat metabolism results in high production of ketones which can no longer be neutralised and a profound metabolic acidosis ensues.

Anion gap: $[Na^+ + K^+] - [Cl^- + HCO_3^-] = 40$ mmol/l.

59 Answer (4 marks)

1. E Subcutaneous salbutamol injections and anaesthetic assessment

The patient has a **severe asthma attack**. The 'normal' pCO_2 in a young patient with 'silent chest' indicates CO_2 retention and failure of the respiratory reserve. Urgent ventilation has to be considered.

60 Answer (2 marks)

1. A Hypertension

A fresh haematoma is seen in the left basal ganglia, a typical site for a hypertensive bleed. The brain otherwise shows some evidence of atrophy with enlarged areas of intra- as well as extracerebral CSF. There is some oedema surrounding the haemorrhage – the increased water content has turned the brain darker.

61 Answers (5 marks)

1. C Relapsing polychondritis
2. A Normal appearances

An elderly patient with a systemic inflammatory disease has evidence of airways obstruction on forced expiration. However, resting lung volumes and gas transfer and saturation are normal. This indicates expiratory airways collapse. In combination with the systemic symptoms, this is highly suggestive of **relapsing polychondritis**. It can affect all cartilaginous structures, most commonly nose, ears and trachea. Biopsy shows a small-vessel necrotising vasculitis.

Episcleritis, arteriopathy and dilation of the cardiac valve rings also occur.

62 Answers (4 marks)

1. C D-dimer levels
2. B Pulmonary embolus

The patient is hypoxic with compensatory hyperventilation. The most likely diagnosis is **pulmonary embolus**. D-dimer levels are likely to be elevated and are the least invasive test. CT angiogram is unlikely to pick up small emboli. If there remains clinical doubt the definitive investigation is a standard pulmonary angiogram.

Pregnancy is not an absolute contraindication to VQ scanning, as the radiation dose to the fetus is low.

63 Answer (2 marks)

1. **E**   Histoplasmosis

Histoplasma capsulatum is endemic in North and South America and, to a lesser degree, in Africa and Australia. It is mainly found in bird and bat droppings ('bat-cave disease') and in soil. Infection may be asymptomatic, but commonly presents with an acute febrile pneumonia. In immunocompromised patients, dissemination may occur. Sputum microscopy is often unhelpful, but lung biopsy usually shows small yeast cells. The lung lesions calcify.

64 Answers (10 marks)

1. **D**   Blood cultures
2. **D**   Traumatic tap
3. **C**   Behçet's disease
4. **B**   Systemic steroids
5. **A**   Superior sagittal sinus thrombosis

Most venereal diseases cause *painless* genital ulcers. Gonorrhoea causes a purulent discharge. However, a systemic infection must be excluded.

The important differential diagnoses of eosinophilia are allergy (drugs!), parasites (including fungi and malaria), vasculitis and Hodgkin's disease.

The combination of painful (oro-) genital ulcers, polyarthritis and iritis should alert you to the diagnosis of **Behçet's disease**. Other features are erythema nodosum, pustular skin rashes and a variety of neurological syndromes (brainstem and cord lesions, aseptic meningitis and encephalitis).

Treatment is with steroids or immunosuppressants. Vascular occlusion is an important complication.

The development of sterile pustules at puncture sites is called 'pathergy' and, although not always seen, is very typical of Behçet's disease.

65 Answers (6 marks)

1. **B**   Small bowel biopsy
2. **D**   Whipple's disease
3. **A**   Tetracycline

Whipple's disease is caused by infection with *Tropheryma whippelii* which can be demonstrated on a PAS stain of a small bowel biopsy as pink material within macrophages. A related polyarthropy or spondylarthropy may precede the gastrointestinal symptoms. A polyserositis similar to FMF can be seen with fever, pleural and pericardial effusions, but presentation in FMF is usually at a young age whereas Whipple's disease classically manifests in men in the 4th or 5th decade. Malabsorption with diarrhoea and steatorrhoea is common.

Therapy is with protracted courses (three to six months) of oral antibiotics.

66 Answers (5 marks)

1. **D** Lyme disease
2. **C** *Borrelia* serology

First described in 1975 in **Lyme**, Connecticut, the disease is caused by *Borrelia burgdorferi* and transmitted by the ixodes tick. If observed, the rash, erythema chronicum migrans, is diagnostic. This may be followed by a variety of neurological symptoms as well as carditis and relapsing arthritis. Treatment should be performed early with penicillin or tetracycline.

67 Answer (2 marks)

1. **D** Chronic lymphocytic leukaemia

The patient is not anaemic but has a surplus of lymphocytes (purple cells, large round nucleus, little plasma). In addition, immature forms, and most importantly 'smudge' cells or 'ghost' cells, are seen. These are fragile cells that have popped when the blood film was made.

68 Answers (4 marks)

1. **A** Drug-induced lupus
2. **C** Alter current medication

Tuberose sclerosis has also been given the acronym EPILOIA as the syndrome is composed of **EPI**lepsy, **LO**w **I**ntelligence and **A**denoma sebaceum. The configuration of autoantibodies indicates a drug-induced lupus and the likely offenders in this context are the anticonvulsants – phenytoin and carbamazepine.

69 Answers (4 marks)

1. **D** Haemochromatosis
2. **B** Liver biopsy

The patient presents with premature osteoarthrosis, mildly deranged liver function tests and diabetes mellitus. Iron overload in **haemochromatosis** is shown by estimating the dry iron content in the liver biopsy, which will also detect associated serotic changes. Chronic hepatic porphyria = porphyria cutanea tarda, the commonest of the porphyrias and found in middle-aged men who drink too much. However, the diagnostic test is porphyrin levels in the urine although a liver biopsy will also be diagnostic. In acromegaly there is premature osteoarthrosis but, due to cartilaginous overgrowth, the joint spaces are characteristically widened.

70 Answers (4 marks)

1. **E** Osteomalacia
2. **E** Chest X-ray

The patient has features of alcoholic liver disease. In the context of hypocalcaemia, a proximal muscle weakness and bone pain is most likely due to **osteomalacia**. Looser's zones are commonly seen in femoral necks, pubic rami, lower ribs and scapulae.

A raised ESR in a malnourished and immunosuppressed patient must alert you to the possibility of active tuberculosis before other causes of infection are excluded.

Paper 2 – Answers

1 Answer (2 marks)

1. D   Mucopolysaccharidosis

The patient has macroglossia. In amyloid (particularly light-chain) the tongue may be bright red and show teeth marks. It is also a feature of glycogen storage disease and the gangliosidoses.

2 Answers (8 marks)

1. C   Coarctation
2. C   Cardiac scintigraphy
3. B   Noonan's syndrome
4. E   Surgery

The patient has **coarctation**, which is one of the main differential diagnoses of hypertension and cardiac failure in a young patient. The post-ductal form is the more benign form presenting in adults. Associated defects are PDA, VSD and bicuspid aortic valve (50%!). Pre- and poststenotic dilatation of the aorta results in the 'figure of three' appearance of the chest X-ray. Collateral formation of intercostal vessels feeding the lower abdominal aorta results in inferior rib notching. Coarctation is commoner in males, and is associated with Turner's and Noonan's syndromes. Antibiotic prophylaxis is required until surgical correction has been performed.

Patients with Klinefelter's and homocysteinuria are of tall stature. Hurler's syndrome is a mucopolysaccharidosis with a poor prognosis and death occurs between 10 and 15 years of age.

3 Answers (6 marks)

1. D   Renal artery stenosis
2. B   Takayasu's arteritis

Takayasu's arteritis is a large-vessel vasculitis resulting in narrowing and occlusion of large aortic branches and the pulmonary artery ('pulseless disease'). It typically affects young women and is commoner in Asian communities. Treatment with steroids is successful in most cases.

Kawasaki disease is a vasculitis which typically affects the coronary arteries, resulting in aneurysm formation. It occurs in children with a severe, systemic flu-like illness.

Pseudoxanthoma elasticum is associated with hypertension, aneurysm formation and ischaemic heart disease.

4 Answers (7 marks)

1. **C**   Echocardiogram
2. **E**   Ebstein's anomaly
3. **B**   AV re-entrant tachycardia

Ebstein's anomaly is characterised by a low insertion of the tricuspid valve resulting in a large atrium and a small, hypoplastic ventricle ('atrialisation' of the right ventricle). The spectrum of the disease is broad, ranging from incidental findings at postmortem to early, severe presentations in childhood. Common associated findings are tricuspid incompetence, atrial septal defect (leading to cyanosis) and accessory conduction pathways. WPW syndrome is found in up to 10%. Supraventricular tachycardias are common, usually due to retrograde conduction through the accessory bundle leading to re-entrant tachycardia. Diagnosis is by transthoracic echocardiogram.

5 Answer (2 marks)

1. **B**   Sputum microscopy and barrier nursing

The patient has consolidation in both lungs with predilection for the apices. In the clinical context this is active tuberculosis until proven otherwise and appropriate precautionary measures have to be taken.

6 Answer (3 marks)

1. **C**   Prinzmetal (variant) angina

There is intermittent ST-segment elevation (at 09.33 and 09.53) as well as ST depression (at 10.13). **Variant angina** is due to coronary spasm, often also associated with atheromatous disease. It typically occurs at night or in the early hours and is more common in women.

7 Answers (5 marks)

1. **E**   Epileptic fit
2. **B**   Electroencephalogram

Cardiac muscle has a much higher AST content than skeletal muscle and in myocardial infarction the levels of AST are usually at least 10% of creatinine kinase levels. An extremely high CK with a relatively low AST indicates damaged **striated** muscle. The estimation of creatinine kinase is being superseded by troponin T, which is more specific and has a higher predictive value for outcome. It may give false negative values in the first 12 hours, however.

8 Answer (3 marks)

1. E Postero-inferior MI

ST elevation in inferior leads is obvious, but in addition there is ST depression in the anterior chest leads, giving the mirror image of a posterior wall infarction.

9 Answer (3 marks)

1. D Aortic stenosis

The ECG shows a mild bradycardia, a normal QRS axis, but marked left ventricular hypertrophy. The Sokolow index ($S_{V2} + R_{V5}$) is over 70 mm. There is descending ST depression in the lateral leads in keeping with left ventricular strain, and the deep T inversion is also suspicious of a recent subendocardial infarct.

Aortic stenosis can go undetected for a remarkably long period of time, as the heart is much better at compensating for a pressure load than a volume load. Cardiomegaly in the chest X-ray ensues with decompensation. Hypertrophic obstructive cardiomyopathy would also have to be considered, although they tend to present earlier and have a strong family history (autosomal dominant).

10 Answers (4 marks)

1 A Left anterior descending artery
2. D Aspirin and rt-PA

The patient has an acute **anterior myocardial infarction**. In a young patient, the thrombolytic agent of choice is rt-PA.

11 Answers (4 marks)

1. E Mobitz type 2 heart block
2. C Sarcoidosis

The ECG shows a **2° AV block** with variable transmission (Mobitz 2). This indicates organic heart disease. Cardiac involvement is rare in **sarcoidosis** (< 5%). Conduction defects, arrhythmias and cardiomyopathy are seen. Polydipsia and polyuria are signs of the associated hypercalcaemia.

12 Answers (4 marks)

1. **B**   Yellow nail syndrome
2. **A**   Lymphoma

In yellow nail syndrome all finger-and toenails grow at a reduced rate leading, to thickening and discoloration. The nails are brittle, with onycholysis. The syndrome may rarely be associated with nephrotic syndrome and penicillamine therapy.

Tylosis has hyperkeratosis of the palms and soles with associated oesophageal carcinoma. The syndrome is autosomal dominant.

13 Answers (10 marks)

1. **C**   Primary hyperparathyroidism
2. **D**   Technetium-MIBI-subtraction scan

Three causes account for 70% of bilateral medullary nephrocalcinosis:
- Primary hyperparathyroidism
- Medullary sponge kidney
- Renal tubular acidosis type I

The patient, besides being hypercalcaemic, also has recurrent duodenal ulcers and evidence of bone resorption, indicating hyperparathyroidism. Assessment of hyperparathyroidism in the first instance is with technetium-MIBI-subtraction scan and ultrasound of the neck. (Cesta-MIBI is taken up by parathyroid as well as the thyroid gland. From this scan a pure thyroid technetium scan is subtracted. Areas of increased activity on the subtraction scan indicate hyperactive parathyroid tissue.)

3. **A**   MR scan of the pituitary and CT of the pancreas
4. **C**   Wermer's syndrome (multiple endocrine neoplasia Type I)
5. **D**   Glucagonoma

Bi-temporal hemianopia indicates compression of the optic chiasm – direct imaging of this area is required.

Unusual rashes are seen with pancreatic tumours. Erythema gyratum repens and wandering thrombophlebitis are paraneoplastic manifestations of carcinoma of the pancreas. However, a migrating necrotising rash is seen typically with glucagonoma.

Patients with **MEN type I** (autosomal dominant) develop a variety of pancreatic tumours, in particular glucagonoma, VIPoma, insulinoma and gastrinoma. The pancreas is best assessed with thin sections of a dynamic contrast-enhanced CT.

The hyperparathyroidism in MEN type I is more often due to parathyroid hyperplasia; in type II it is more often due to parathyroid adenoma, but variation is considerable.

MEN type IIa consists of phaeochromocytoma, hyperparathyroidism and medullary carcinoma of the thyroid. This may be associated with marfanoid habitus and skin neurinomata reminiscent of neurofibromatosis and is then termed MEN type IIb.

376

14 Answers (8 marks)

1. **B** Primary hypothyroidism
2. **E** Chest X-ray
3. **A** Increased TRH production
4. **C** Oral thyroxine

The patient has multiple clinical stigmata of **hypothyroidism**, including a macrocytic anaemia and evidence of a pericardial effusion. This is supported by the biochemistry which indicates primary thyroid failure with a raised TSH as the pituitary is trying to stimulate thyroxine production. The presence of thyroid antibodies confirms the autoimmune aetiology.

Long-standing, untreated hypothyroidism will lead to hyperplasia of the pituitary, which can lead to compression of the optic chiasm and, rarely, to secondary pituitary failure. However, there is no other evidence of end-organ failure and gonadotrophins and cortisol are normal. Increased release of thyrotrophin from the hypothalamus also stimulates release of prolactin from the anterior pituitary. Thyroid replacement therapy will remove the stimulus to the pituitary, which will reduce in size, and prolactin levels will drop.

15 Answer (2 marks)

1. **C** Self-administration of insulin

The patient has a raised insulin in the presence of hypoglycaemia. C-peptide, which is produced by cleavage of pro-insulin, is reduced, however, indicating that the insulin present is exogenous insulin. In sulphonylurea overdose, pro-insulin, C-peptide and insulin are raised which can make differentiation from an insulinoma difficult.

16 Answer (1 mark)

1. **B** Peutz-Jeghers' syndrome

The barium enema shows 'apple core' appearance of a carcinoma.

Adenomatous polyps of the colon may undergo malignant transformation, the risk of which is related to the size of the polyps. The polyps in Peutz-Jeghers' syndrome are hamartomatous polyps, which in themselves have virtually no risk of neoplasia. There is, however, a small independent risk of developing malignancy, in particular of the stomach and ovary.

17 Answers (4 marks)

1. **D**   Peripheral diabetes insipidus
2. **A**   No change

The patient has a plasma osmolality that rapidly rises with water deprivation above normal levels, while the urine osmolality remains inappropriately low. The patient is losing water which indicates diabetes insipidus (DI).

In the context given, the patient is *most likely* to have drug-induced (i.e. lithium) **peripheral diabetes insipidus** where there is resistance of the kidney to endogenous (and exogenous) antidiuretic hormone. In this case, injection of synthetic ADH will also have no significant effect on the urine osmolality. Other causes for nephrogenic DI include chronic hypokalaemia and hypercalcaemia, other drugs, such as demeclocycline, amphotericin B and a rare X-linked recessive form which requires early treatment to prevent mental and physical impairment.

In central diabetes insipidus, there is failure of the posterior pituitary to produce ADH. The patients equally fail to retain water and, under water deprivation, the serum plasma osmolality rises above 300. However, after injection of DDAVP, there is an increase in the urine osmolality of > 15%. DDAVP can be administered therapeutically as a nasal spray. Psychogenic polydipsia is not a differential diagnosis as the patient starts with a high normal plasma osmolality (normal 270–295 mOsm/kg) and, by definition, has therefore not caused any dilution himself.

18 Answers (5 marks)

1. **B**   Prolactinoma
   F   Panhypopituitarism
2. **C**   Synacthen® test
   F   MR scan of the pituitary

GH fails to increase by 15 mU/l to rise above 20 mU/l despite adequate hypoglycaemia (2.2 mmol/l or less). TSH is low and does not show a sustained elevation (30-min peak should be 5 mU/l or more above baseline, 60-min value at least 60% of 30-min value). LH is low and shows poor response. Prolactin is in diagnostic range (> 4000 mU/l) for **prolactinoma** and shows only minimal increase after TRH. It is vital to assess the adrenal axis, as steroids will have to be replaced before thyroxine in order to prevent an acute addisonian crisis.

19 Answers (6 marks)

1. **B** ACTH levels
   H Chest X-ray
2. **A** Hypokalaemia
   E Hypercortisolism

Neoplastic excretion of ectopic ACTH usually occurs with small cell carcinoma of the bronchus. Plasma cortisols are very high, the circadian rhythm is lost and there is no suppression with dexamethasone. This produces myopathy, diabetes mellitus, skin pigmentation, hyperkalaemia and secondary alkalosis. The hoarse voice indicates recurrent laryngeal nerve palsy and inoperability.

The weakness in Eaton-Lambert syndrome is due to impaired release of acetylcholine and *improves* with exercise.

20 Answers (6 marks)

1. **C** Blood cultures and urine antibody studies

The patient has a severe infectious disease, characterised by high fever, diarrhoea and hepatorenal failure with coagulopathy. Although abdominal ultrasound is sensible and a brain scan should be considered, liver biopsy and lumbar puncture would be contraindicated.

2. **A** Leptospirosis

The occupational history should alert you to the possibility of leptospiral infection.

Leptospirosis or **Weil's disease**, is caused by the spirochaete *Leptospira interrogans*, serotype *icterohaemorrhagiae*. It is usually seen in patient groups that have a high exposure to animals and their urine, particularly rodents. Most common in veterinarians, abattoir workers and farmers, it is also found in sewage workers. Often taking a benign, self-limiting course, the onset can, however, be brutal with severe cardiovascular collapse. Generalised myalgia is typical. Serology is positive in blood and urine. Cultures from blood or CSF are only positive in the first ten days. Severe hepatitis and renal failure may ensue. Antibiotic treatment is only effective if given within the first five days.

21 Answer (10 marks)

1. **D** X-linked recessive
2. **B** Psoas haematoma
3. **E** Liver cirrhosis
4 **A** Abdominal ultrasound
   C Hepatitis serology

The combination of flank pain and inability to extend the hip indicates irritation of the psoas muscle, a common site for haemorrhage. The patient has additional evidence of liver failure, with deranged LFTs and a raised INR. The deficiency of factor VIII does not affect the extrinsic pathway of the clotting cascade and the prothrombin time should be normal. The raised INR indicates established liver damage. Although a liver biopsy is desirable in a patient with chronic hepatitis, a noninvasive method has to be chosen in the first instance. The young age of the patient is against hepatitis B, as serological tests for blood components were available in the 1980s, however Hepatitis C was not described then. Up to 20% of patients with **Hepatitis C** develop cirrhosis.

22 Answers (6 marks)

1. **C** Gilbert's syndrome
2. **A** Autosomal dominant
3. **E** Nicotinic acid test

The hereditary hyperbilirubinaemias are characterised by an increase in unconjugated bilirubin (Gilbert's and Crigler-Najjar = inconjugated) or conjugated bilirubin (Dubin-Johnson and Rotor). Conjugated bilirubin is water soluble and is excreted in the urine and these two syndromes are excluded by the normal Dipstix. **Gilbert's syndrome** has an excellent prognosis and is often discovered incidentally. It is characterised by a mild elevation of bilirubin which shows a slow rise in the nicotinic acid test, with a high and delayed peak at 2–3 hours (usually around 40–60 µmol/l). Peak levels in normal individuals are reached at 90 minutes (usually less than 25 µmol/l). An increase in bilirubin is also provoked by three days of fasting (less than 400 kcal/day).

23 Answer (2 marks)

1. **E** Systemic lupus erythematosus

The patient has a complete right-sided facial nerve palsy. The loss of wrinkles over the forehead indicate a lower motor neurone lesion and the patient has had a lateral tarsorrhaphy. Likely levels are at the cerebellopontine angle, which would be associated with damage to the right vestibulocochlear nerve or within the facial canal, which would be associated with hyperacusis and loss of taste of the anterior two-thirds of the tongue. The commonest cause is idiopathic (Bell's palsy); others are vestibular schwannoma (acoustic neuroma), Ramsay Hunt syndrome, parotid tumour and/or surgery.

24 Answers (6 marks)

1. **B** Chronic pancreatitis
2. **B** Alcohol abuse
    C Gallstones
3. **B** Small bowel biopsy
    D ERCP

Faecal fat excretion is high (> 30 g in 3 days) but xylose absorption and excretion is normal. This excludes malabsorption and small bowel causes for steatorrhoea. The most likely diagnosis is chronic pancreatitis either due to gallstones or alcohol. Other causes for chronic pancreatitis include haemochromatosis, hyperlipidaemia, primary biliary sclerosis and sclerosing cholangitis. Amylase levels will only be elevated in acute exacerbations.

25 Answers (5 marks)

1. **A** HELLP syndrome
2. **E** Delivery of the baby

Pre-eclampsia is defined as hypertension developing in the last three months of pregnancy, with associated oedema and proteinuria. The aim is to control the blood pressure. Whereas eclampsia is characterised by hypertension, proteinuria, oedema, coagulopathy and focal necrosis of the liver, **HELLP** is defined as the syndrome of **H**aemolysis, **E**levated **L**FTs and **L**ow **P**latelets. Either condition requires urgent delivery.

Acute fatty liver of pregnancy occurs after 30 weeks. It consists of acute fatty degeneration of the liver, hepatorenal failure, DIC and encephalopathy. It resolves with delivery. Cholestasis (intrahepatic) of pregnancy also occurs in the third trimester and presents with pruritus and jaundice and may lead to premature labour and postpartum haemorrhage. It also resolves spontaneously, within two weeks after delivery.

26 Answers (5 marks)

1. **B** Pseudomyxoma peritonei
2. **D** Krukenberg metastases

Gelatinous ascites is seen with **mucinous adenocarcinomas** of the ovary and GI tract. The past history suggests intraperitoneal metastases (Krukenberg metastases). These spread gravitationally, through the pouch of Douglas to the ovaries.

27 Answer (3 marks)

1. **C** Surgery

The patient has a hyper-acute right extradural haematoma. In its centre the clot contains dark areas, indicating active bleeding. The basal cisterns are effaced, indicating imminent coning.

28 Answers (9 marks)

1. **C** Blood cultures and standard blood film
2. **A** Resuscitation and iv penicillin
3. **B** Pneumococcal vaccination
4. **E** Viral infection

A young black patient with a suspicious deficit in family history (Beware – the adopted child!) presents with features of a lobar pneumonia. In addition, he has a macrocytic anaemia (reticulocytosis) with changes in the skeleton. In combination, the features suggest **sickle cell crisis** complicated/precipitated by pneumococcal pneumonia. Treatment is with aggressive rehydration, analgesia and antibiotics suitable for the organism as well as the patient (a child).

As homozygous patients with sickle cell disease will develop splenic atrophy due to infarction, pneumococcal vaccination is mandatory. Hyposplenism is evident on re-admission due to the presence of Howell-Jolly bodies (nuclear residues within erythrocytes).

Infection with parvovirus B19 (fifth disease, slapped-cheek disease), which otherwise is a benign self-limiting viral infection, can lead to aplastic crisis in patients with haemolytic anaemias.

Other complications include infarction of other organs, in particular bone and the development of *Salmonella* osteomyelitis.

Diagnosis is by blood film and haemoglobin electrophoresis which shows replacement of glutamine by valine in the beta chain. Homozygous patients will have approximately 80% HbS and 20% HbF.

29 Answers (9 marks)

1. **D** Bone marrow biopsy
2. **B** Myelodysplastic syndrome
3. **B** Tuberculosis
   I Invasive aspergillosis
4. **A** Acute myeloid leukaemia

The patient has a bicytopenia with an excess of blasts and the presence of ring sideroblasts. This indicates a **myelodysplastic syndrome** (MDS) (FAB classification **RAEB, r**efractory **a**naemia with **e**xcess of **b**lasts). However, the diagnosis of MDS requires exclusion of leukaemia and aplastic syndromes and more benign conditions, such as B_{12} or folate deficiency, drug-induced and post-infectious marrow suppression. Therapy is supportive and good results have been achieved with stimulators of haemopoiesis, such as erythropoietin and GM-CSF. CMML is one end of the spectrum of MDS. MDS can transform into acute myeloid leukaemia or acute myelomonocytic leukaemia. The latter is a cause of gingival (gum) hyperplasia (also phenytoin).

Invasive aspergillosis, a cavitating infection, can occur in any form of immune-compromise. This has to be distinguished from mycetoma, which is a fungus ball in a pre-existing cavity and from allergic bronchial pulmonary aspergillosis (ABPA) which is a hypersensitivity reaction to the ubiquitous fungus. This typically occurs in young asthmatic men. ABPA leads to proximal bronchiectasis.

30 Answers (6 marks)

1. **A** Bleeding time
2. **D** Symptomatic therapy only
3. **D** Autosomal dominant

A young boy has a bleeding disorder suggestive of platelet dysfunction. The platelet count is normal, ruling out idiopathic thrombocytopenic purpura. The associated regenerating anaemia is most likely due to the previous surgery.

Haemophilia is excluded as the patient, being male, would be homozygous (X-linked recessive) and the clotting results would be markedly abnormal. In addition, petechial haemorrhages indicate a platelet problem.

There is a mild reduction in factor VIII concentration which, on its own, is unlikely to be symptomatic (concentrations over 50% are usually not clinically important). However, the combination of platelet dysfunction and mild factor VIII reduction indicates **von Willebrand's disease**. This autosomal dominant condition (variable penetrance) is characterised by a deficiency in the large molecular fraction of factor VIII (F VIII vWF) which is responsible for platelet aggregation. The bleeding time is prolonged and diagnosis is made by factor VIII vWF assay.

31 Answers (4 marks)

1. **D**   AV re-entrant tachycardia
2. **B**   24 h ECG

The patient has **Wolff-Parkinson-White syndrome type B** as indicated by a short PR interval and a slurred early upstroke of the QRS complex (delta wave). In type A the accessory bundle conducts earlier activity from the left atrium to the left ventricle resulting in a relative right bundle branch block (with a positive QRS complex in V1). In type B the accessory bundle is on the right, resulting in a relative left bundle branch block (negative QRS in V_1).
WPW type *A*: QRS in V_1 *Above* the baseline
WPW type *B*: QRS in V_1 *Below* the baseline

32 Answers (4 marks)

1. **C**   Multiple myeloma
2. **B**   ESR

The patient has several features of **myeloma**: osteoporosis with vertebral collapse, polyuria (hypercalcaemia), normochromic anaemia (and low white cells and platelets). None of these features are diagnostic, although the rouleaux formation on the blood film suggests an increase in blood protein.

A bone scan is not helpful for myeloma as this only assesses increased osteoblastic activity. Approximately two-thirds of patients with myeloma have Bence-Jones proteins (light chains) in their urine but a small proportion do not excrete abnormal protein. The anaemia is a poor prognostic factor and, in combination with the hypercalcaemia, makes Waldenström's very unlikely.

Tuberculous spondylitis typically affects more than one vertebral segment, is unlikely to cause the blood changes and would show up on the bone scan.

A raised ESR would not necessarily differentiate between infection, myeloma or metastatic disease.

33 Answers (5 marks)

1. **B**   Direct Coombs' test
2. **C**   Delayed transfusion reaction

Delayed transfusion reactions occur in patients previously exposed to 'foreign red cell antigens' such as previous transfusions or pregnancy. A positive direct Coombs' test will confirm that the transfused red cells are laden with antibodies. (An indirect Coombs' test only confirms the presence of free antibodies.)

The patient requires re-testing of her serum against standard red cells to identify the antibodies produced. Antibodies frequently exist against multiple epitopes. In addition, the patient needs to be re-crossmatched against the units received which would also be useful for an estimate of how many of the units received are likely to have haemolysed.

34 Answers (4 marks)

1. **C** Red cell mass
2. **B** Stop smoking

The patient fulfils virtually all the criteria for **stress polycythaemia** (Gaisböck's syndrome). He is a hypertensive smoker on diuretics with a relative increase in red cell volume. The absolute red cell mass is not increased which distinguishes it from polycythaemia rubra vera. Blood viscosity, however, is increased with the risk thromboembolic episodes. The most important factor is to stop smoking. Venesection may be required. Chronic hypoxia in a smoker will be evident in arterial blood gases and leads to a secondary increase in erythropoietin. Carboxyhaemoglobin levels are increased up to 15% in smokers.

35 Answer (2 marks)

1. **A** Autoantibody screen

The patient has a low calcium and PTH, indicating **primary hypoparathyroidism**. This may be autoimmune (idiopathic), post-thyroid surgery or congenital (DiGeorge syndrome).

36 Answers (5 marks)

1. **B** Minimal change nephropathy
2. **A** Corticosteroids

The patient has nephrotic syndrome as indicated by heavy proteinuria, hypoalbuminaemia and oedema. IgA nephropathy is excluded by the absence of haematuria. Poststreptococcal immune complex nephritis usually presents within two to three weeks of an upper respiratory tract infection. Membranous and crescentic glomuleronephritis can be diagnosed on light microscopy. **Minimal change nephropathy** usually presents in early childhood but can be found in adults. The patients present with nephrotic syndrome but otherwise normal urine and are not usually hypertensive. Electron microscopy reveals fusion of the podocytes. Prognosis is good with oral steroids.

37 Answers (6 marks)

1. B Medullary sponge kidney (MSK)

MSK is characterised by bilateral medullary nephrocalcinosis which is caused by formation of small stones in the dilated distal tubules.

2. A Wegener's granulomatosis
3. B Anti-neutrophil cytoplasmic antibodies

The patient has a **pulmonary-renal syndrome**. The differential diagnosis includes Goodpasture's syndrome, most vasculitides (in particular polyarteritis nodosa, Wegener's and Churg-Strauss) and a primary pulmonary cause (i.e. pneumonia) with secondary renal impairment.

A combination of cavitating pulmonary nodules, a high ESR and crescentic (rapid progressive) glomerulonephritis is virtually diagnostic of **Wegener's granulomatosis**. The main differential diagnosis is Goodpasture's syndrome with pulmonary haemorrhage (in which case, the CO-transfer factor would be increased). Pulmonary cavitation is not a feature and patients tend to be men under the age of 40.

In polyarteritis nodosa, the lung changes seen on radiography are usually of pulmonary congestion and oedema, rarely due to focal infiltrates, although cavitation can be seen. p-ANCA is positive as opposed to c-ANCA in Wegener's. Angiography invariably shows small saccular aneurysms of small- and medium-sized arteries in all affected organs.

38 Answers (4 marks)

1. E Haemolytic uraemic syndrome
2. C *Escherichia coli* infection

HUS is a childhood syndrome characterised by intravascular haemolysis (micro-angiopathic haemolysis), thrombocytopenia and acute renal failure. Precipitating causes are respiratory tract infections and gastroenteritis with *E. coli* O157. The prognosis is usually very good.

Aplastic crises in children with congenital haemogloblinopathies (i.e. sickle cell) occur after infection with parvovirus B19 (fifth disease, slapped-cheek disease).

39 Answer (2 marks)

1. A Acute myeloid leukaemia

There is a reduced number of red cells and immature myeloid precursors are seen (large cells with under-segmented nucleus and large amount of cytoplasm). In the central cell the pathognomonic Auer rods are present.

40 Answer (3 marks)

1. A Wilms' tumour

Nephroblastoma is a malignant childhood tumour of the kidney, with the main differential diagnosis being a neuroblastoma of the sympathetic chain (frequently arising in the adrenal gland). Infection as a complication of horseshoe kidney or vesico-ureteric reflux is excluded by the absence of protein and white cells in the urine.

41 Answers (6 marks)

1. C Bilateral renal vein thrombosis
2. A Warfarin

Thrombotic episodes are common in **nephrotic syndrome**, in particular in the context of membranous glomerulonephritis. In membranous nephropathy, up to 30% undergo spontaneous remission, but progression to end-stage renal failure occurs in the majority of patients.

Thrombosis classically affects the renal veins – urinary loss of antithrombin III has been implicated. If there is venous infarction of the kidney, this is associated with loin pain, as well as haematuria and increased proteinuria. If adequate collateral circulation is present, the event may be subclinical. Rapid deterioration of renal function indicates bilateral venous occlusion.

If the patients are considered to be at high risk of pulmonary embolism anticoagulation is required. Heparin may be ineffective, however, as anti-thrombin III, which is a mediator of its effect, is usually low. Warfarin, as is it largely protein-bound, has to be administered with great care.

42 Answers (4 marks)

1. **E** Urine cytology and radio-isotope bone scan
2. **A** Transitional cell carcinoma (TCC)

Occupational diseases of the chemical worker are **transitional cell carcinoma** due to aniline dyes and haemangiosarcoma of the liver due to PVC poisoning (this also causes resorption of the mid-portions of the terminal phalanges in the hands). TCC presents with haematuria and features of renal obstruction. They are best demonstrated by cystoscopy and retrograde pyelography. However, urine cytology and an IVU for demonstrating the level of obstruction should be performed first, and this patient also has evidence of metastatic bone disease.

43 Answer (2 marks)

1. **B** Mixed mitral valve disease

There is global cardiomegaly, but predominantly enlargement of both atria. The left main bronchus is elevated with splaying of the carina and there is a double right heart border.

44 Answers (8 marks)

1. **A** Chest X-ray
2. **C** Von Hippel-Lindau syndrome
3. **D** Bilateral renal cell carcinoma
4. **C** 40–50%

Von Hippel-Lindau syndrome (retinocerebellar haemangioblastosis) is characterised by haemangioblastoma formation in the eye, the cerebellum and, less commonly, in other organs. Cysts are frequently found in the liver, spleen and kidneys. Large, benign angiomyolipomas can be found in the kidneys, but the combination of hypertension and haematuria is very suggestive of the commonly found (up to 40%) renal cell carcinoma. The tumours are frequently multicentric and commonly bilateral.

Although staging with CT of the abdomen will be required, exclusion of metastases with a chest X-ray is more important in the first instance.

Polycythaemia is found in a significant minority – erythropoietin is produced by the hypernephroma as well as the cerebellar haemangioblastoma.

The defect is localised in chromosome 3 and transmission is autosomal dominant with 80–90% penetrance, so the patient's children have a 1:2 chance of acquiring the defect with a very high likelihood of this being expressed.

45 Answers (8 marks)

1. **E** Paraneoplastic syndrome
2. **D** Response to exercise
3. **C** Ectopic ACTH secretion
4. **A** Chest X-ray

A complex picture, but the neurological problem can be classified as a lower motor neurone deficit affecting the peripheral system symmetrically, but also involving the cranial nerves. Being better in the evening suggests improvement with exercise which is strongly suggestive of **Eaton-Lambert syndrome**, a myasthenic myopathic syndrome which is a paraneoplastic manifestation of small cell carcinoma of the bronchus. It is characterised by a defect in release of acetylcholine and is an important differential diagnosis to myasthenia gravis (it *improves* with repetition). In addition, the patient has evidence of ectopic ACTH secretion with diabetes, high sodium, low potassium and truncal obesity. A Cushingoid state may also cause a proximal myopathy, but this does not improve with exercise.

Ectopic PTH secretion (or PTH-related hormone) is usually found with *squamous cell carcinoma*.

Hypertrophic pulmonary osteoarthropathy (HPOA) is normally found with squamous and adeno-carcinoma.

Small cell carcinoma is aggressive and spreads quickly, even with a small primary tumour, but is the one tumour that responds well to chemotherapy.

46 Answers (4 marks)

1. **E** Drug screen
2. **B** Periodic paralysis

An acute presentation of a generalised lower motor neurone syndrome involving the bulb. The patient is not dehydrated, which would suggest a 'rave' party; myasthenic crisis cannot be excluded but is unlikely; McArdle's syndrome (myophosphorylase deficiency) causes fatiguability but myoglobin is found in the urine which tests falsely positive for blood on Dipstix.

The striking hypokalaemia in a young patient should alert you to **hypokalaemic periodic paralysis**, an autosomal dominant trait presenting in childhood with remission in the third decade. Attacks last several hours, are usually self-limiting but respond to administration of potassium.

A hyperkalaemic form has also been described.

47 Answer (2 marks)

1. **C** Vestibular schwannoma (acoustic neuroma)

The patient has a deficit of both components of the 8th cranial nerve with marked sensorineural hearing loss and vertigo. Deafness is not a common feature of the other causes of vertigo. MR scanning of the posterior fossa should be performed. Rinne's test in the affected ear would still show normal findings, with air conduction better than bone conduction.

48 Answers (5 marks)

1. **E** Pneumococcal meningitis
  H Sickle cell disease
2. **A** Cefotaxime + 100% O_2
3. **C** Pneumococcal vaccination
  F Notification of Public Health

Asplenia in sickle cell disease or after splenectomy requires pneumococcal vaccination. In children additional anaphylactic prophylaxis is recommended. Clinically, the main differential diagnosis is meningococcal meningitis, although these are Gram-negative diplococci. Treatment of choice is currently cefotaxime (*BNF*, vol 44, September 2002). Meningitis is a notifiable disease.

49 Answers (6 marks)

1. **D** Listeriosis
2. **A** Blood cultures
3. **B** iv erythromycin

Listeria monocytogenes is a ubiquitous facultatively anaerobic bacillus which is heat-resistant to 60 °C (unpasteurised milk!). It becomes invasive in immune-suppressed patients and pregnancy when it causes meningitis, septicaemia and abortion. It is classically transmitted in blue cheeses but can be found in most poorly prepared foodstuffs.

Treatment is either with a combination of broad-spectrum penicillin and gentamicin, alternatively erythromycin or 4-quinolones.

Viral infection and SLE would cause lymphocytosis.

50 Answers (5 marks)

1. **B**   Right optic atrophy
2. **E**   Multiple sclerosis

The patient has a **right afferent pupillary defect**. This indicates damage to the right optic nerve as the light shone in the right eye does not cause ipsilateral or contralateral pupillary constriction.

Associated with walking difficulties in a young woman it is most likely due to **demyelination**.

Neurosyphilis causes a small irregular pupil that constricts on convergence but not to light (Argyll-Robertson pupil).

The pale retinal tumours of tuberose sclerosis can also cause blindness. Other features are epilepsy, low intelligence, adenoma sebaceum (hence the acronym EPILOIA) and the other rashes, ash-leaf macule and shagreen patch.

A Holmes-Adie pupil is a large pupil with sluggish reaction to light and accommodation. It is of no clinical significance other than its association with reduced tendon reflexes in young women.

51 Answer (2 marks)

1. **B**   Multiple myeloma

The patient has reduction of all protein fractions except for an increase in the α_2 band. The appearances are of established nephrotic syndrome. Myeloma may cause nephrotic syndrome, but an increase in the γ band would be expected in this.

52 Answers (9 marks)

1. **E**   *Pneumocystis carinii* pneumonia (PCP)
2. **C**   HIV infection
3. **A**   Sputum microscopy
     J   High-resolution CT scan
4. **B**   iv cotrimoxazole

A small pneumothorax of this size in a young male should not cause respiratory compromise to this degree. In addition, the patient has features of infection as well as immune compromise (pancytopenia). The social history strongly points towards **PC-pneumonia in HIV infection**.

AIDS testing must not be performed without counselling and sneaky ways of establishing CD4 counts are unethical.

Other differential diagnoses in chest infection, i.e. atypical mycobacteria, other fungi and CMV also need to be considered.

PCP typically presents with bilateral hazy mid-zone shadowing although the chest X-ray may be normal. A pneumothorax is present in up to 10%. It is a marker disease for HIV. Proof is by silver staining of sputum or lung biopsy. High-resolution CT scanning is very sensitive, but not as specific.

53 Answers (7 marks)

1. **E**   Chest X-ray
2. **D**   Kartagener's syndrome
3. **A**   0%

Kartagener's syndrome (described by Max Kartagener, Swiss physician, in 1933), or immotile ciliae syndrome, is characterised by the recurrent upper (sinusitis) and lower respiratory tract infections leading to bronchiectasis. The defect in ciliary motility affects the bronchial escalator as well as the motility of sperm and the male patients are *infertile*. It is associated with dextrocardia/complete situs inversus as indicated by the ECG findings.

54 Answers (6 marks)

1. **B**   Autoantibody screen
2. **E**   Cryptogenic fibrosing alveolitis
3. **A**   Autoimmune chronic active hepatitis

The patient has a severe, restrictive lung defect with radiographic evidence of active alveolitis (ground-glass). **Cryptogenic fibrosing alveolitis** usually presents insidiously in middle-aged men, although a rare fulminant form has been described (Hamman-Rich syndrome). It is associated with other autoimmune conditions, such as chronic active hepatitis (CAH), coeliac disease and inflammatory bowel disease. Diagnosis can usually be made on a combination of the clinical findings and thin-section CT, although broncho-alveolar lavage or lung biopsy may be required.

CAH is characterised by an increase in hepatic transaminases and markedly raised immunoglobulins. Liver biopsy gives the diagnosis.

55 Answer (2 marks)

1. **C**   Short Synacthen® test

The patient has haemochromatosis, as indicated by the hyperpigmentation, which is diffuse rather than limited to skin creases (c.f. Addison's disease). Ultrasound will assess the state of the liver and possible portal hypertension. Blood clotting needs to be estimated prior to liver biopsy and the presence of diabetes needs to be excluded. The increased iron content of the liver may also be confirmed with magnetic resonance scanning.

56 Answers (4 marks)

1. **E**   Extrapulmonary restriction
2. **B**   Ankylosing spondylitis

Reduced lung volumes with a normal FEV_1/FVC coefficient indicate a restrictive defect. The normal transfer factors indicate that this is not due to parenchymal disease. Apical cavitation is a late, but typical manifestation of ankylosing spondylitis.

Upper lobe lung disease:
Progressive massive fibrosis (silicosis)
Ankylosing spondylitis
Sarcoid
TB
Extrinsic allergic alveolitis (chronic)
Mnemonic **PASTE**

57 Answers (4 marks)

1. **D**   Bone marrow biopsy
2. **B**   Chronic lymphocytic leukaemia (CLL)

The diagnosis of **CLL** requires a lymphocytosis of $> 10 \times 10^9/l$ and $> 30\%$ lymphocytes in bone marrow. Presentation is usually insidious with lymphadenopathy and/or hepatosplenomegaly. It is a leukaemic form of a low-grade non-Hodgkin's lymphoma.

58 Answers (4 marks)

1. **B**   Allergic bronchopulmonary aspergillosis (ABPA)
2. **A**   Sputum microscopy

ABPA is a hypersensitivity reaction to the ubiquitous fungus. Hyphae are present in the sputum; proximal bronchiectasis is a late complication. Diagnosis can also be made on serum precipitins, skin prick test and high-resolution CT, although this may be non-specific in the early stages. Occupational asthma and vasculitis are unlikely to produce sputum and should show some response to bronchodilators.

59 Answers (4 marks)

1. **C**   Left atrial enlargement
2. **E**   Prothrombin time

The patient has a mitral valve replacement. The oesophagus is compressed and displaced by the enlarged left atrium. As this is a metallic valve replacement the patient must be on warfarin.

60 Answer (3 marks)

1. E Arterial blood gases and iv erythromycin

Infection with **Legionella pneumophila** is characterised by signs of a chest infection (usually in smokers or patients with pre-existing lung disease) with systemic involvement. The classic MRCP-triad consists of hyponatraemia, abdominal pain and haematuria. Treatment is with macrolide antibiotics.

61 Answer (3 marks)

1. D Drug side-effects

The prophylactic treatment for thrombosis in antiphospholipid syndrome is **aspirin**. This is confirmed by the prolonged bleeding time. The prolongation of the APTT is a false-positive result as the lupus anticoagulant interferes with the test.

Causes for pulmonary eosinophilia include a number of drugs (commonest are antibiotics and NSAIDs), fungal and parasite infections, vasculitis, more rarely asthma and the benign, self-limiting idiopathic Loeffler's syndrome.

62 Answers (5 marks)

1. B Carbon monoxide (CO) poisoning
2. B Exchange transfusion

CO poisoning occurs acutely in attempted suicide (running car engine) or chronically with malfunctioning heating appliances. CO has a 250 times greater affinity to haemoglobin than O_2. Central cyanosis occurs with O_2 saturations of < 80% due to the dark colour of deoxyhaemoglobin. However, carboxyhaemoglobin has a cherry-red colour, disguising the hypoxia clinically as well as on pulse oximetry. The treatment of choice is hyperbaric oxygen, but in practice the availability is very limited. Removal of carboxyhaemoglobin in an emergency situation can be achieved by exchange transfusion.

63 Answer (2 marks)

1. B Diabetes insipidus

The patient has a plasma osmolality of (Na+K) × 2 + Urea + Glucose = 312 mOsm/l.

64 Answers (7 marks)

1. **B** Creatinine kinase
2. **E** Polymyositis
3. **B** Barium enema

Polymyositis is a systemic disease of striated muscle characterised by perivascular lymphocytic infiltration. It causes a myopathy which may be painful and dysphagia and myocarditis. It is commoner in women (x 2) and is associated with HLA-B8 and HLA-DR3.

If associated with skin changes (i.e. vasculitic changes of hands and fingers) and the notorious periorbital rash and oedema (a heliotrope is a small purple flower), it is termed 'dermatomyositis'. The majority of cases are idiopathic, but 10% are associated with underlying malignancy (GI tract, thyroid, breast, lymphoma). It is also found in mixed connective tissue diseases.

Painful proximal myopathy is characteristic and the diagnosis is made by EMG and/or muscle biopsy. Muscle enzymes (CK, AST, LDH) are markedly elevated. Anti-nuclear antibodies are positive in 60%, anti-Jo1 antibodies positive in 30%.

Differential diagnoses are polymyalgia rheumatica (slight elevation of CK only), myasthenia gravis (marked eye signs) and familial myopathies. Therapy is with steroids and treatment of any underlying malignancy.

In this case, the presence of the microcytic anaemia and abnormal liver should alert you to a possible underlying carcinoma of the colon.

65 Answers (6 marks)

1. **E** Churg-Strauss syndrome
2. **D** Anti-neutrophil cytoplasmic antibodies (ANCA)
3. **A** Degree of renal involvement

The patient has a multisystem disease with predominant renal involvement. The features are most consistent with a vasculitis and the presence of asthma-like symptoms and eosinophilia indicate **Churg-Strauss syndrome**. It is a granulomatous vasculitis affecting small- to medium-sized vessels. Clinical presentation is similar to polyarteritis nodosa (PAN) (= non-granulomatous). All organs can be affected; prognosis is determined by the progression of the renal failure; lung involvement is more common than with PAN.

Treatment is with steroids and immunosuppressants.

66 Answers (4 marks)

1. **C** Diffuse systemic sclerosis
2. **D** Blood pressure measurement

The distribution of autoantibodies is typical of **diffuse systemic sclerosis**. The limited cutaneous form (formerly CREST) typically shows antibodies against centromere. Raynaud's phenomenon and the skin stigmata are a prominent feature of the cutaneous form, but may be absent or preceded by systemic symptoms in the diffuse disease.

The main prognostic factor is currently lung involvement and the investigation of choice is high-resolution CT. Monitoring of the blood pressure is mandatory as the patient may develop a renal crisis.

The pulmonary fibrosis is typically in a basal distribution as with all the other connective tissue diseases.

67 Answer (2 marks)

1. **D** Thrombolysis

The patient has acute antero-inferior changes indicative of an acute MI. In addition he has developed third-degree heart block as seen in the rhythm strip. However, the QRS complex is not widened and there is no bradycardia and pacing is not indicated at this stage.

68 Answers (4 marks)

1. **B** Chest X-ray
2. **D** Loefgren's syndrome

Loefgren's syndrome (acute sarcoidosis) typically occurs in young women. The classic triad comprises (ankle) arthritis, erythema nodosum and bi-hilar adenopathy. It is associated with pyrexia, cough and raised acute-phase proteins. A positive rheumatoid factor is present in approximately 15%; hyperuricaemia can also be seen in up to 25%.

ACE levels are useful for monitoring disease activity but as an unspecific marker of lung disease are not diagnostic for sarcoid.

69 Answers (6 marks)

1. **A** Paget's disease
2. **D** Congestive cardiac failure
3. **E** Pelvic X-ray

An elderly gentleman presents with evidence of massively increased bone turnover, but a normal calcium and normal full blood count. This is associated with bone pain and increased osteoblastic activity in the pelvis. The features are of **Paget's disease of the bone**.

The biochemistry is not of osteomalacia. The borderline-high prostate-specific antigen is perfectly consistent with prostatic hyperplasia. It does not exclude prostatic carcinoma, but there are no biochemical indicators of malignancy. A normal ESR essentially rules out myeloma.

The mildly raised liver function tests are in keeping with hepatic congestion due to the high-output cardiac failure which also explains the shortness of breath.

70 Answers (3 marks)

1. **D** Gonococcal arthritis
2. **A** Blood cultures

An acute monoarthritis in a young man, even without the pustular rash and the tenosynovitis, is strongly suspicious of **gonococcal arthritis**. Other complications include epididymitis, meningitis, pelvic inflammatory disease and peri-hepatitis (Fitz-Hugh and Curtis syndrome).

Diagnosis is with urethral swabs and blood cultures; joint aspirates may be culture negative. Treatment is with penicillin, ciprofloxacin or tetracycline. Penicillin has the advantage of also covering syphilis; tetracycline also covers *Chlamydia*.

Paper 3 – Answers

1 Answers (4 marks)

1. **B** Renal tubular acidosis type I
2. **A** Abdominal X-ray

The patient has ECG evidence of hypokalaemia. This is unusual to be combined with a metabolic acidosis. Flank pain and haematuria indicate renal stones. The diagnosis is **distal renal tubular acidosis (type 1)**. The most sensitive way of detecting stones is a simple X-ray. Confirmation is with an acid-load challenge, the ammonium chloride test. The kidneys will fail to acidify the urine below a pH of 5.4.

2 Answers (6 marks)

1. **D** Pericardial effusion
2. **B** Gout
3. **E** Thyroxine

The patient has clinical, cardiac, haematological and biochemical manifestations of **hypothyroidism**. Pericardial effusions in myxoedema respond well to thyroxine replacement and should not be drained. Postviral pericardial effusion has to be considered; tuberculous and lymphomatous effusions are unlikely. Uraemia may cause pericardial effusion in end-stage disease; gout does not.

3 Answers (10 marks)

1. **D** Echocardiogram, blood cultures and CT brain
2. **B** iv antibiotics and iv furosemide (frusemide)
3. **A** Endocarditis
4. **B** Cerebral abscess

Prophylaxis for **bacterial endocarditis** is currently recommended for high-risk patients (prosthetic valve, previous endocarditis) undergoing instrumentation of the GI, GU and respiratory tract as well as dental procedures (prophylaxis for barium enema is no longer recommended): iv amoxicillin and iv gentamicin pre-procedure and oral amoxicillin post-procedure are currently regarded as adequate. Prophylaxis with oral amoxicillin only is adequate for patients with uncomplicated valvular lesions, septal defects and PDA undergoing simple dental procedures. Septic emboli to the brain are a serious complication that can lead to abscess formation.

4 Answers (7 marks)

1. **A** Vertebro-basilar embolus
2. **C** Atrial myxoma

Atrial myxoma is a benign, gelatinous tumour arising from the septum. It is three times more common on the left side and is frequently associated with a raised ESR and raised globulins and may have associated systemic symptoms. Embolisation is common and treatment is by surgical resection. Echocardiogram shows an echogenic tumour in the atrium. During diastole it partially prolapses through the valve, resulting in a third heart sound, 'tumour plop'.

Infarction of the occipital cortex is a consequence of occlusion of the basilar artery or its branches and results in occlusion, and results in the failure of processing of the visual input. The patient may not be aware of the visual deficit, as the memory of vision is retained. It is, however, frequently associated with other neurological or behavioural disturbances.

5 Answers (5 marks)

1. **D** Cardiac failure
2. **B** INR

There is consolidation in both lungs, in the typical peri-hilar distribution ('bat wing') of cardiogenic pulmonary oedema. In addition the patient has both an aortic and a mitral valve replacement. The immediate differential diagnoses are myocardial infarction or valve failure. Besides assessment for myocardial infarction, a prothrombin time or INR must be performed as the valves may have thrombosed.

6 Answer (2 marks)

1. **D** Fallot's tetralogy

The pressure in the right ventricle is higher than in the left ventricle but however pulmonary artery pressure is normal. There must be pulmonary stenosis. A right-to-left shunt is required to cause cyanosis – the most likely explanation is **Fallot's tetralogy** (pulmonary stenosis, right ventricular hypertrophy, ventricular septum defect with the aortic root overriding the VSD).

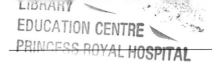

7 Answers (5 marks)

1. **E** Patent ductus arteriosus (PDA)
2. **D** Angiographic embolisation

PDA may be an isolated defect and, if small, may be discovered as an incidental finding. Large PDAs without pressure reduction result in secondary pulmonary hypertension and shunt reversal if untreated. Compensating PDAs (i.e. with associated pulmonary stenosis/atresia) may represent a life-saving left-to-right shunt and closure may be prevented by prostaglandin E1. Prostacyclin inhibitors (NSAIDs) may be used as a conservative treatment for closure of a PDA, particularly in premature babies. All PDAs require endocarditis prophylaxis.

8 Answers (5 marks)

1. **C** Wolff-Parkinson-White type A
2. **E** Left-sided accessory bundle

There is a short PR interval and a slurred upstroke of the R wave (Δ wave). In addition there is RBB pattern in V_1 and V_2 with an M-shaped, positive deflection indicating **WPW type A**. (Type $\underline{A}$ = QRS $\underline{a}$bove baseline). This occurs because the left-sided Kent bundle excites the left ventricle before the right, the appearance being of a relative conduction delay to the right ventricle (RBB). Conversely, in type B there is normal appearance in V_1 (Type $\underline{B}$ = QRS $\underline{b}$elow baseline) with a LBB pattern, because the right-sided Kent bundle triggers the right ventricle prior to the left.

9 Answer (2 marks)

1. **C** Hereditary spherocytosis

There is a profound anaemia in an asymptomatic patient, indicating a long-standing/congenital process. Besides hypochromic cells, the blood film shows microspherocytes. In the full blood count absolute figures for MCV and MCH would be reduced but the ratio (MCHC) is increased, which is virtually pathognomonic of the disease.

10 Answer (2 marks)

1. C Carotid dissection

Electromechanical dissociation ('normal' ECG without output) can be caused by the following mechanisms – massive haemorrhage and hypovolaemia, cardiac outflow obstruction (massive PE, air embolism, failing prosthetic valve), cardiac tamponade, tension pneumothorax, hypothermia and drug overdose.

Carotid dissection can occur after trivial trauma to the neck and is one of the leading causes of stroke in young patients.

11 Answer (3 marks)

1. B Limb lead reversal

There is a complete inversion of the trace in lead I and AVL with normal appearances in the chest leads. The P axis is in the region of 110–120° without evidence of abnormal atrial conduction.

12 Answers (5 marks)

1. D Hypertrophic obstructive cardiomyopathy
2. B Friedreich's ataxia

The relentlessly progressive **Friedreich's ataxia** manifests in childhood or adolescence with progressive ataxia. Inheritance is autosomal recessive. Pes cavus, the mixture of lower and upper motor neurone signs and marked cerebellar signs are typical. Cardiac involvement results in cardiomyopathy, HOCM, arrhythmias and left ventricular hypertrophy.

13 Answer (1 mark)

1. C Atenolol

Raynaud's phenomenon, besides being a part of the connective tissue diseases, is also seen in cryoglobulinaemia and as a side-efffect of vasoconstrictors and beta-blockers.

14 Answers (9 marks)

1. A Impaired glucose tolerance

There is a slow rise in the glucose which does not reach diabetic levels, but remains higher than 8 mmol/l at two hours.

2. C Adrenal adenoma and ectopic ACTH secretion

The baseline cortisol is raised. It does not suppress in the extended (high-dose) dexamethasone test. These are the features of either a **primary adrenal tumour** or **ectopic ACTH secretion**. Pituitary-driven (Cushing's disease) and hyporthalamic-driven hypercortisolism both suppress in the high-dose dexamethasone test. Factitious cortisol administration cannot be excluded on the basis of this test, but the history indicates that this is a long-standing process and no suitable combination of answers is available.

3. E Serum ACTH levels

Adrenal adenoma and ectopic ACTH secretion are easily distinguished by estimating the serum ACTH which would be extremely low in the case of an adrenal adenoma or carcinoma, as the pituitary would be suppressed by the high levels of cortisol.

Ectopic ACTH secretion and pituitary-driven hyperadrenalism can also be distinguished by the CRH test which leads to a further increase in plasma ACTH in the central form, whereas with ectopic ACTH secretion the pituitary is completely suppressed and will not respond to CRH.

Long-term therapy with systemic steroids will, of course, also suppress endogenous ACTH and cortisol production.

4. C Acute adrenal failure

The patient is in addisonian crisis, as the endogenous ACTH/cortisol production will have been chronically suppressed by either an adenoma or ectopic ACTH secretion.

15 Answers (7 marks)

1. **A** Congenital adrenal hyperplasia
2. **E** Increased mineralocorticoids
3. **E** ACTH

Hypertension in the presence of hypokalaemia in a young patient should always alert you to the possibility of Conn's syndrome. However, the fact that the patient has evidence of virilisation and the unusual endocrine tests suggests an alternative diagnosis.

The patient has excess testosterone with suppression of the gonadotrophins. In addition, there is evidence of hyperaldosteronism with high Na, low K and a suppressed renin.

Congenital adrenal hyperplasia, CAH (also adreno-genital syndrome, AGS) is an inherited enzyme defect in the production of corticosteroids in the adrenal gland. The two main sites are at the level of the 21-betahydroxylase (90%) and one step further down in the synthesis at 11-betahydroxylase (5%). In the commoner form, no functional precursors are produced and, as well as features of hypocortisonalism, the patients have evidence of salt wastage. In the second form, a functioning mineralocorticoid precursor (11-deoxycorticosterone) is produced leading to functional hyperaldosteronism.

The absence of glucocorticoids leads to a reactive increase of ACTH secretion which stimulates the attempted production of the hormones. As all the corticoid precursors accumulate, there is further increase in androgen synthesis. This results in pseudopubertas praecox in boys and virilisation in girls. The patients are initially tall but, due to premature fusion of the epiphyses, end up with a reduced body height. Treatment is with substitution of the missing hormones, aiming to suppress ACTH production and remove the stimulus to the adrenal. Family screening is also required as some forms can remain subclinical.

16 Answers (5 marks)

1. **E** Acromegaly
2. **D** Compression of the pituitary stalk

The patient has *manifest* diabetes and shows a paradoxical rise of growth hormone in the oral glucose tolerance test, indicating **acromegaly**.

The excretion of prolactin is regulated by secretion of prolactin-inhibiting hormone (PIH = dopamine). Suprasellar extension of a pituitary tumour may compress the pituitary infundibulum and PIH cannot reach the anterior pituitary which results in an uninhibited production of prolactin.

17 Answer (2 marks)

1.   C   Pseudoxanthoma elasticum

The ECG shows an acute infero-lateral infarct.

Pseudoxanthoma elasticum not only has the well-known cutaneous and fundoscopic features but is associated with widespread vascular changes due to abnormal elastic tissue in arterial walls. Buerger's disease typically occurs in young male smokers; thrombocythaemia presents at a more advanced age with venous thrombotic episodes.

18 Answers (4 marks)

1.   E   Still's disease
2.   B   Upper lobe pulmonary fibrosis

A young patient with clear evidence of rheumatoid disease as well as two renal transplantation scars in the right iliac fossa. This is **Still's disease** complicated by amyloidosis and renal failure. Pulmonary fibrosis in the context of connective tissue disease has a predilection for the lung *bases*. Intrathoracic complications of rheumatoid arthritis include pleural effusions (commonest), basal fibrosis, rheumatoid nodules and drug-induced changes. Osteoporosis may occur locally due to the inflammation and systemically, due to steroid therapy and renal failure.

19 Answer (3 marks)

1.   D   Familial hypocalciuric hypercalcaemia

This is an autosomal dominant condition, characterised by increased renal absorption of calcium and magnesium. A mild hypermagnesaemia is seen in approximately 50%. The parathormone level is reduced, the other electrolytes are normal. Other causes of hypercalcaemia and renal tubular acidosis show an increased urinary calcium.

20 Answers (5 marks)

1. **D** Cushing's syndrome
2. **E** Long-term steroid therapy

In the short Synacthen® test, plasma cortisol should rise by 200 nmol/l to exceed 550 nmol/l. The impaired response is consistent with primary, secondary or tertiary **adrenal insufficiency** or steroid therapy. In Cushing's syndrome/disease clearly the cortisol should be high.

In the long Synacthen® test, primary adrenal failure will show no significant response. Adrenals, however, that have been deprived of their stimulus for a long period of time, either due to pituitary or hypothalamic failure, or due to suppression by exogenous steroids, will show a delayed response.

21 Answers (5 marks)

1. **D** Polycystic ovary syndrome (PCO)
2. **C** Ultrasound scan of the pelvis

PCO (Stein-Leventhal) syndrome is a syndrome of secondary virilisation of genetically normal women. A spectrum of signs is found, the most prominent being hirsutism, menstrual irregularities and primary or even secondary (!) infertility. The patients are frequently obese and on ultrasound the ovaries are enlarged with multiple cysts. Serum testosterone is frequently elevated, as is the LH to FSH ratio (> 3).

Although the ultrasound scan is very suggestive, cystic ovarian changes can also be seen in the other main differential diagnoses, which are congenital adrenal hyperplasia and Cushing's syndrome. In the case given, the U&Es are against hypercortisolism and the normal hydroxyprogesterone is against congenital adrenal hyperplasia.

Patients with testicular feminisation never have periods as genetically they are men.

22 Answer (2 marks)

1. **B** Normal-pressure hydrocephalus

There is dilatation of the ventricles out of proportion to any atrophy seen on the brain surface. However CT may be inconclusive. The main differential diagnosis of the presentation is a chronic subdural haematoma.

23 Answers (8 marks)

1. **A** Endoscopy and small bowel biopsy
2. **E** Coeliac disease

Coeliac disease is a hypersensitivity to gluten, the protein contained in cereals. It is characterised by (subtotal) villous atrophy of the small bowel, resulting in malabsorption. Symptoms are slow in onset and can present late in life, usually with malaise and abdominal symptoms. Diarrhoea, recurrent stomatitis and sequelae of malabsorption, i.e. osteomalacia, polyneuropathy and macrocytic anaemia, are seen. Patients frequently show eosinophilia. Antigliadin and anti-reticulin antibodies are found in the majority of patients but can be normal. It is associated with dermatitis herpetiformis, an intensely itchy polymorphic skin rash. 10–20% show a familial incidence with variable expression.

3. **C** Poor diet

The condition usually responds to a gluten-free diet, with the risk of relapse as the patient becomes asymptomatic.

4. **B** Small bowel carcinoma

There is an associated risk of small bowel malignancy. The risk of developing small bowel lymphoma is greatly reduced by a strict diet, as indicated in the history, but the risk of developing small bowel carcinoma is not affected by avoidance of gluten, making this the more likely cause in this context.

24 Answers (10 marks)

1. B Stool microscopy and culture

The acute onset in two family members suggests **food poisoning**. Most of these have an incubation period of less than one week, indicating a source other than traveller's diarrhoea. The commonest pathogens would be *Escherichia coli*, *Salmonella*, *Shigella* and *Staphylococcus*. *Campylobacter* and viral infection may also have to be considered.

2. E Erythema nodosum

Painful red-to-purple nodules erupt over the extensor surfaces of the upper and lower limbs. In 50% this is idiopathic. It is associated with granulomatous diseases (TB, sarcoid, leprosy), inflammatory bowel disease, infections (*Streptococcus*, *Salmonella*, *Yersinia*) and a number of drugs (penicillin, sulphonamides, oral contraceptive pill).

3. A X-ray of both wrists and pelvis
4. C Reiter's syndrome

The patient has developed an asymmetrical polyarthritis of large joints, probably associated with a sacroiliitis. Breathlessness may be due to associated pericarditis or pleuritis/pleural effusion. Other features include uveitis, keratoderma blenorrhagica (an exfoliative process of palms and soles), and a circinate balanitis (a well-demarcated rash of the glans of the penis). The latter two are more common in **Reiter's syndrome** following non-specific urethritis.

Septic arthritis may occur after some earlier infection, but it would be most unusual to be polyarticular. Immune complex vasculitis (type III hypersensitivity) may be observed after chronic low-grade infection. There is no specific test for Reiter's disease. If severe, characteristic X-ray changes with erosions and a fluffy periosteal reaction may be seen.

5. A Non-steroidal anti-inflammatory drugs

Treatment is symptomatic.

25 Answers (4 marks)

1. **E** Anti-mitochondrial antibodies
2. **C** Primary biliary cirrhosis (PBC)

A middle-aged woman presents with generalised pruritus, steatorrhoea and evidence of sicca syndrome. Her globulins are elevated (markedly raised IgM).

PBC is a chronic, aseptic destructive cholangitis. It accounts for approximately 1% of liver cirrhosis. 90% are of women in their fifth decade. Pruritus precedes jaundice, biliary obstruction leads to maldigestion. It is associated with Sjögren's syndrome, polyarthralgia, autoimmune thyroiditis and hypercholesterolaemia. Antimitochondrial antibodies are found in over 90% – of the several subtypes, anti-M_2 are specific. Titres are elevated above 1:100.

26 Answers (4 marks)

1. **C** Inappropriate ADH secretion
   G Dilutional hyponatraemia

On admission the patient is dehydrated with serum osmolality at the upper limit of normal, which is treated to abnormally low levels (267 mOsm/kg). Prolonged regimes of iv glucose and insulin result in the effective administration of pure water. Causes of inappropriate ADH secretion (SIADH) include head injury, raised intracranial pressure, intracranial haemorrhage, tumours and cerebral abscess.

27 Answers (4 marks)

1. **C** Blind loop syndrome
2. **E** Radiocarbon (C14) breath test

The likely treatment for ulcers at that time would have been a partial gastrectomy either with anterograde anastomosis between the stomach and the duodenum (Billroth 1 gastrectomy) or a side-to-side anastomosis with the jejunum (Billroth 2 or Polya gastroenterostomy). The delayed onset of the symptoms is against dumping syndrome – this is excluded by the normal oral glucose tolerance test (dumping syndrome should show a sharp drop in the one-hour value to hypoglycaemic levels). The macrocytic anaemia suggests bacterial overgrowth in a blind-ending afferent loop. This could be confirmed by endoscopy and aspiration or a hydrogen or radiocarbon breath test (increased bacterial activity breaks down the radioactive compound leading to increased excretion of radioactive gas through the lungs).

28 Answers (6 marks)

1. **D** Proton pump inhibitor therapy
2. **B** Chronic atrophic gastritis
   D *Helicobacter* gastritis
3. **E** Gastroscopy and biopsy

Causes for elevated gastrin levels include Zollinger-Ellison Syndrome (ZES), atrophic gastritis, pernicious anaemia, *Helicobacter* gastritis, previous antrectomy and therapy with proton pump inhibitors. However, pernicious anaemia does not present with relapsing ulcers and the patient has not had previous surgery. ZES is characterised by a paradoxical *increase* of gastrin after administration of secretin, by at least 100%.

29 Answers (6 marks)

1. **B** Abdominal ultrasound
2. **A** Streptococcal liver abscess
3. **E** Percutaneous drainage

The patient has features of chronic sepsis with a normocytic anaemia, low albumin, raised globulins, raised ESR and intermittent pyrexia. This is localised to the right upper quadrant. The history of left iliac fossa irritation is suggestive of either diverticular disease/diverticulitis or carcinoma of the colon. The most likely diagnosis is a ***Streptococcus milleri* abscess** which accounts for over 75% of liver abscesses. Most of these are secondary to a predisposing cause relating to the GI tract.

30 Answer (2 marks)

1. **C** Change medication

The patient has **renal papillary necrosis (RPN)**, which is indicated by the blunted, but not dilated calyces. The filling defects are blood clots and sloughed papillae. In addition, the patient has a 'bamboo spine'. Besides long-term non-steroidals, causes for RPN include diabetes, chronic obstruction, alcohol and any cause of ischaemia, including sickle cell disease.

31 Answers (9 marks)

1. **C** Blood film
2. **E** α-interferon
3. **B** Renal vein thrombosis
4. **C** Essential thrombocythaemia

The patient has dramatic elevation of the platelet count with mild associated leucocytosis. In addition, he has a microcytic anaemia which may either be due to chronic GI blood loss or depletion of iron stores by associated polycythaemia. The patient has a raised urate indicating increased cell turnover. Thrombocytosis to this degree is highly suggestive of **essential thrombocythaemia** which has an association (up to 30%) with gastroduodenal ulceration. Philadelphia chromosome is absent, and the LAP is increased (differential diagnosis, CML). The blood film shows megakaryocytes and the diagnosis can be confirmed by marrow biopsy. Complications include thromboembolism (main cause of death), haemorrhage (deficit in platelet function) and transformation to acute leukaemia (10%). The patients affected are usually over 50 years; mean survival time is 10 to 15 years.

Therapy is successful in the majority of cases with α-interferon; second-line treatment is myelosuppressant therapy (5-hydroxyurea). In acute thrombotic crises, thrombocytapheresis may be required. Anti-platelet drugs are contraindicated.

32 Answers (7 marks)

1. **C** Angiodysplasia
2. **A** Right hemicolectomy

The patient has a microcytic anaemia with a history of blood loss. The normal barium enema in combination with the abnormal angiogram suggests **angiodysplasia of the colon**. Angiodysplasia is a common finding and it can be difficult to decide whether it is responsible for a GI bleed. Acute haemorrhage may be controlled by embolisation, but this carries a risk of bowel necrosis. Treatment is usually by resection.

3. **D** Benign monoclonal gammopathy

The most important differential diagnosis is multiple myeloma. However, the normal calcium, alkaline phosphatase, and renal function and, in particular, the low levels of bone marrow plasma cells (< 10%) are against myeloma, although this is not entirely excluded. Further investigations would require a more detailed investigation of the gamma band and a skeletal survey.

33 Answers (6 marks)

1. **E**   Sickle cell trait
2. **C**   β-thalassaemia minor
3. **B**   25%

A women with haemoglobin S who remains asymptomatic into the first trimester must be heterozygous. In the homozygous form, HbS is greater than 90%.

The father has a mild anaemia, but no reduction in red cells and a severe microcytosis. The presence of HbF ($\alpha_2\gamma_2$), and increased HbA$_2$ ($\alpha_2\delta_2$) over 5% indicates a problem with the β-chains. However, the haemoglobin being above 100 g/l again indicates a heterozygous constellation.

The child has a 1 : 4 chance of each the following haemoglobin arrangements:
- Normal haemoglobin
- Sickle cell trait
- β-thalassaemia trait
- Sickle thalassaemia

The first three conditions are not associated with serious problems (see parents). However, sickle thalassaemia is a true sickling syndrome which, in its manifestations, can approach homozygous sickle cell disease.

34 Answer (2 marks)

1. **D**   Calcium substitution

The patient has short 4th and 5th metacarpals and skin calcification suggesting a diagnosis of **pseudohypoparathyroidism**. The syndrome consists of end-organ resistance to endogenous PTH with resulting hypocalcaemia, hyperphosphataemia, short stature, soft tissue calcification, and learning difficulties. PTH levels are normal or increased.

35 Answers (5 marks)

1. **E** Lead poisoning
2. **A** Abdominal X-ray

Lead intoxication is becoming rare since the withdrawal of lead-containing paints. However, neglected children especially may still present after chronic ingestion = pica syndrome (Lat. *pica* = magpie). Lead residue is well demonstrated on X-ray if still present within the bowel.

Pallor is caused by anaemia as well as vasospasm. Other features are lead-lines on the gums, constipation, neuropathy and encephalopathy. δ-aminolaevulinic acid is increased in blood and urine.

The differential diagnosis of sideroblastic anaemia includes hereditary causes, myeloproliferative disorders, toxins (lead, alcohol, anti-TB drugs), leukaemia and connective tissue diseases.

A dimorphic film indicates two erythrocyte populations of different ages, such as seen after blood transfusion, treated iron deficiency, combined iron and B_{12} deficiency and sideroblastic anaemia.

36 Answers (4 marks)

1. **C** Gold
2. **D** Blood film

In rheumatoid arthritis, all types of anaemia can be found. Most are **drug-induced**, but there are associated autoimmune conditions, such as pernicious anaemia and hypothyroidism, and there is the anaemia of chronic disease and hypersplenism (Felty's syndrome).

Chronic GI bleeding is found with non-steroidal anti-inflammatory drugs; methotrexate is a folate antagonist; sulfasalazine causes intravascular haemolysis with compensatory reticulocytosis which can raise the MCV.

Gold and D-penicillamine, however, cause aplastic anaemia.

37 Answers (8 marks)

1. **F** Carpal tunnel syndrome
   G Secondary hyperparathyroidism
2. **C** Nerve conduction studies
   F Parathormone levels
3. **B** Median nerve decompression
   G Increased calcium and vitamin D supplements

The patient has evidence of a sensory and motor neuropathy of the left median nerve. The most likely cause for this is **compression at the carpal tunnel** due to β2-microglobulin deposition in the flexor retinaculum. The fistula is not at a site where it can compress the median nerve and a localised pressure effect from the brown tumour in the metacarpal would not cause a sensory deficit in the index finger. Treatment is by splitting of the flexor retinaculum.

In addition, the patient has radiological features of **hyperparathyroidism**, with the hallmark subperiosteal bone resorption. This is usually best seen at the radial aspects of the middle phalanges. However, the calcium is on the low side, indicating that this is secondary to inadequate replacement and has not yet become autonomous (tertiary hyperparathyroidism). The treatment at this stage is with a replacement to remove the stimulus of hypocalcaemia to the parathyroid glands.

38 Answer (2 marks)

1. **B** Forced expiratory volume in the first second (FEV_1)

The patient has **chronic obstructive pulmonary disease** (FEV_1 markedly reduced, and a slow-rising curve which does not even plateau). FEV_1 can be used as a predictor for mortality and relates best to the patient's dyspnoea. PEFR cannot differentiate between obstructed or restricted air flow and is more variable in testing than FEV_1. For the latest guidelines see the website of the British Thoracic Society.

39 Answers (9 marks)

1. **C**   Serum electrophoresis
   G   Skeletal survey
2. **E**   Multiple myeloma
3. **E**   Acute tubular necrosis
4. **C**   Presence of light chains

Two of the three following cardinal features have to be present for the diagnosis of **myeloma**:

1. Presence of monoclonal immunoglobulins in plasma/urine
2. Increase of plasma cells within bone marrow > 10% (normal < 8%)
3. Well-defined osteolytic (punched out) bone lesions

The presence of anaemia, hypercalcaemia and renal failure are poor prognostic factors in myeloma. Light chains (kappa & lambda) are present in up to 60% of IgG and IgA myelomas, and 100% in pure light chain myeloma. These are excreted in the urine and can obstruct the tubules. Administration of iv contrast is contraindicated! Bence-Jones proteins precipitate if urine is heated to 50 °C and dissolve again on further heating.

The well-defined bone lesions are caused by osteoclastic activity with virtually no sclerotic response unless a pathological factor occurs. The uptake of Technetium-labelled diphosphonate during a bone scan, however, is dependent on the activity of osteoblasts and false negative results are usually obtained.

40 Answers (2 marks)

1. **B**   Combined respiratory and metabolic acidosis

The patient is clearly acidotic. O_2 tension is decreased; CO_2 tension is increased, indicating respiratory failure in keeping with chronic COAD. However, there is no compensatory increase of the bicarbonate which is reduced below normal levels, indicating an associated metabolic acidosis. The oxygen saturation of > 80% indicates an arterial sample. (Conversion from kiloPascal to millimetres of Hg is done by multiplying by an approximate factor of 7.5 (10 kPa = 75 mmHg)).

41 Answers (4 marks)

1. **A**   Aplastic anaemia
2. **D**   Drug-induced glomerulonephritis

The patient has a pancytopenia and heavy proteinuria. The renal biopsy is consistent with the **membranous glomerulonephritis**. Both features can either be due to therapy with gold or penicillamine. Methotrexate, as a folate antagonist, can cause macrocytic anaemia.

42 Answer (2 marks)

1. B Pulmonary function tests (PFT)

The patient has extensive calcified pleural plaques and an area of round atelectasis ('folded lung') in the right lower lobe, indicating previous asbestos exposure. There is no circumferential pleural encasement to account for the dyspnoea, and asbestosis (pulmonary fibrosis) has to be excluded. This may be done with a thin-section (high-resolution) CT scan or with spirometry and transfer factor. As the patient is entitled to compensation, quantification with PFT is the best answer.

NB. The peak incidence of asbestos-related lung disease is expected between 2010 and 2020.

43 Answers (5 marks)

1. C Renal artery stenosis
2. D Isotope renogram

The patient has raised baseline aldosterone and renin. The aldosterone drops to normal values after captopril, indicating a **secondary hyperaldosteronism**. In Conn's syndrome, the aldosterone levels are not affected. An increase in renin concentration by up to 50% can be seen in essential hypertension and this is non-specific. However, an increment of more than 100% is highly suggestive of renal artery stenosis. A renogram will quantify residual function, an angiogram will assess suitability for angioplasty or surgery.

44 Answers (5 marks)

1. B Allergic interstitial nephritis
2. E Withdrawal of all medication

The symptoms described are of osteoarthritis and not of an inflammatory arthropathy. Her GP would have treated her with simple analgesics or non-steroidal anti-inflammatory drugs (NSAIDs). One month later, she has heavy proteinuria as well as glycosuria, indicating both glomerular and tubular damage.

NSAIDs are a common cause of **allergic interstitial nephritis**, as are antibiotics. Other features may include fever, arthralgia, eosinophilia, haematuria and acute renal failure. The diagnosis can be confirmed by renal biopsy showing interstitial lymphocytic infiltrates. Withdrawal of the offending drug will usually lead to spontaneous resolution; in severe cases steroids may be required.

45 Answers (7 marks)

1. **B** Guillain-Barré syndrome (GBS)
2. **C** Pulmonary function tests
3. **B** Ventilation

The patient has a distal neuropathy which is also involving both facial nerves. This is associated with a sensory neuropathy affecting the spinothalamic tracts as well as the dorsal columns (soft touch).

This is of fairly acute onset and the CSF shows a characteristically high protein with normal microscopy. This can cause communicating hydrocephalus due to impaired reabsorption of CSF.

The reduction in nerve conduction is typical for a demyelinating polyneuritis.

Treatment of **GBS** is mainly supportive; respiratory depression may require ventilation.

Tetanus and botulism affect the motor endplates only (as does myasthenia gravis); herpes encephalitis may cause UMN signs but not a peripheral neuropathy.

46 Answer (3 marks)

1. **E** Surgery

A young patient with hypertension and a low potassium must alert you to the diagnosis of **Conn's syndrome**. The renogram shows normal, sharp uptake and prompt excretion in both kidneys with a symmetrical distribution, indicating normal renal perfusion.

417

47 Answers (9 marks)

1. **A**   Botulism
2. **B**   Arterial blood gases
3. **E**   Antitoxin
4. **D**   Admit to intensive care and inform Public Health

The acute onset of a global neurological syndrome characterised by paralysis is suggestive of an acute infection or toxic effects. The absence of focal symptoms and normal blood parameters essentially exclude a cerebral abscess. Tetanus is characterised by tonic seizures in a conscious patient; rabies has a protracted onset with features of encephalitis.

Organophosphate poisoning is characterised by strong cholinergic/ muscarinic effects and not by a flaccid paralysis.

Spores of **Clostridium botulinum** are found in soil. Under anaerobic conditions (home canned meat, pickled vegetables, home-made wine) the most potent toxin known to man is produced. It is destroyed by heat, the earliest manifestations, besides diarrhoea and vomiting, are diplopia. The eye muscles, in particular lateral rectus, are the best innervated muscles in the body and the most sensitive to toxic effects. Treatment is with anti-toxins and supportive measures, if the patient survives the respiratory paralysis, outcome is usually good.

48 Answers (5 marks)

1. **B**   Cerebral sarcoid
2. **A**   Chest X-ray

The patient has a lower motor neurone palsy of the facial nerve associated with CSF lymphocytosis and mildly raised protein. The features are consistent with **cerebral sarcoidosis**. The facial nerves are directly affected and both sides can be involved simultaneously. Involvement of the parotid glands may indicate Heerfordt's syndrome (uveoparotid fever). Ophthalmology referral for assessment of uveitis should be considered. A benign pleomorphic adenoma of the parotid does not cause CSF changes.

49 Answers (6 marks)

1. **D**   Impaired glucose tolerance
2. **B**   Hypergonadotropic hypogonadism
3. **A**   Myotonic dystrophy

The combination of diffuse lower motor neurone lesion, cardiac conduction defects and a visual problem not corrected by glasses (cataract!) should alert you to **myotonic dystrophy**.

An autosomal dominant condition associated with impaired glucose tolerance, primary hypogonadism and impaired intellectual function.

The patient is too old for Friedreich's ataxia; Kallmann's syndrome is characterised by reduced gonadotrophins and anosmia, but no neuromuscular problems.

50 Answer (2 marks)

1. **B**   Atrial septal defect

There is cardiomegaly with predominant enlargement of the atria and the pulmonary outflow tract. In addition there is enlargement of the central arteries with peripheral pruning indicating the onset of pulmonary hypertension.

51 Answers (4 marks)

1. **D**   Hereditary sensorimotor neuropathy
2. **A**   Normal fundi

The patient has a neuropathy affecting sensory and motor systems. There is no evidence of upper motor neurone signs, making SACD and neurosyphilis unlikely. Friedreich's ataxia is unlikely due to the absence of cerebellar signs, and involvement of the lateral spinothalamic tracts is not usually seen.

52 Answers (6 marks)

1. **A** Wegener's granulomatosis
2. **C** Lateral chest X-ray
3. **B** iv cyclophosphamide

The patient has a systemic disease affecting eyes, chest and kidneys. In addition, 9% of the differential is unaccounted for which is likely to represent eosinophils. Of the vasculitides, pulmonary nodules are typical for **Wegener's granulomatosis**. These frequently cavitate.

Renal biopsy and estimation of c-ANCA is required. In view of the occupation, extrinsic allergic alveolitis has to be excluded. Lateral chest X-ray will not provide any further information. The nasal passage and the sinuses are usually involved and diagnosis can also be made on biopsy from this site. Eye involvement and retrobulbar granulomata are common.

Treatment is with cyclophosphamide and additional steroids if required.

53 Answers (7 marks)

1. **B** Serum phosphate
2. **A** Squamous cell carcinoma of the lung
3. **E** Forced diuresis and chest X-ray

Hyperparathyroidism occurs as a paraneoplastic manifestation of **squamous cell carcinoma of the lung**. This is due to secretion of parathormone-related peptide (PTH-rp). Its effect is confirmed by a low phosphate. Bone metastases and Paget's disease are essentially excluded by the normal bone scan; multiple myeloma is extremely unlikely in the presence of a normal (< 8%) plasma cell count in the bone marrow. The hypercalcaemia of ectopic PTH secretion does not suppress as well in the *steroid suppression test* as sarcoidosis, myeloma, Addison's disease or hypervitaminosis D. Treatment in the first instance is with aggressive rehydration and added diuretics. Removal of the primary tumour usually results in a dramatic drop of the serum calcium within 48 hours.

54 Answers (8 marks)

1. **A** Myasthenia gravis
2. **F** Acetylcholine receptor antibodies
   J Spiral CT of the chest
3. **E** Pyridostigmine
4. **C** Midazolam
   H Curare derivatives

Myasthenia gravis is associated with a thymoma in 10% and there is a risk of malignant change. Thymectomy must be offered, but this is the surgical option. The Tensilon® test is less specific than acetylcholine receptor antibodies and carries a high risk of acute respiratory failure. Benzodiazepines and muscle relaxants have to be used with extreme caution.

55 Answers (6 marks)

1. **A** Chronic myeloid leukaemia in blast crisis
2. **C** Cytomegalovirus
3. **B** Isolation and sputum examination

The patient has **CML in blast transformation**. She is susceptible to atypical and fungal infections. Besides TB and *Mycobacterium*, invasive aspergillosis has to be considered as a further cause of cavitating pneumonia. *Staphylococcus* and *Klebsiella* are bacterial causes of cavitating pneumonia.

Pneumocystis carinii, CMV and varicella pneumonitis tend to be diffuse and bilateral and do not cavitate.

56 Answers (4 marks)

1. **D** Allergic bronchopulmonary aspergillosis (ABPA)
2. **A** Sputum microscopy and culture

Differential diagnosis of a **pulmonary-renal syndrome** can be split into systemic diseases (i.e. Goodpasture's syndrome, vasculitides), primary pulmonary pathology (carcinoma, infection) which may cause secondary renal impairment or glomerulonephritis, and primary renal pathology with secondary lung involvement (pulmonary oedema, embolism, metastasis).

ABPA is a hypersensitivity reaction to the fungus characterised by mucoid plugs and central bronchiectasis. It typically affects young asthmatic men.

57 Answers (4 marks)

1. **D** Re-breathing from a paper bag
2. **A** Hyperventilation

The patient is hypocapnic without evidence of hypoxia or tachycardia. In the absence of these, the most likely cause is **hyperventilation**, with pulmonary embolus being the main differential diagnosis although this is less likely in the first trimester.

58 Answers (2 marks)

1. **B** Biochemical profile
   C Intravenous urogram

The patient has **medullary nephrocalcinosis**. The three predominant causes for this are:
- Primary hyperparathyroidism
- Renal tubular acidosis type 1 (distal)
- Medullary sponge kidney

IVU will demonstrate any possible obstruction as well as the dilated distal tubules of MSK; calcium levels as well as the renal function need to be assessed. Nephrocalcinosis may also rarely occur with other causes of prolonged hypercalcaemia, including sarcoidosis, although in practice this is extremely rare.

59 Answers (4 marks)

1. **A** Emphysema
2. **D** α_1-antitrypsin deficiency (α_1-ATD)

A young patient has increased lung volumes, reduced CO transfer coefficient and an obstructive pattern. The features are of **emphysema**. In a patient of this age, **α_1-ATD** has to be excluded.

60 Answers (4 marks)

1. **B** Pulmonary haemorrhage
2. **D** Hereditary haemorrhagic telangiectasia (HHT)

HHT (Osler-Weber-Rendu syndrome) is an autosomal dominant condition with telangiectatic changes mainly throughout the GI tract (lips!) but with associated pulmonary AV malformation. The patients present with recurrent haemorrhage and iron deficiency anaemia. Increase in transfer coefficient (KCO) is seen in pulmonary haemorrhage, polycythaemia and increased blood flow through the lungs and asthma. KCO is the amount of CO taken up by the lungs (TCO) corrected for lung volume.

61 Answers (4 marks)

1. **A** Barium swallow
2. **D** Whipple's disease

The patient has a microcytic anaemia and dysphagia – the upper GI tract needs to be assessed. Causes of basal lung fibrosis include all the connective tissue diseases, cryptogenic fibrosing alveolitis, asbestosis, drug-induced fibrosis and causes of **chronic aspiration**. Systemic sclerosis is less likely with a normal CRP and a microcytic anaemia. Tylosis is an autosomal dominant syndrome of hyperkeratosis of the palms and soles of the feet which is associated with carcinoma of the oesophagus.

Whipple's disease has associations with sacroiliitis, sero-negative arthropathy, clubbing and erythema nodosum, but not pulmonary fibrosis.

62 Answers (4 marks)

1. **I** Chronic lymphocytic leukaemia (CLL)
    J Autoimmune haemolysis

The diagnosis of CLL is based on a markedly raised peripheral blood count of lymphocytes (often $> 40 \times 10^9$/l), 'smudge' cells in the blood film and marrow infiltration of $> 50\%$. The lymphocytes seen in the blood film are predominantly mature (as opposed to ALL). 'Smudge' cells (also smear or ghost cells) are fragile lymphocytes that burst during the preparation of the blood films. Lymphadenopathy and splenomegaly may be found.

A proportion of cases of CLL are complicated by the development of warm-antibody autoimmune haemolytic anaemia. This is diagnosed by an anaemia with evidence of haemolysis and an increased reticulocyte count ($> 2\%$). The direct Coombs' test would be positive as the direct test detects antibodies which have bound to red cells *in vivo*. Anaemia in CLL may also be caused by marrow failure, folate deficiency, hypersplenism and bleeding due to thrombocytopenia.

63 Answers (4 marks)

1. **B** Bronchoscopy and biopsy
2. **B** Alveolar cell carcinoma

Alveolar cell carcinoma accounts for 2–3% of lung tumours. Chest X-ray may show a solitary nodule, but a diffuse area of consolidation is common and these tumours can produce large amounts of mucoid secretion. The pneumonic form has a poor prognosis.

64 Answers (9 marks)

1. **C** Systemic lupus erythematosus
2. **E** Renal biopsy
3. **A** Avascular necrosis
4. **B** Nephrotic syndrome

A young woman with a multisystem disorder affecting the CNS (supra- and infra-tentorial), joints and kidneys. There is a significant occupational history, although the normal CRP is strongly against an infective cause, which would also not explain her pancytopenia.

HIV has to be considered but would not readily explain the impaired renal function and heavy proteinuria.

Systemic lupus erythematosus typically shows a discrepancy between a raised ESR and a normal CRP and also causes a falsely positive VDRL (the test incorporates cardiolipin as part of the antigen in the immune assay).

The patient has cerebral lupus and renal impairment. The joints are frequently affected in the acute phase and avascular necrosis is a rare, but well-described complication, in particular if the patient has been on long-term steroid therapy.

Renal involvement may be due to minimal change, proliferative or membranous glomerulonephritis, and often determines the outcome of the disease. A lumbar puncture may show an increased amount of protein, though this will by no means be diagnostic, and the renal biopsy is going to be abnormal in the presence of hypertension and proteinuria.

65 Answers (9 marks)

1. **C**   Electrocardiogram
   G   ASO titres
2. **A**   Rheumatic fever
3. **E**   Chorea minor (Sydenham's)
4. **B**   Seven years of oral penicillin

Rheumatic fever is a hypersensitivity reaction following two to three weeks after an infection with β-haemolysing group A streptococci. It affects heart (peri-, myo- or endocarditis), joints (polyarthritis), CNS (chorea minor) and skin and subcutaneous tissues. A typical rash is erythema marginatum (pink annular rash over the trunk), but erythema nodosum can also be seen.

Prognosis is determined by the extent of endocardial involvement leading to valve defects (80% mitral, 20% aortic), which is a late manifestation. In the acute phase, an ECG is more important than an echocardiogram to demonstrate the prolonged PR interval, while valvular defects have not developed. Pericardial effusions, however, may be seen.

The diagnosis of rheumatic fever is made by the prescence of a combination of two major or one major and two minor Duckett Jones criteria (American Heart Association) with evidence of a preceding streptococcal infection.

Major criteria	Minor criteria
1. Carditis	1. Fever
2. Polyarthritis	2. Arthralgia
3. Chorea minor	3. Raised ESR/CRP
4. Subcutaneous (Aschoff) nodules	4. Prolonged PR interval
5. Erythema marginatum/annulare	5. Previous history of rheumatic fever

Haemolytic group A streptococci usually cause pharyngitis which, in the acute phase, can be demonstrated by throat swab; in the subacute phase a rising antibody titre is the examination of choice. Systemic infection causes scarlet fever. Treatment of rheumatic fever is with antibiotics to the age of 20.

66 Answer (2 marks)

1. E   Gastroscopy

The patient has a dilated oesophagus which tapers into a narrow cardia, although barium is seen to pass through to the stomach. These are the appearances of **achalasia**. The differential diagnoses of a peptic stricture or a carcinoma need to be excluded.

67 Answers (4 marks)

1. D   Reactive amyloidosis
2. B   Renal biopsy

Reactive (secondary) **amyloidosis** is found in conditions with chronic infection (e.g. bronchiectasis), chronic inflammation (e.g. inflammatory bowel disease) and some malignancies. Renal involvement leading to nephrotic syndrome or chronic renal failure and hepatosplenomegaly are typical, although in this patient the underlying lymphoma may account for the latter.

Diagnosis is with biopsy, showing the amorphous amyloid deposits which stain red with Congo red and fluoresce green under polarised light.

68 Answers (4 marks)

1. E   Sjögren's syndrome
2. C   Symptomatic therapy only

The positive autoantibodies (> 1:80) indicate an autoimmune disease. The absence of double-stranded DNA antibodies is strongly against SLE. The normal hand X-ray does not rule out rheumatoid arthritis, but the presence of Ro and La antibodies suggest **primary Sjögren's syndrome**.

In the Schirmer test, strips of blotting paper are placed with one end under the lower eyelids and the distance soaked with tears after five minutes is measured, normal is wetting of > 10 mm in five minutes; < 5 mm in five minutes is diagnostic of defective tear production.

Mikulicz's syndrome is infiltration of salivary and tear ducts in lymphoma or CLL.

Heerfordt's syndrome (uveoparotid fever) is an extrapulmonary manifestation of sarcoid with bilateral uveitis in the eyes and parotid gland infiltration which is occasionally associated with a lower facial nerve palsy.

69 Answers (4 marks)

1. **E** Takayasu's arteritis
2. **C** Arch-aortogram

A young woman with systemic inflammatory disease. This does not apply for coarctation – in the proximal form the blood pressure should be higher in the *right* arm anyway.

She is too young for polymyalgia or tertiary syphilis. Polymyositis does not affect the large vessels.

Takayasu's arteritis ('pulseless disease') is a granulomatous vasculitis affecting large vessels in young women. Arteriography will show wasting or occlusion of the aorta and its major branches.

70 Answer (2 marks)

1. **D** Alcohol

Additional hepato toxic drugs or enzyme-inducing drugs increase the relative hepatotoxicity. Difficulties arise when the ingestion has occurred over a long period of time. For further details see the *British National Formulary (BNF)*.

Paper 4 – Answers

1 Answer (3 marks)

1. E   Echocardiogram

Septic emboli are seen on the soles of both feet. The most important differential diagnosis lies between Gram-negative meningitis and bacterial endocarditis. As a lumbar puncture is required for the diagnosis of meningitis and Down's syndrome has a high incidence of congenital heart disease (in particular VSD), this is the most appropriate answer.

2 Answers (7 marks)

1. B   DC shocks, intubation and cardiac compressions
2. C   Romano-Ward syndrome
3. D   Torsade-de-pointes tachycardia

Romano-Ward syndrome is one of the two congenital syndromes of prolonged QT interval, which is autosomal dominant with normal hearing (Jervell and Lange-Nielsen has recessive inheritance and neural deafness). Torsade-de-pointes arrhythmias are usually repetitive and self-terminating, but they can establish into VF. The QRS axis varies through the paroxysm. Acquired causes of QT prolongation include hypokalaemia, hypomagnesaemia, antihistamines, tricyclic antidepressants and some anti-arrhythmics (amiodarone, sotalol, flecainide).

Torsades-de-pointes is resistant to DC shock and best treated with iv magnesium (1 ampoule, 8 mmol).

Wolff-Parkinson-White (WPW) and Lown-Ganorg-Levine are syndromes of accessory pathways. WPW is characterised by slurred R upstrokes (delta waves). In Type **A** the QRS complex is above the baseline in V_1 (RBB pattern); in Type **B** the QRS complex is below the baseline (LBB pattern).

3 Answers (10 marks)

1. **B**   Aortic dissection
2. **A**   Myocardial infarction
    G   Left common carotid occlusion
3. **A**   Hand X-ray
4. **E**   Marfan's syndrome

Dissection of the aorta may ascend from the root to involve the great vessels as well as the coronary arteries. The dilatation of the ascending aorta causes aortic incompetence by dilatation of the valve rings.

The patient has an inferior infarction. The raised JVP may be due to compromise of the right ventricle or haemorrhage into the mediastinum. Normal heart sounds and jugular venous waveform are against pericardial haemorrhage. The cardiac complications account for the reduced life expectancy in **Marfan's syndrome** – the patients often die in their forties. Other features include upper dislocation of the lens of the eye, angioid streaks, increased armspan and arachnodactyly, high arched palate and recurrent pneumothoraces. Arachnodactyly, as defined by long, slender metacarpal bones, is of no diagnostic value.

4 Answers (8 marks)

1. **B**   Nephroblastoma (Wilms' tumour)
2. **B**   Urinary catecholamines
3. **E**   iv rehydration and alpha-blockade

Only approximately 50% of patients with **phaeochromocytoma** present with episodic hypertension – 50% of adults and up to 90% of children present with sustained hypertension which may remain unnoticed for a long period of time. Drug abuse may result in hypertensive crises, but is unlikely to result in left ventricular hypertrophy. Ten percent of phaeochromocytomas are malignant/bilateral/familial/extra-adrenal. Thoracic phaeochromocytomas tend to secrete noradrenaline only. The patients require alpha-blockade prior to surgery to prevent a hypertensive crisis and aggressive rehydration to prevent postoperative hypotension. Fibromuscular renal artery stenosis may present in younger patients, as may Conn's syndrome, the key feature being hypokalaemia. Nephroblastoma is a malignant embryological tumour of the kidney which usually presents before the age of five with a large renal mass and haematuria.

5 Answer (2 marks)

1. **A**   Cystic fibrosis

The chest X-ray shows cystic bronchiectases. All answers given are a recognised cause for this but at this age cystic fibrosis is the least likely.

6 Answers (5 marks)

1. **E** Coarctation and bicuspid aortic valve
2. **B** Chromosomal analysis

The patient has **Turner's syndrome**. Over one-third of patients have coarctation and this is associated with a bicuspid aortic valve. Diagnosis can simply be made on a buccal smear which shows the absence of a Barr body. A hand X-ray may show short 4th and 5th metacarpals, which is also a feature of pseudohypoparathyroidism and pseudo-pseudohypoparathyroidism.

7 Answer (2 marks)

1. **A** Cholangiocarcinoma

The patient is jaundiced with a vascularised and ulcerated nodule. This proved to be a skin metastasis of a bile duct tumour.

8 Answers (5 marks)

1. **A** Dilating (congestive) cardiomyopathy
2. **E** Alcohol abuse

The patient has cardiomegaly with a poor ejection fraction ('a large floppy heart'). HOCM and aortic stenosis show concentric hypertrophy of the myocardium with dilatation only in the final stages. Restrictive cardiomyopathy is a rare condition with endocardial fibrosis, the main differential diagnosis being constrictive pericarditis.

Causes of **dilating cardiomyopathy** include autoimmune, post-viral, drug-induced (cytotoxic and tricyclic antidepressants) and alcohol. The patient has macrocytic anaemia which tips the balance towards a social cause.

9 Answers (4 marks)

1. **D** Mitral stenosis
2. **C** Pulmonary hypertension

There is increased pressure in the left atrium, the lungs and the right heart. The gradient between the atrial pressure and the diastolic pressure in the left ventricle indicates **mitral stenosis**. There is also a significant pressure gradient across the pulmonary capillary bed. The pulmonary vascular resistance (PVR) can be calculated as the mean pressure difference between pulmonary artery and left atrium, divided by the cardiac output. In this case it is $24/3 = 8$. Normal PVR is < 1; values > 8 indicate high risk for surgery.

10 Answer (3 marks)

1. B Bendroflumethiazide (bendrofluazide)

In terms of long-term beneficial effects there is not much difference in the major classes of antihypertensive. Choice therefore needs to take into account co-existing problems such as right heart failure (diuretics), diabetic nephropathy (ACE inhibitors), ischaemic heart disease (beta-blockers) etc. Bendroflumethiazide (bendrofluazide) is currently the first-line antihypertensive of choice in the absence of any complicating factors.

11 Answers (5 marks)

1. E Complete heart block
2. A Thrombolysis

The patient has pain, early enzyme rise and acute complete heart block, consistent with an **acute inferior infarction**. Prognosis of this is usually good with recovery within two weeks. Unless the patient is haemodynamically compromised, pacing should be withheld.

12 Answer (2 marks)

1. A Lateral skull X-ray

The patient has the facial features of **acromegaly**. This is confirmed by high growth hormone levels, which fail to suppress in the oral glucose test. The size of the adenoma needs to be assessed with an MR scan of the pituitary – the lateral skull X-ray is useless for this purpose. Functional assessment is best made with a combined pituitary function test, which also assesses the function of the residual normal pituitary. Other important complications include hypertension, cardiac failure, diabetes and nerve entrapment (i.e. carpel tunnel syndrome).

13 Answer (2 marks)

1. E Eisenmenger's complex

The patient has a step-down of saturation in the left ventricle with a slight increase in left-sided pressures. Eponyms should be generally avoided, but Eisenmenger's *complex* indicates shunt reversal associated with VSD. Eisenmenger's *syndrome* denotes the reversal of a left-to-right shunt due to the development of pulmonary hypertension without specifying the underlying cause. At this stage, the patients are inoperable.

14 Answer (3 marks)

1. C   Sarcoidosis

The patient has a restrictive lung defect with reduction in FVC and FEV_1, but a preserved ratio (86%). Other complications of sarcoid to be borne in mind for MRCP are facial nerve involvement, pituitary involvement, bone involvement and hypercalcaemia.

15 Answers (8 marks)

1. C   Radio-isotope bone scan
2. D   Metastatic carcinoma
3. A   Leucoerythroblastic film due to bone marrow invasion
4. A   iv saline

The patient presents with symptoms of hypercalcaemia. The following causes usually suppress to normal levels with oral steroids: sarcoidosis, myeloma, hypervitaminosis and Addison's disease. Ectopic PTH production and bone metastases suppress to a variable degree; hyperparathyroidism is not affected.

Hyperparathyroidism is also ruled out by the normal phosphate. The low globulin fraction (total protein – albumin) and low ESR are against myeloma.

The patient has erythroid and myeloid precursors in the bloodstream indicating bone marrow invasion or myelofibrosis, but there is no hepatosplenomegaly.

In combination, this makes a **metastasised carcinoma** with bone metastases (the patient has back pain) and bone marrow invasion the most likely cause. In a female of that age, the likely primaries are breast and bronchus.

Treatment of hypercalcaemia is with hyperhydration with intravenous saline – cardiac and renal function allowing. Addition of loop diuretics such as furosemide (frusemide) will increase renal excretion of calcium.

Treatment with diphosphonates is a further option. Steroids can be used in hypercalcaemia due to myeloma.

16 Answers (7 marks)

1. **E**   Hereditary vitamin D-dependent rickets
2. **C**   Vitamin D levels
3. **B**   Autosomal recessive

The results are of a hypocalcaemia with secondary hyperparathyroidism (in primary hyperparathyroidism, there would be elevation of the calcium). The radiograph is typical for rickets. The family history suggests a congenital, possibly a familial disorder (confirmed by the third question). The history also leads away from common causes of vitamin D deficiency, such as poor diet, malabsorption and drug-induced.

The differential diagnosis now lies between vitamin D-dependent rickets (autosomal recessive) and familial hypophosphataemic rickets (X-linked dominant). **Vitamin D-dependent** rickets has two types. The much more common type I has a failure of 1-hydroxylation of cholecalciferol in the kidney. Serum levels of $1,25\text{-}(OH)_2\text{-}D$ are <u>low</u>. There is excellent response to small doses of exogenous vitamin D and $1\alpha\text{-}OH\text{-}D$. In the rarer type II, there is end-organ resistance to $1,25\text{-}(OH)_2\text{-}D$ and serum levels are high.

In familial hypophosphataemic rickets (vitamin D-**resistant** rickets) there is profound renal tubular loss of phosphate with a relatively normal calcium. The parathormone is normal. Treatment here is with oral phosphate, as well as vitamin D. Due to the calcium/phosphate imbalance, there is secondary end-organ resistance to vitamin D.

Assuming the data given are correct, the disease has been passed with male-to-male transmission from grandfather to grandson, skipping a generation. Skipping a generation indicates a recessive disorder, which suggests that both parents are carriers of the faulty gene. Male-to-male transmission excludes an X-linked condition.

17 Answers (4 marks)

1. **B** Klinefelter's syndrome
2. **E** Testosterone replacement

The presence of Barr bodies in a man indicates an extra X chromosome, in keeping with **Klinefelter's syndrome** (47 XXY). This is confirmed by an increased lower/upper body segment ratio (normal less than one). The patient would also have gynaecomastia and underdeveloped external genitalia. Patients with Klinefelter's syndrome patients are infertile. There is a deficiency of androgens leading to an increased growth of long bones. The result is a eunuchoid growth pattern with increased armspan and long legs. Testicular biopsy shows fibrosis and hyalinisation of the seminiferous tubules which results in small, firm testes and azoospermia, but this is not diagnostic of the condition. Some patients may show a mosaic pattern in the chromosomal analysis/mixture of (46 XY and 47 XXY) leading to a milder expression of the disease with preserved fertility in some individuals. Treatment is with depot injections of testosterone which will produce virilisation and prevent osteoporosis, but fertility cannot be restored.

Testicular feminisation is an end-organ resistance to androgens leading to completed development of secondary female characteristics. The patients grow up normally as girls until investigations for amenorrhoea reveal the male genome (46 XY).

18 Answer (2 marks)

1. **D** Oral nimodipine

The patient has a cystic lesion with a blood fluid level within it and further blood anterior to it. These are the appearances of a haemorrhagic metastasis (i.e. from a hypernephroma, melanoma or bronchial carcinoma). The less likely differential diagnosis is of a haemorrhagic brain abscess. Nimodipine is of use in the initial treatment of subarachnoid haemorrhage.

19 Answers (5 marks)

1. **F** Neck ultrasound
    G Parathormone levels
2. **E** Multiple endocrine neoplasia (MEN) type 2

MEN type II (Sipple syndrome) is an autosomal dominant syndrome of primary hyperparathyroidism (more commonly adenoma), phaeochromocytoma and medullary carcinoma of the thyroid (J.H. Sipple, US chest physician). If associated with marfanoid habitus and multiple neurinoma of skin and mucous membranes, it is termed 'type IIb'. Medullary carcinoma of the thyroid on its own is also transmitted as an autosomal dominant trait.

MEN type I (Wermer's syndrome), also autosomal dominant, is a combination of primary hyperparathyroidism (more commonly hyperplasia), variable pancreatic tumours (gastrinoma, glucagonoma, insulinoma, etc.) and pituitary tumours.

20 Answer (2 marks)

1. **D** Renal cell carcinoma

The patient has neurofibromatosis type I. Renal cell carcinoma, particularly bilateral, is a complication of von Hippel-Lindau syndrome.

21 Answers (5 marks)

1. **B** Renal tubular acidosis (RTA) type I
2. **A** Plain abdominal radiograph

The patient is unable to acidify his urine after an acid load. This is combined with a metabolic acidosis and a paradoxical hypokalaemia. The features are of **renal tubular acidosis type I**. It is a defect of proton excretion in the distal tubule, as opposed to proximal bicarbonate wastage in RTA type II. In type II the urine shows a normal depression of pH to < 5.4 in the ammonium chloride test.

There is a high incidence of renal stones and a sensitive way of detecting these is with the plain X-ray.

22 Answers (5 marks)

1. **A**   Hypogonadotrophic hypogonadism
2. **C**   Craniopharyngioma

The patient has low gonadotrophins which show a delayed response to GN-RH. This indicates a functioning but chronically understimulated pituitary, in keeping with a hypothalamic syndrome. In addition, the patient is hyperosmolar (plasma osmolality 305 mOsmol/kg) in the presence of dilute urine, suggesting associated diabetes insipidus.

The combination of adiposity, central diabetes insipidus, hypogonadism and dwarfism has also been termed as 'dystrophy adiposo-genitalis' and is part of a syndrome caused by a **craniopharyngioma**. This benign tumour of Rathke's pouch can cause variable symptoms of pituitary compression or hypothalamic dysfunction. Fifteen percent occur within the pituitary fossa, they usually manifest themselves after the sixth year, but up to 50% remain asymptomatic until the third decade.

The patient may also present with headaches, bi-temporal hemianopia and suprasellar calcification on radiographs/CT. Besides hormone replacement, the patients frequently require surgery as the tumour is not radiosensitive.

23 Answer (2 marks)

1. **C**   Emphysema

The patient has a large-volume chest with initial sharp rise in expiratory flow, but subsequent airways collapse. Spirometry is explained in detail on the website of the British Thoracic Society.

24 Answers (8 marks)

1. **C**   Primary sclerosing cholangitis
2. **E**   Abdominal ultrasound
3. **B**   Metastasised carcinoma of the colon
4. **E**   CT of the abdomen

In addition, the findings are suspicious of an extrinsic compression of the bile duct at the porta hepatis. This is most likely due to a nodal mass. With a history of active ulcerative colitis greater than ten years, a metastasised carcinoma of the colon has to be considered. The CT would assess the large bowel as well as the liver and the extrahepatic bile duct. Other complications of ulcerative colitis include amyloid, seronegative arthritis, erythema nodosum, pyoderma gangrenosum and uveitis and episcleritis. Fistulae and abscesses are features of Crohn's disease caused by transmural inflammation of the bowel.

25 Answers (12 marks)

1. **C** Blood glucose
   F Serum ferritin
2. **B** Haemochromatosis
3. **A** Liver biopsy
4. **A** Autosomal recessive inheritance
5. **B** Portal hypertension
   G Hepatocellular carcinoma

The patient has the key features of skin pigmentation, hepatomegaly, degenerative joint disease and features of diabetes mellitus. **Haemochromatosis** is an inherited disease characterised by excessive iron deposition throughout the body. This is exacerbated by excess alcohol intake. Expression is milder in women due to the menstrual blood loss.

An iron stain (e.g. Pearl's) will demonstrate the increased iron content in the liver (which incidentally is also seen on MR scanning).

Up to one-third of patients who develop liver cirrhosis progress to development of hepatoma. The presence of cirrhosis in this patient is indicated by the reduction in hepatic size and splenomegaly.

As with most inborn errors of metabolism, haemochromatosis is an autosomal recessive trait. This pattern of inheritance is characterised by the fact that not every generation is affected and that male-to-male transmission occurs.

26 Answers (4 marks)

1. **B** Zieve's syndrome
2. **E** Spurious hyponatraemia

The patient has a combination of hypercholesterolaemia and haemolytic anaemia, as indicated by the increased reticulocyte count (greater than 2%) and increased unconjugated bilirubin. Haptoglobin estimation would show this to be reduced. On the social background given, alcoholism has to be assumed and the triad of these features is known as **Zieve's syndrome** (alcoholism, hypercholesterolaemia and haemolytic anaemia). Sodium that low indicates that the patient is either very ill, or that there has been error in the estimation. In hyperlipidaemia the sodium is mainly contained within the aqueous phase of the blood sample, whilst the blood sample volume is increased by the lipid phase, giving a falsely low reading. Hyperaldosteronism secondary to liver cirrhosis may lead to hypernatraemia.

27 Answer (2 marks)

1. **C** Spirometry and reversibility

The patient is most likely to have obstructive airways disease and formal lung functions tests are indicated. Depending on the results, differential diagnoses of extrinsic allergic alveolitis and fibrosing alveolitis may need to be considered.

28 Answers (3 marks)

1. **C** Whipple's disease
2. **D** Polymerase chain reaction (PCR) from duodenal biopsy

Whipple's disease is caused by *Tropheryma whippelii*, a bacterium that can be identified within macrophages under the electron microscope. The identification of PAS-positive glycoproteins within macrophages in the lamina propria of the small bowel is diagnostic; PCR techniques will allow direct identification of the rod. Typically affecting middle-aged men, it presents with diarrhoea, abdominal pain and malabsorption. Extraintestinal manifestations include fever, polyarthritis, polyserositis, lymphadenopathy and skin pigmentation. Therapy is with prolonged (3–6 months) antibiotics (e.g. tetracycline).

29 Answers (5 marks)

1. **E** Hydatid disease
2. **E** CT brain

The history suggests a rupture of a **hydatid liver cyst**, as indicated by an allergic reaction, fever and bilirubinuria. Cerebral hydatid cysts have to be excluded in view of the fit.

30 Answers (6 marks)

1. **C** Lag storage
2. **E** Wilson's disease
3. **D** Ceruloplasmin levels

Lag storage curves are also seen in renal failure, gastrectomy and some normal patients. **Wilson's disease** (hepatolenticular degeneration) is an autosomal recessive defect of copper excretion. Ceruloplasmin, the serum transport and storage protein, is markedly reduced. Biliary excretion of copper is impaired, leading to increased renal excretion and deposition of copper throughout the body. Deposition in liver, CNS, cornea (Kayser-Fleischer ring), renal failure/type 2 renal tubular acidosis, cardiomyopathy and haemolytic anaemia can be seen. Renal excretion is increased with the chelating agent D-penicillamine, which is the therapy of choice.

31 Answer (3 marks)

1. **D**   ACE inhibitor

The patient will also require optimising of glucose control as the HbA_1c is raised. However, the best added therapy is with an ACE inhibitor.

32 Answers (10 marks)

1. **D**   Anti-phospholipid antibodies
2. **B**   Autoimmune haemolytic anaemia
3. **E**   Autoantibody screen
4. **A**   Retinal vein branch occlusion
5. **B**   Aspirin

A young woman has recurrent thromboses. This suggests a hypercoagulable state but may also be due to a red cell defect (HbC, HbS) or an increase in red cells or platelets.

The APTT, however, shows a paradoxical prolongation which does not correct after addition of normal plasma. This suggests an active inhibiting factor, such as anti-phospholipid antibodies. The antibodies interfere with the test, giving a false result. In addition, the patient has evidence of an autoimmune haemolytic anaemia with a positive Coombs' test (the red cells are laden with autoantibodies) and a compensatory reticulocytosis.

Subsequently, the patient developed renal impairment and hypertension. The patient has **systemic lupus erythematosus**.

Venous occlusion and haemorrhage has occurred in the eye (arterial occlusion would lead to a pale (anaemic) area in the fundus). Longstanding significant hypertension is excluded by the absence of hypertensive changes. The treatment for this is aspirin – more aggressive anticoagulation will exacerbate the retinal haemorrhage.

33 Answers (4 marks)

1. **C** Fibrin degradation products (FDP)
2. **B** Amniotic fluid embolus

The patient has **disseminated intravascular coagulation (DIC)** as evidenced by intravascular haemolysis (red cell fragmentation), thrombocytopenia and abnormal clotting, in particular the thrombin time indicating consumption of the clotting factors.

The most likely cause is an obstetric complication, as it would be unusual for infection to cause this degree of disease within such a short period of time, and the white cell count is relatively low for extensive septicaemia. Multiple tests are appropriate in this scenario, but FDP levels and blood cultures are the most sensible combination, as one test confirms the diagnosis whereas the other one excludes an important differential diagnosis.

In DIC the thrombin time is prolonged by a) consumption of fibrinogen and b) the presence of FDP which interfere with the formation of crosslinked fibrin. This is partially corrected for by the addition of protamine sulphate, although this is not a test required to make the diagnosis.

There are many causes of DIC, the commonest being sepsis. In a young woman other causes would include abruptio placentae, septic abortion and toxic shock syndrome.

The most important step in the management is treatment of the underlying condition. Severe haemorrhage may require fresh frozen plasma.

34 Answers (5 marks)

1. **C** Immune electrophoresis
2. **C** Cold haemagglutinin disease

The absence of a blanching phase preceding purple discoloration in the hands exposed to cold indicates that this is not true Raynaud's syndrome.

The patient has delayed haemolysis of one blood sample after cooling and re-warming. This is essentially the basis of the Donath-Landsteiner reaction which confirms the presence of cold haemagglutinins. These are found in **chronic cold haemagglutinin disease** where there are complement-fixating monoclonal antibodies of IgM class against red cells. It is a condition of the elderly which may precede lymphoma. Chronic haemolysis leads to pigment gallstones.

A similar picture is found following infection in children where it is called **paroxysmal cold haemoglobinuria**. It is seen in congenital syphilis and after viral infections, such as measles, mumps or chickenpox. The antibodies, however, are polyclonal IgG.

35 Answer (2 marks)

1. B Bronchoscopy

The patient has pleural calcification with a 'holly leaf' on the left and over both diaphragmatic surfaces indicating asbestos exposure. A diffuse density over the right thorax without loss of volume is strongly suspicious of a pleural-based mass. Confirmation of this cannot be done with a bronchoscopy. A full respiratory work-up is required to assess the respiratory reserve and coexistent restrictive defects and asbestosis.

36 Answer (1 mark)

1. B Haemolysis

An old favourite!

The discrepancy is between the fact that the patient is, by definition, reasonably well (as he is an outpatient) and the grossly abnormal biochemical profile which, if correct, suggests that the patient is probably unconscious, if not dead. The answer lies in **delayed processing** of a sample which was left uncentrifuged on the shelf overnight and has haemolysed.

37 Answers (9 marks)

1. B Left sensorineural deficit
2. E Lenticonus
3. D Alport's syndrome
4. C Progressive renal failure

Alport's syndrome is a rare, inherited condition primarily affecting males. Inheritance is usually X-linked recessive although other traits have been described. The typical ocular abnormality is a conical deformity of the anterior aspect of the lens which may present as an apparent dark spot on fundoscopy. Sensorineural nerve deafness is well described. The condition presents with haematuria and nephritis in childhood or adolescence. The renal failure is progressive.

38 Answers (8 marks)

1. **C** Haemorrhage into a cyst
2. **A** Adult polycystic disease
3. **D** *Pneumocystis carinii* pneumonia (PCP)

The patient is at high risk for HIV infection. The combination of bilateral mid-zone infiltrates with or without cyst formation and desaturation on exercise are typical of PCP.

4. **E** Subarachnoid haemorrhage

For the purpose of the exam, a history of adoption or foster parents should raise the suspicion about an inherited condition.

Adult polycystic disease is an autosomal dominant condition with a gene defect on the short arm of chromosome 16. Small cysts are formed in infancy which increase in size throughout life. Manifestation is usually in the second or third decade with renal failure, hypertension or clinical signs of haemorrhage into a cyst (loin pain or haematuria). It can affect all parenchymatous organs, in particular, the liver, pancreas and spleen, but huge cystic masses of both kidneys are the typical finding. The patients have an increased incidence of berry aneurysms of the circle of Willis (in 20–25%) with the associated risk of subarachnoid haemorrhage. A normal brain scan does **not** exclude SAH!

The autosomal recessive condition of infantile polycystic kidney disease is not a realistic differential diagnosis as these present either antenatally or within the first five years of life. There is an associated risk of hepatic fibrosis and portal hypertension. Patients rarely reach the second decade. In both conditions, genetic counselling is essential.

In APKD there is also a risk of hypertensive stroke which has to be differentiated from a subarachnoid haemorrhage. Other complications include renal calculi, UTI and rupture or infection of cysts.

39 Answers (2 marks)

1. **E** Myotonic dystrophy
2. **A** Cardiomyopathy

Besides muscle weakness, fatiguability and cataracts, the patient may also display frontal balding, ptosis and subnormal intelligence. Myotonic dystrophy affects the heart, causing cardiomyopathy and conduction defects. It is autosomal dominant with onset in the 3rd and 4th decade and slow progression.

40 Answers (4 marks)

1. **C** Right ventricular infarction
2. **A** Thrombosis of right coronary artery

The right ventricular filling pressure is high, while left ventricular filling pressure (pulmonary capillary wedge pressure) is low. This indicates that the right ventricle is predominantly affected. The sinus node is supplied by a branch of the right coronary artery.

41 Answers (4 marks)

1. **A** Rhabdomyolosis
2. **E** Electric shock

The discrepancy between the elevation of urea/creatinine and ALT/AST indicate that these changes are secondary to damage to striated muscle and not to hepatic or renal failure. The extensive tissue damage from electrocution also causes hyperkalaemia and calcium levels may be low.

42 Answers (5 marks)

1. **C** Salt-wasting nephropathy
2. **E** Renal tuberculosis

The patient clearly has **salt wastage**, which is an unspecific indicator of tubular damage. Causes include analgesics, chronic infection (including TB!) and obstruction, heavy metals (including Wilson's disease), amyloid, recovering acute tubular necrosis, and nephrocalcinosis.

Sterile pyuria (> 10 white cells/μl) is strongly suggestive of **TB**, but may also be seen in stone disease, interstitial nephritis and papillary necrosis.

43 Answer (2 marks)

1. **E** Isotope renogram

The patient has a short left renal artery stenosis. This is asymmetric and close to the origin, indicating this to be an atheromatous plaque. The artery is only 50–60% stenosed suggesting this is not clinically relevant. A MAG-3 renogram will quantify the respective renal function.

44 Answers (4 marks)

1. **D** *Treponema pallidum* haemagglutination test (TPHA)
2. **B** Jarisch-Herxheimer reaction

For the purpose of the exam, a travelling salesman and the Far East equal an infectious, usually venereal, disease. The clinical features are of **secondary syphilis** which can produce aseptic meningitis. The 'snail track ulcers' are infective, but microscopy and culture are unreliable. TPHA is a useful screening test, FTA (fluorescence-treponema-antibody-absorption test) is more specific and confirms active infection. The VDRL test is non-specific but a reasonable monitor of disease activity.

The Jarisch-Herxheimer reaction is caused by release of large amounts of endotoxins due to a good response to antibiotics. It usually occurs within 24 hours and can be ameliorated by concomitant prednisolone cover.

Treatment of syphilis is with intramuscular depot penicillin (1.2 g/day) for two weeks.

45 Answers (7 marks)

1. **B** Duchenne muscular dystrophy (DMD)
2. **E** Creatinine phosphokinase (CPK) levels
3. **B** Death as a teenager

DMD is an X-linked recessive disorder with some spontaneous mutations and an incidence of 1:3000. The boys manifest the disease within five years, become disabled within 10 years and die before 20 years of age. Clinically, there is a progressive proximal myopathy, the boys become unwilling to run and play and they need to 'climb up their legs' to an erect position (Gower's sign).

An associated cardiomyopathy is frequently found, CPK levels are raised one hundred- to two hundred-fold and the EMG shows evidence of myopathy. Muscle biopsy (second-line test in a four-year-old) shows necrosis with regeneration, disorganisation and fatty replacement.

The main differential diagnosis is with Becker's dystrophy which manifests in later childhood (5–10), leads to disability in the 20s and death occurs in middle-age. Cardiac involvement is unusual; inheritance is also X-linked recessive.

46 Answers (9 marks)

1. **E** Left-sided thoracic tumour
2. **C** Superior orbital fissure meningioma
3. **A** Right sensorineural deficit
4. **D** Neurofibromatosis type II

The patient has features of **Brown-Séquard syndrome**. A unilateral lesion causes an ipsilateral upper motor neurone deficit and ipsilateral posterior column signs. As the spinothalamic fibres cross in the spine at segmental level, deficits to sharp pain and temperature are found on the contralateral side below the level of the lesion. Hyperaesthesia at the costal margin indicates a lesion in the mid-thoracic spine. A disc problem would not cause posterior column signs.

The motor deficit in the left eye affects the 3rd as well as the 6th cranial nerve; the lack of parasympathetic drive (mydriasis) indicates nerve compression. The 3rd, 4th and 6th cranial nerves run together in the lateral wall of the cavernous sinus and enter the orbit in the superior orbital fissure. Cavernous sinus thrombosis is a dramatic event with chemosis and proptosis of the affected side.

In **Weber's test**, the tuning fork placed centrally on the forehead is appreciated louder in an ear with conduction deficit (the background noise from the environment is reduced and the sound conducted through the skull to the functioning nerve is appreciated louder). In a sensorineural problem the sound is conducted less well through the damaged nerve and, therefore, lateralisation is to the normal side.

In **Rinne's test**, a middle ear problem causing a conduction deficit will lead to bone conduction through the mastoid being appreciated louder than air conduction. With a neural deficit, both modalities are reduced equally, air conduction still being appreciated better.

The patient has multiple defects at different sites caused by nerve compression. The most likely cause is multiple benign tumours as seen in type II (central) neurofibromatosis. Bilateral acoustic neuromas are the classical presentation, transmitted on chromosome 22 with autosomal dominant inheritance. The patients rarely have skin manifestations and there is no association with phaeochromocytoma/MEN or the other typical features of NFI (autosomal dominant; chromosome 17). The two are separate entities; NFI is nine times more common.

47 Answers (3 marks)

1. **D** Left oculomotor palsy
2. **C** HbA$_{1c}$

The patient is unable to fully adduct the left eye as indicated by the eccentric light reflex in the pupil. In addition there is mydriasis indicating a complex lower motor neurone lesion of the left 3rd cranial nerve. The patient is alert and co-operative and a mononeuritis multiplex (i.e. diabetes) is the most sensible of the given answers.

48 Answer (2 marks)

1. C Erythropoietin

If the patient was on haemodialysis, blood transfusion would be the more appropriate treatment for symptomatic anaemia. Intravenous administration of iron chelates is associated with a very high risk of adverse reactions.

49 Answers (6 marks)

1. C Subarachnoid haemorrhage (SAH)
2. C Sturge-Weber syndrome
3. E MR Scan of the brain

The xanthochromia indicates that blood was present in the subarachnoid space prior to the traumatic lumbar puncture. Xanthochromia (yellow staining) of CSF occurs 2–4 hours after haemorrhage.

The usual cause for this is a ruptured berry aneurysm (75%); occasionally other vascular abnormalities. A normal brain CT does not exclude a SAH. Intravenous contrast *does not improve* visualisation of subarachnoid blood.

The capillary angiomata found in **Sturge-Weber syndrome** on the leptomeninges cause seizures, focal cerebral atrophy and calcification, in a serpiginous pattern ('tramline'). Rupture is rare and incidental aneurysms need to be excluded.

50 Answers (3 marks)

1. A CT scan of the brain
2. E Benign intracranial hypertension

The young woman is overweight and on the Pill, two risk factors for benign intracranial hypertension, which is confirmed by lumbar puncture. The ventricular system is most likely to show normal appearances on CT scan. The importance of the CT scan is to exclude an obstructing lesion and this should be done prior to LP. Treatment is required to prevent blindness. If weight reduction and stopping the Pill fails, repeated lumbar punctures or a shunt may be required. The condition may be primary or secondary.

51 Answers (6 marks)

1. **E** Wernicke's syndrome
2. **C** iv thiamine
3. **B** Oral chlordiazepoxide

The macrocytic anaemia and chronic subdural haemorrhage in a vagrant suggest chronic alcohol abuse. The rapid onset of the typical triad of ataxia, confusion and nystagmus are diagnostic of **Wernicke's encephalopathy**. The chronic thiamine deficiency is acutely exacerbated by the high carbohydrate intake with hospital food. This results in haemorrhagic necrosis in the limbic system, particularly the mamillary bodies and the brainstem. Intravenous thiamine or combined vitamin B compounds need to be given with great care due to possible anaphylaxis.

The impaired clotting due to liver damage forbids intramuscular injections. Administration of hypertonic saline can result in central pontine myelinolysis.

52 Answer (3 marks)

1. **D** Neurosurgical referral

The patient has freshly clotted blood in the subarachnoid space, seen as hyperdense (white) outline of the brain surface and the sulci. This is apparently centred over the right sylvian fissure and the most likely bleed is therefore from an aneurysm at the trifurcation of the right middle cerebral artery. Patients with a Glasgow Coma Scale score of < 9 should be intubated and are therefore not suitable for oral medication.

53 Answers (7 marks)

1. **D** High-resolution CT Scan
   G 24 h ECG
2. **B** Sarcoidosis
3. **D** Systemic steroids
   E Cardiac pacing

A young Afro-Caribbean woman presents with a systemic disease characterised by a restrictive pulmonary defect, lymphadenopathy, polyarthralgia and a cardiac conduction defect. In the presence of hypercalcaemia, the diagnosis is **sarcoidosis**.

The ECG findings indicate a bi-fascicular block (RBBB plus left-anterior hemi-block) with an associated first-degree AV block. This heralds a tri-fascicular block/complete AV block and pacing must be considered. Acute sarcoidosis responds well to steroids. Chronic pulmonary sarcoid and cardiac involvement have a poor prognosis.

54 Answers (8 marks)

1. **C** Urinary protein and acetylcholine receptor antibodies
2. **D** Drug-induced myasthenia
3. **C** Stop penicillamine
4. **A** Rheumatoid lung

A woman with autoimmune disease (RA, thyrotoxicosis) develops diplopia and proximal weakness with fatiguability. She is on penicillamine and has evidence of recognised side-effects (thrombocytopenia, hypoproteinaemia with renal impairment). **Drug-induced myasthenia** is more likely than myasthenia gravis, although primary MG cannot be excluded on the basis of the findings given. Patients with HLA-BW35 and DR1 are said to have a higher incidence of drug-induced myasthenia; patients with HLA-DR3 generally show a higher side-effect rate with penicillamine.

Lung changes found in rheumatoid arthritis are pleural effusions, pulmonary nodules, basal fibrosis and infection secondary to immune suppression.

Causes for **basal fibrosis** include cryptogenic fibrosing alveolitis, asbestosis, connective tissue diseases and drug side-effects (bleomycin, cyclophosphamide, nitrofurantoin).

55 Answers (5 marks)

1. **G** Bronchoscopy
   I Contrast-enhanced CT of the thorax
2. **A** Bronchial carcinoid

Bronchial carcinoid (bronchial adenoma) is a low-grade malignant tumour of the APUD system which may produce serotonin or ACTH. The other end of the spectrum is represented by small cell carcinoma. These tumours are usually endobronchial and present with haemoptysis or localised obstruction. The serotonin secretion may produce local pulmonary fibrosis or endocardial/valve fibrosis of the left heart. Full-blown carcinoid syndrome is rare. The benign, class I carcinoid is ten times commoner in females and the five-year survival rate is 95%. Therapy is by resection. High-resolution CT of the chest is exclusively used for the assessment of interstitial lung disease and is unsuitable for assessment of focal lesions due to the large gaps between the thin slices.

56 Answer (2 marks)

1. C Thyrotoxicosis

The patient has elevated T3 and T4 with suppressed TSH, indicating true hyperthyroidism. Viral thyroiditis (de Quervain's) presents as a flu-like illness. Inflammation of the gland tends to liberate the thyroxine stores with a sequence of hyperthyroidism, through to hypothyroidism and recovery in most cases.

Riedel's fibrosis of the thyroid leads to progressive hypothyroidism, whereas Hashimoto's presents with an acute inflammatory-type reaction of the thyroid.

The commonest cause of thyrotoxicosis is Graves' disease with stimulating receptor antibodies. Important differential diagnosis for the exam is factitious thyroxine administration.

57 Answer (2 marks)

1. B Occupational asthma

The patient has evidence of mild airway obstruction at rest, with increased reactivity in the methacholine test. A hyper-reactive system should have normal values unless provoked.

Other differential diagnoses for a 'veterinarian' for MRCP include brucellosis, extrinsic allergic alveolitis, psittacosis, rabies and Orf.

58 Answers (5 marks)

1. C *Mycoplasma* pneumonia
2. A Direct Coombs' test

In *Mycoplasma* infection, the presence of cold agglutinins results in haemolysis. This occurs *in vivo* with cooling of the blood in the periphery. Blood samples also frequently show haemolysis by the time they arrive in the lab. There is often a discrepancy between dramatic changes on the chest X-ray and relative well-being of the patient. Treatment is with macrolide antibiotics (erythromycin).

59 Answer (2 marks)

1. C Myasthenia gravis

The patient has alveolar hypoventilation. Associated with diplopia, this indicates a neuromuscular disorder. The likeliest is **myasthenia gravis**; possible differential diagnoses include botulism or overdose of muscle relaxants. Guillain-Barré syndrome would produce sensory signs and more extensive peripheral involvement before affecting the ocular muscles.

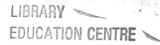

60 Answer (2 marks)

1. **E** None

A consultation with the anaesthetist would probably be appropriate, although the potassium is only mildly elevated and patients with chronic renal failure are relatively tolerant to hyperkalaemia. Intravenous fluids would be a bad option in terminal renal failure.

61 Answers (4 marks)

1. **C** Arterial blood gases
2. **D** Pulmonary fibrosis

The patient presents subacutely after being started on **non-steroidal anti-inflammatory treatment**. Complications of this include precipitation of asthma, GI bleed, deterioration of renal function, sodium and fluid retention, and allergic reaction. ESR would be useful to confirm a flare-up of the disease, whereas the blood gases are unlikely to provide any further information in the context of normal pulse oximetry and pulmonary function tests. A single normal lung function measurement does not exclude bronchospasm, which may be intermittent.

Drugs that induce pulmonary fibrosis are nitrofurantoin and immune suppressants (bleomycin, cyclophosphamide and busulfan). This is a *long-term* complication. Rheumatoid arthritis may cause lower lobe fibrosis, but the lung function tests show no evidence of it.

62 Answers (5 marks)

1. **E** O_2 administration
2. **D** iv doxapram

The patient has **type II respiratory failure**. The main respiratory drive in this context is hypoxia. The commonest cause for removing the respiratory stimulant is administration of high concentrations of oxygen, either directly or during nebulising of bronchodilators, which will cause acute worsening of the respiratory failure. Intravenous respiratory stimulants have to be administered with close monitoring and great caution. Intubation in type II failure is controversial and usually only recommended if there is an immediate correctable cause.

63 Answers (4 marks)

1. **C** Extrinsic allergic alveolitis (EAA)
2. **A** Apical fibrosis

EAA is a hypersensitivity reaction, usually to fungi (farmers, malt workers, cheese workers, the list is endless) or animal protein (pigeons). The *acute* form presents with fever and flu-like symptoms shortly after exposure to the allergen. *Chronic* exposure causes fibrosis of the upper aspects of the lungs. Causes of apical fibrosis include tuberculosis (calcification!), sarcoidosis (usually mid-zone), ankylosing spondylitis (often cavitating), EAA and other inhaled agents, except for asbestos. Mnemonic **PASTE: P**MF, **A**nkylosing spondylitis, **S**arcoid, **T**B, **E**AA.

64 Answer (2 marks)

1. **B** Coal dust inhalation

The patient has basal fibrosis with reticular shadowing and loss of distinction of the cardiac contour ('shaggy heart').

Coal miners' pneumoconiosis typically shows numerous well-defined nodules while the patients are relatively asymptomatic. The causes for basal fibrosis are: fibrosing alveolitis, asbestosis, connective tissue diseases and drug side-effects (cytostatics, amiodarone, nitrofurantoin).

65 Answers (7 marks)

1. **D** Sarcoidosis
2. **E** Skull X-ray and urine osmolality
3. **C** Central diabetes insipidus

Eosinophilic granuloma is the benign end of the spectrum of *Langerhans cell histiocytosis* (formerly histiocytosis X), usually presenting in early adulthood with respiratory problems. Most of the patients are smokers. The typical findings are reticulo-nodular changes which, if progressive, result in cyst formation and honeycombing. The cysts may rupture and pneumothorax is common. The lung volumes are usually preserved. It may affect other parts of the body, notably the bones where the commonest site is the parietal bone in the skull. The classic appearance is of punched-out lesions with a bevelled edge. Involvement of the pituitary may cause central diabetes insipidus. (The patient has a serum osmolality of 305 mOsmol/kg and polyuria). The disease is often self-limiting and treatment with steroids is sometimes effective. Aggressive forms of the childhood disease (Hand-Schüller-Christian disease) and the progressive form of infancy (Letterer-Siwe disease) carry a poor prognosis, and are associated with more systemic features, such as skin involvement, lymphadenopathy and hepatosplenomegaly.

Tuberose sclerosis and neurofibromatosis may also lead to cystic changes in the lungs.

Lymphangio-leiomyomatosis is a progressive hyperplasia of smooth muscles in the lymphatics, leading to lymphatic obstruction. This is also associated with lung cysts. It is virtually limited to women and the prognosis is poor unless pulmonary transplantation is performed. Sarcoidosis may cause pulmonary fibrosis, not pneumothorax. Lung cysts and pneumothoraces are not a feature of sarcoidosis.

66 Answers (5 marks)

1. **C** Acute gout
2. **D** Joint aspiration and polarised light microscopy
3. **B** Diclofenac

The sudden onset of a monoarthritis in somebody who has been started on cytotoxic therapy for a condition with increased cell turnover is very suggestive of an **acute gout attack**. Chondrocalcinosis is a descriptive term which can be caused by a variety of different substances deposited in the cartilage. It occurs in the context of degenerative change, pseudogout, hyperparathyroidism, haemochromatosis and acromegaly, gout and Wilson's disease.

Gout crystals are negatively and calcium paraphosphate crystals positively bi-refringent. Treatment of acute gout is with non-steroidals.

67 Answers (4 marks)

1. **E**   Still's disease
2. **E**   Ophthalmology referral

Pauciarticular **Still's disease** and adult Still's disease are often misdiagnosed for chronic sepsis due to the absence of rheumatological markers and the frequently present swinging pyrexia.

The systemic form seen in young children is associated with lymphadenopathy and splenomegaly and a characteristic macular erythema which is brought out by warmth and in the evening. In most forms the joints are less swollen and painful than in rheumatoid arthritis. The chronic iritis seen in the pauciarticular form is a sight-threatening condition.

68 Answer (2 marks)

1. **B**   Benzhexol

The patient has an acute dystonic reaction. Metoclopramide is frequently administered during barium follow-through. It is also a treatment for gut motility disorders. *Emergency* treatment for dystonic reactions is usually with procyclidine; biperiden may also be used.

Haloperidol may *induce* dystonic reactions.

69 Answers (4 marks)

1. **B**   Pseudoxanthoma elasticum (PXE)
2. **C**   Acute myocardial infarction

PXE is an inhomogeneous group of inherited disorders of elastic tissue. It affects skin, blood vessels, eyes and the heart. Although easily diagnosed by its lax skin which fails to recoil and a characteristic 'plucked chicken skin' appearance, the systemic complications are too often neglected. Intermittent claudication, angina and severe GI haemorrhages occur at an early age. Inheritance varies, but family screening and counselling is vital. Breaks in Bruch's membrane behind the retina causes *angioid streaks* (other causes include Marfan's, Ehlers-Danlos disease and sickle cell).

70 Answer (3 marks)

1. **A**   Acute renal failure

This is the high-arched (Gothic) palate of a patient with **Marfan's syndrome**. Complications of this autosomal dominant connective tissue disease include pneumothorax, aortic dissection, aortic incompetence, degenerative changes of the mitral valve and a variety of skeletal abnormalities.

LECTURE NOTES

LABORATORY TESTS IN GENERAL MEDICINE

The following are only guidelines to the principle of each test. There is a great variation between hospitals, refer to your own lab before embarking on a physiological adventure. Several tests (i.e. insulin stress test and Tensilon test) are dangerous, particularly in the elderly and must only be performed with resuscitation facilities readily available. Many contraindications exist and these must be carefully excluded. Some tests are becoming obsolete in clinical practice.

Ammonium chloride acidification test   Renal tubular acidosis I

Principle: Oral administration of ammonium chloride results in a metabolic acidosis which is corrected by the kidneys and results in an acidic urine (pH < 5.4). In type I RTA the kidneys cannot excrete the acid load and the urine pH will fail to drop. Excretion is preserved in RTA type II

Criteria: Plasma bicarbonate must drop by at least 4mmol/l within 2 hours. Patient must not vomit during the test.

- Overnight fast, good hydration
- Baseline urine pH, if < 5.4 test not required
- 0.1 g/kg NH_4Cl is given orally
- Hourly urine pH-measurements for 8 hours

Positive if: urine pH does not fall < 5.4

Anion gap   Metabolic acidosis

Principle: Not actually a test as such, estimation of the anion gap is a useful way of estimating whether extra acidic substances (i.e. lactic acid, ketones, salicylates, methanol, ethylene glycol) are responsible for the acidosis.
Normal: 10–18 mmol/l, accounted for by phosphate and some organic acids

- $[Na^+ + K^+] - [HCO_3^- + Cl^-]$

<u>NB</u>. With a high anion gap the chloride is usually low (hypochloraemic acidosis). Chloride is not a standard test, as soon as it appears in the data, calculation of the anion gap is required!

Lactic acidosis type A: **A** for **A**noxia
secondary to tissue hypoxia (shock, burns, hypoxia)
Lactic acidosis type B: **B** for **B**oisons
biguanides (metformin, phenformin)
= second cause for high anion gap in diabetics besides ketoacidosis, liver failure, poisoning (paracetamol, alcohol), lymphoma/leukaemia

Arginine infusion test   **Growth hormone deficiency**

Principle: Intravenous administration of arginine stimulates the excretion
                  of GH
                  Combined pituitary function test is usually preferred.
Dose: 30g arginine iv over 30 minutes
Positive if: GH-rise less than 15 mU/l

Breath Tests   **Bacterial overgrowth/Malabsorption**
1.   Hydrogen breath test

                  The only source of hydrogen in mammals is bacterial
                  metabolism of carbohydrates in the gut. This normally occurs
                  in the colon and up to 20% is absorbed into the blood and
                  excreted via the lungs. In overgrowth of anaerobic bacteria in
                  the small bowel an oral load of 75g of glucose (or 15g of
                  lactulose) results in an early increase in hydrogen in the
                  expired air as the sugar is already broken down before it
                  reaches the colon.

2.   Radiocarbon breath test

                  The patient is given 1g of xylose labelled with radioactive ^{14}C.
                  Normally xylose is absorbed to > 25% in small bowel, but not
                  significantly metabolised.
                  In bacterial overgrowth the compound is broken down and
                  radioactive $^{14}CO_2$ develops as a byproduct, which again is
                  excreted via the lungs.

Bromsulphthalein excretion test   **Dubin-Johnson syndrome**

Principle: iv BSP is conjugated and excreted in the bile.
                  Normally < 5% of injected dose present at 45 min.
                  In any form of liver dysfunction this level remains high, in
                  Dubin-Johnson syndrome it is said that after an initial drop the
                  serum levels at 120 min. are higher than at 45 min. The test is
                  risky and probably obsolete.

Captopril Test   **Hyperaldosteronism**

Principle: Renin (an enzyme produced in the juxtaglomerular apparatus)
                  cleaves angiotensinogen to angiotensin 1 which is converted in
                  the lungs to angiotensin 2 by A-1 converting enzyme (ACE). A-2
                  is not only the most potent (known) vasoconstrictor, but also
                  stimulates the secretion of aldosterone in the adrenals. Blockade
                  of ACE results in a drop of aldosterone in healthy individuals and
                  secondary (RAS and idiopathic) hyperaldosteronism.
                  In primary hyperaldosteronism (Conn's syndrome) the
                  aldosterone levels are unaffected and baseline renin is low.
                  In renal artery stenosis (RAS) there is an exaggerated increase
                  in renin following ACE-inhibition, as the compromised kidney
                  is being starved even further of its compromised blood supply.
Criteria: Baseline aldosterone should be raised (>400 pmol/l)

- After bed-rest from at least midnight 08.00 am blood sample for baseline renin and aldosterone is taken in *supine* position
- 25 mg captopril orally
- After 120 min (*supine*) take further sample for renin and aldosterone

Normal: Aldosterone level below 400 pmol/l with further drop after captopril

Conn's: Aldosterone > 400 pmol/l, no drop after ACE inhibition

RAS: Aldosterone high, drops after captopril.

Renin doubles (or more) after captopril. In essential hypertension and increase of up to 150% of baseline may be seen.

Combined pituitary function test   Hypopituitarism

Principle: Combination of
- insulin stress test for GH and cortisol
- TRH test for thyroid axis
- GN-RH test for gonadotrophic axis

Criteria: Evidence of hypopituitarism rather than end-organ failure. Hypoglycaemia of < 2.2 mmol/l must be achieved, ideally with patient being symptomatic (iv glucose must be immediately available, if this needs to be given continue the test, as hypoglycaemic stress was adequate to induce hormone release). Many contraindications (see *insulin stress test*).

- iv cannula sited at least 30 min prior to test to reduce stress of blood sampling
- After 30 min. baseline samples for GH and cortisol, TSH, LH and FSH and glucose
- Start test with injection of 0.15 U/kg soluble insulin i.v., 200 µg TRH and 100 µg GN-RH
- Repeat blood samples from cannula at 30, 60, 90 and 120 min.

Positive if: 1.   GH rise < 15mU/l / GH peak < 20 mU/l

               2.   Cortisol rise < 200 nmol/l (basal level should double)/ Cortisol peak < 550 nmol/l

               3.   TSH response
                    exaggerated (1° hypothyroidism)
                    reduced (2° hypothyroidism)
                    delayed (3° hypothyroidism)
                    absent (hyperthyroidism)
                    → see *TRH test* for details
                    Gonadotrophin response (see *GN-RH test*)

Corticotrophin releasing hormone test   Cushing's disease vs. syndrome

Principle: Intravenous CRH stimulates the secretion of ACTH by the anterior pituitary resulting in an increase in cortisol.
A pituitary adenoma will respond by releasing an overshoot of ACTH resulting in a marked increase in serum cortisol = **Cushing's disease**, pituitary driven adrenal hyperplasia

An autonomous adrenal adenoma or ectopic ACTH secretion will not be influenced by additional ACTH = **Cushing's syndrome**

Dexamethasone suppression test   Cushing's disease vs. syndrome

Principle: Dexamethasone, a potent synthetic steroid should suppress ACTH secretion resulting in a drop in serum cortisol. The feedback mechanism is impaired in pituitary driven hypercortisolism (Cushing's disease) and absent in adrenal adenoma and ectopic ACTH production.

Criteria: Basal serum cortisol must be high to begin with, otherwise a high ACTH is secondary to adrenal failure
All cortisol samples should be taken between 8.00 and 9.00 a.m.

• The cortisol levels in a normal person should drop by more than 50%.

a. low dose dexamethasone test

Dose: 2 mg/day orally for 48 hours (either single dose at night or 0.5 mg qds)

Positive if: Serum cortisol fails to suppress below 50% of baseline / below 125 nmol/l

NB: this does not differentiate between a pituitary or adrenal/ectopic cause

b. high dose dexamethasone test

Criteria: Abnormal low dose dexamethasone test
Often this follows immediately on from the low-dose test on day three

Dose: 8 mg/day orally for 48 hours (either single dose at night or 2 mg qds)

Positive if: serum cortisol fails to suppress below 50% of baseline / below 125 nmol/l
→ this is in favour of adrenal/ectopic production, as most (2/3) of pituitary adenomas suppress on the high dose test

Dicopac® -Test   Pernicious anaemia

Principle: The body is saturated with an im injection of vitamin B_{12}. A mixture of ^{58}Co-labelled B_{12} and a compound of ^{57}Co labelled B_{12}/intrinsic factor is given orally. In pernicious anaemia there will be differential excretion of the two isotopes in the urine (i.e. the former will be abnormally low). In other causes of B_{12} deficiency (i.e. terminal ileal disease, bacterial overgrowth) urinary excretions of both substances will be low. For full details see *Schilling-test*.

Positive if: Excreted dose of radioactive B_{12} < 8% (24hr urine collection)

Ellsworth-Howard test   **Pseudo-/Hypoparathyroidism**

PTM increases urine phosphate excretion. This is mediated via the intracellular second messenger cyclic-AMP, which also appears in the urine.

Normal excretion: urinary PO_4^{3-} 13–42 nmol/day,
                    urinary c-AMP 0.5 nmol/mmol creatinine

Principle: Hypoparathyroidism (reduced/absent endogenous parathormone): The infusion of parathormone results in a 10–20 fold increased urinary excretion of PO_4^{3-} and c-AMP.

Pseudohypoparathyroidism (end-organ resistance): endogenous parathormone is present, but ineffective. Administration of exogenous PTH makes no difference → no increased PO_4^{3-} excretion in the urine. Two types:

- Type 1: receptor defect results in complete failure of target cell response
  → no c-AMP is produced in the cell, no urinary increase of c-AMP or PO_4^{3-}
- Type 2: receptor intact, but c-AMP ineffective
  → rise in urinary c-AMP, urinary PO_4^{3-} unaltered

Faecal fat excretion   **Steatorrhoea**

Principle: Normal daily fat excretion is less than 7 g/day. Steatorrhoea can be due to maldigestion (pancreas) or malabsorption (small bowel). The reliability of the test is impaired by daily variation of diet and difficulties collecting all the samples. Usually an average over 5 consecutive days is obtained.

Criteria: Normal diet containing 50–100 g fat/day (no more!) for at least three days prior to test.

Positive if: Total faecal fat > 10 g/d (> 30 g in 3 days)

Glucose suppression test   **Acromegaly**

Principle: Growth hormone (GH) levels should drop in response to an increasing blood sugar. (See also OGTT)

- Overnight fast
- iv cannula sited at least 30 min. prior to test to reduce stress of blood sampling
- Basal glucose and GH-levels are taken
- 75g of glucose or equivalent carbohydrates are given orally in 250–300ml of fluid within five minutes
- Further glucose and GH levels at 30, 60, 90 and 120 minutes

Positive if: GH fails to suppress below 4 mU/l

False positive: severe hepatic or renal failure, drug addicts, levodopa therapy

Gonadotrophin releasing hormone (GN-RH) test   **Amenorrhoea**

Principle: GN-RH should result in release of LH and FSH from the pituitary. Normal values vary greatly throughout the female cycle and between hospitals and normal ranges are usually given in the exam. Both values should roughly rise by more than 5 U/l into double figures. In primary ovarian failure basal gonadotrophins will be high, in pituitary failure there will be no response to GN-RH, in hypothalamic dysfunction there will be a normal or delayed response analogue to the TRH test.

Criteria: Low gonadotrophin levels, otherwise primary ovarian failure is present.

- Basal levels
- 100 µg GN-RH
- FSH and LH levels at 30, 60, 90 and 120 min.

Hypothalamic dysfunction: normal response
Pituitary failure/anorexia: absent/reduced response

Ham's test   Parox. nocturnal haemoglobinuria
Principle: Acquired sensitivity of red cells to activated complement results in intravascular haemolysis. Haemolysis occurs during sleep (reduced oxygen tension) with dark urine in the morning. *In vitro* this manifests as a reduced tolerance to acidic media resulting in haemolysis at higher pH (less acidic) than normal erythrocytes.

Insulin stress test   Growth hormone (GH) deficiency
Principle: Hypoglycaemia causes a physiological increase in the 'diabetogenic' hormones GH and cortisol.
Usually performed as part of the *combined pituitary stimulation test*.
Contraindicated in ischaemic heart disease, epilepsy and the frail and elderly!

- iv cannula sited at least 30 min. prior to test to reduce stress of blood sampling
- Baseline GH and glucose
- 0.15 U/kg soluble insulin iv
- Repeat samples at 30, 60, 90 120 min.

Criteria: Blood glucose < 2.2 mmol/l, ideally patient should be symptomatic (iv Glucose must be drawn up & ready, if it needs to be given, *continue sampling!*) If poor response, test can be repeated with 0.3 U/kg
Positive if: GH increases by less than 15 mU/l/peak value < 20 mU/l

Joint Aspirate

	Normal	Septic arthritis	Rheumatoid	(Pseudo-) Gout	OA
Colour	straw clear	yellow-grey pus	yellow-green turbid	yellow clear/turbid	yellow clear
Viscosity	high	very low	very low	low	high
pH	7.3–7.6		6.8–7.4		7.2–7.5
Protein [g/l]	11–22	30–60	> 40	> 40	normal
Glucose	> 60% of blood	< 40%	40–60%	normal	
LDH [U/l]	< 200	> 300	> 200	> 200	normal
Lymphocytes	< 200/µl	> 100 000/µl	10–50 000/µl	5–20 000/µl	< 5 000/µl
Polymorphs	none				

Lactose tolerance test   Lactose intolerance

Principle: The disaccharide lactose is split by lactase into galactose and glucose which is absorbed in the small bowel.

- Basal blood glucose
- 50 g of oral lactose
- Blood glucose should rise more than 1 mmol/l

Lumbar Puncture

	Normal	Bacterial	Viral
Colour	clear	pus	clear/turbid
Pressure	10–16 cm H_2O	$\leftrightarrow/\uparrow$	$\leftrightarrow$
Protein	0.2–0.4 g/l	0.5–5 g/l	0.4–1 g/l
Glucose	> 60% of blood	< 40%	normal
Red cells	none	no	no
Lymphocytes	< 5/µl	<50/µl	10–100/µl
Polymorphs	none	300–3000/µl	occasional

	TB	SAH	traumatic tap
Colour	turbid, sticky	Xanthochromia after 4 hrs	blood
Pressure	$\uparrow$	$\leftrightarrow/\uparrow$	$\leftrightarrow$
Protein	0.5–3 g/l	0.2–0.5 g/l	0.2–0.5 g/l
Glucose	< 40%	normal	$\leftrightarrow/\uparrow$
Red cells	no	yes	yes
Lymphocytes	100–300/µl	occasional	occasional
Polymorphs	0–200/µl	occasional	occasional

Methacholine provocation test — Hyperreactive bronchial tree/asthma

Principle: Inhaled methacholine causes bronchoconstriction. The concentration required to produce a reduction in FEV1 of >20% is an indicator of the (hyper-) responsiveness of the bronchial tree.

	Methacholine concentration
Normal	> 4 mg/ml
Mild hyper-responsiveness	4 mg/ml
Moderate asthma	0.5 mg/ml
Severe asthma	0.1 mg/ml

Nicotinic acid test — Gilbert's syndrome

Principle: Unconjugated bilirubin levels rise (5–10 μmol/l) after administration of nicotinic acid to a peak (average 15–20 [mu]mol/l) at *90 min* in normal persons.
In Gilbert's the peak is higher (45–50 μmol/l) and occurs at *2–3 hours*.
Baseline is usually 20–25 μmol/l
A 1.5–2 fold increase is also seen on fasting (< 400 kcal/d for 3 days), normal levels < 25 μmol/l.

* 50 mg nicotinic acid iv
* Bloods at 60, 90, 120 and 360 min

Oral glucose tolerance test (OGTT) — Diabetes mellitus

Random plasma glucose > 11mmol/l or fasting plasma glucose > 8 mmol/l DM present, **OGTT not required**
Random plasma glucose < 8 mmol/l or fasting plasma glucose < 6 mmol/l DM excluded, **OGTT not required**

Principle: Oral glucose load leads to an abnormal increase in plasma glucose levels in DM.
A mixture of glucose and its oligosaccharides is preferred to pure glucose as this is less osmolar, the patient is less likely to vomit and absorption is more reliable

* Patient on normal diet, overnight fast
* Basal plasma levels are taken
* 75g of glucose or equivalent carbohydrates are given orally in 250–300ml of fluid within five minutes, patient should sit or walk, if patient must lie down this should be on the right side in order to allow gastric emptying
* Further glucose levels at 30, 60, 90 and 120 minutes

Results:

Impaired glucose tolerance:	2 hr glucose > 8mmol/l, but <11mmol/l (normal fasting levels)
Diabetes mellitus:	2 hr glucose > 11mmol/l
'Lag storage curve':	Peak plasma glucose reached early (can be > 11mmol/l) 2 h glucose normal/lower than baseline often delayed hypoglycaemia (→ late samples required) Seen in: 'dumping syndrome' following gastric surgery, liver disease, some normals
Flat response:	Levels do not rise above 7mmol/l Seen in: patient lying on the left during test, vomiting, malabsorption, pituitary/adrenal failure

Osmolality (plasma)   Fluid overload/SIADH

Principle: Useful normal value, particularly in combination with urine osmolality (see water deprivation test) The sum of the major electrolytes (for ease of calculation the cations are added and doubled to account for the corresponding anions) is added to the two major organic molecules.

Normal: 280–295 mosm/kg

* $[Na^+ + K^+] \times 2 + [Urea] + [Glucose]$

Osmotic resistance/fragility   Hereditary spherocytosis

Principle: Due to an inherited membrane protein defect the cells 'swell' from a saucer to a spherical shape, thus reducing their cross-section (→ microcytosis). When introduced into an increasingly hypotonic medium the already 'swollen' cells tolerate the further influx of water less than normal cells and lyse earlier.
This corrects with the addition of glucose.

Pentagastrin test   Abnormal gastric acid output

Principle: Pentagastrin stimulates gastric secretion analogue to gastrin. In Zollinger-Ellison syndrome there is an overshoot 'peak acid output' (PAO), pernicious anaemia shows a reduced response.

* NG tube sited, collection of gastric secretions over 1 hour (basal acid output, BAO: < 5 mmol/h))
* 6 μg/kg pentagastrin s.c.
* gastric aspiration at 15, 30, 45 and 60 min.

Positive if: PAO > 60 mmol/h → Z-E syndrome
                (also BAO > 15 mmol/h)
                PAO < 10 mmol/h → pernicious anaemia,
                H_2-blockers, vagotomy, hypothyroidism

Peak acid output is defined as the two subsequent aspirates with the highest values.

Pleural aspirate

	Transudate	Exudate	RA
Colour	clear	turbid	turbid
Protein [g/l]	< 30	> 30	> 30
Albumin	< 60% of serum	> 60% of serum	> 60% of serum
Glucose	> 60% of blood	< 40% of blood	< 20% of blood
pH	7.3–7.5	< 7.3	< 7.2
Lactate [mmo/l]	1–5	5–20	> 5
			RF positive, LDH ↑

Schilling Test   Vitamin B_{12} deficiency

Principle: Dietary B_{12} is absorbed in the terminal ileum in the presence
                of intrinsic factor produced in the gastric mucosa.

1st part   After saturation of the body stores by an im injection of 1mg
                normal B_{12} a dose of radioactive ^{58}Co-labelled B_{12} is given
                orally. As the body is saturated by the injection, more than
                10% of the radioactive dose should be excreted in the
                following 24hr urine collection

2nd part   If this is not the case the test is repeated with the addition of
                intrinsic factor. If excretion normalises, pernicious anaemia is
                confirmed.
                If excretion still low, then there is either terminal ileal disease
                or overgrowth of bacteria metabolising the B_{12}. The latter is
                confirmed by repeating the test after oral antibiotics or by
                hydrogen breath test or small bowel aspiration for culture.

                Both parts can be performed at the same time with a mixture
                ^{58}Co-labelled B_{12} and a compound of intrinsic factor and B_{12}
                which is labelled with ^{57}Co (Dicopac®-Test). In pernicious
                anaemia there will be differential excretion of the two isotopes,
                in other pathology both urinary excretions will be low.

Positive if: Excreted dose of radioactive B_{12} < 8% (24hr urine collection)

Secretin suppression test   Zollinger-Ellison syndrome

Principle: Gastrin levels are normally suppressed by secretin. In Z-E a
                paradoxical rise of greater than 100% occurs after injection
                of secretin.

Steroid suppression test   Hypercalcaemia

Principle: Hypercalcaemia due to **sarcoidosis**, myeloma,
                  hypervitaminosis D and Addison's disease (rare manifestation)
                  suppress with high doses of steroids. Ectopic PTH suppresses
                  to a lesser extent. Hyperparathyroidism (primary or tertiary) is
                  unaffected. Metastatic bone involvement suppresses in 50%.

- Hydrocortisone 40 mg tds for ten days

Positive if: Ca2+ levels suppress to normal levels (< 2.55 mmol/l).
                  The clinical context decides between sarcoid, vitamin D
                  effects or myeloma.

Synacthen® test   Hypoadrenalism/Addison's disease

Principle: Synthetic ACTH stimulates the adrenals and results in
                  increased serum cortisol.
                  Failure of cortisol to rise in the short test can be due to primary
                  adrenal failure (Addison's disease), adrenal suppression (i.e.
                  steroid therapy) or longstanding hypopituitarism. The latter
                  two are excluded by prolonged adrenal stimulation with the
                  long test.
Criteria: Low serum cortisol

a. short Synacthen® test:
- Basal cortisol levels
- 250 µg tetracosactrin i.m.
- Cortisol levels at 30 and 60 min.

Positive if: Cortisol < 550nmol/l at 30 min, < 650 nmol/l at 60 min If the
                  test positive proceed to

b. long Synacthen® test
- Following short test 1 mg tetracosactrin depot is given i.m.
- Cortisol levels after further 24hr

Delayed response: hypopituitarism or exogenous steroids; no response:
Addison's disease.

Tensilon® test   Myasthenia gravis

Principle: Injection of a cholinesterase inhibitor increases the
                  concentration of acetylcholine at the motor endplate by
                  inhibition of its breakdown. Increase in muscle power (i.e.
                  resolution of bilateral ptosis on upward gaze) occurs within
                  seconds lasting several minutes.
                  This type of drug is used in Anaesthetics as a depolarising
                  muscle relaxant, it can cause severe bronchospasm or syncope
                  and resuscitation facilities must be at hand.

- Edrophonium test dose 1 mg iv
- Edrophonium 10 mg iv bolus
- As the test is subjective, several observers should be present, control injection with saline can be performed if in doubt

TRH-test (Thyrotropin releasing hormone)   Hypothyroidism

Principle: Assessment of hypothalamic-pituitary-thyroid axis
                    After TRH the normal TSH should peak at 20 min (5–20 mU/l, increase > 2 mU/l over baseline) and drop steadily (60 min. value no lower than 1/3rd of 20 min peak).

- Basal TSH levels
- 200 µg TRH iv
- TSH levels after 20 and 60 min.

Results: **1° hypothyroidism:**
                    basal TSH high, exaggerated and prolonged response to TRH
                    2° hypothyroidism (pituitary failure):
                    low baseline, minimal increase at 20 min (< 2 mU/l), back to baseline at 60 min.
                    3° hypothyroidism (hypothalamic dysfunction):
                    delayed rise in TSH with low 20 min and high 60 min value
                    hyperthyroidism:
                    flat response, no increase in TSH

Water deprivation test   Diabetes insipidus

Principle: Test for investigation of polyuria/suspected defect in urinary concentration.
                    Restriction of water intake stimulates ADH-secretion resulting in increasing urine osmolality but maintained serum osmolality.

In **diabetes insipidus** ADH is absent (central form) or ineffective (nephrogenic form) and the kidneys fail to retain water. If the baseline plasma osmolality is low, DI is excluded. On fluid deprivation the plasma osmolality rises > 300 mosm/kg while the urine fails to concentrate.

If there is evidence of DI the administration of synthetic ADH (DDAVP, Vasopressin) will correct the defect in the central form, but will make no difference in the peripheral form as there is a receptor defect in the kidney.

Psychogenic polydipsia is easily distinguished as the plasma osmolality is low to begin with and will not rise above normal values. DDAVP is not required. Frequently the concentration gradient has been washed out of the kidney and prolonged fluid restriction is required. The patient may also secretly continue drinking during the test.

- Overnight fast
- Baseline weight and urine and plasma samples → if urine > 800 mosm/kg the kidneys can concentrate normally and the test can be stopped

- No food or water for 8 hours, 2-hourly measurements
- The test is stopped, if the urine > 800 mosm/kg or the patient has lost 5% of their body weight
- If urinary concentration does not occur in the presence of haemoconcentration 4µg DDAVP are given im

Results after 8hr fluid deprivation:

	Normal	Central D.I.	Nephrogenic D.I.	Polydipsia
Serum	280–295	305–320	305–320	270–295
Urine	800–1500	100–300	100–300	200–700
Urine after DDAVP	–	increased by > 10%	Unchanged as ineffective	–

Xylose absorption test   Malabsorption

Principle: D-xylose is rapidly absorbed and largely excreted in the urine. A 5g dose is usually preferred to 25 g as less osmotic side-effects. It is an unspecific and not very sensitive test for small bowel absorption

Normal: > 25 % of oral dose excreted within five hours (> 12 % after two hours)

- Empty bladder
- 5 g (25 g) D-xylose in 200 ml water
- Urine collection of first two and further three hours

FAMILY TREES

Family trees are confusing, but not that difficult.
Two questions need to be answered:
1. Is every generation affected?   = dominant
2. Is there male-to-male (father-to-son) transmission = autosomal

Autosomal Dominant Inheritance

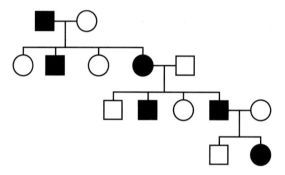

Key Features
- Male-to-male transmission
- All generations are affected
- Both sexes are equally affected
- The transmission stops with an unaffected person

Risks for offspring
- One parent heterozygous: 1:2 (50%) chance of being affected
- Both parents heterozygous: 1:2 (50%) chance of being heterozygous
                                and affected
                                1:4 (25%) chance of being homozygous
                                1:4 (25%) chance of normal genes

- One homozygous parent: all children will affected (heterozygous)
- One homozygous and one   all children affected, 50%
  heterozygous parent: heterozygous, 50% homozygous

Examples:

Acute intermittent porphyria

Adult polycystic kidney disease

α1-Antitrypsin deficiency

C_1-esterase deficiency

Familial intestinal polyposis/Peutz-Jeghers syndrome

Hereditary spherocytosis

Hereditary telangiectasia

Huntingdon's chorea

Marfan's syndrome/Osteogenesis imperfecta tarda

Medullary carcinoma thyroid/Multiple endocrine neoplasia

Neurofibromatosis/Tuberose sclerosis/von-Hippel Lindau (Sturge-Weber sporadic)

Rotor's disease

von Willebrand's disease

Autosomal Recessive Inheritance

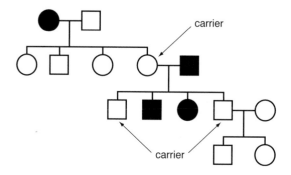

carrier

carrier

Key Features:
- <u>Male-to-male transmission</u>
- <u>NOT every generation is affected</u>
- Both sexes are equally affected
- Unaffected persons can transmit the abnormal gene = heterozygous carriers

<u>Risks for offspring</u>:
- One parent carrier: 1:4 (25%) of being a carrier
- One affected parent (homozygous): 100% ofl children are carriers
- Both parents carriers: 1: 2 (50%) chance of being a carrier
                                                        1:4 (25%) chance of being affected,
                                                        1:4 (25%) chance of normal genes
- One affected parent, one carrier: 1: 2 (50%) chance of being <u>either</u> a
                                                        carrier or being affected

<u>Examples</u>:
Cystic fibrosis
Haemochromatosis/Wilson's disease
Infantile polycystic disease
Dubin-Johnson syndrome/Gilbert's syndrome
Congenital adrenal hyperplasia
Sickle cell disease/â-thalassaemia
Hurler's disease

<u>Most metabolic disorders</u>:
Fructose intolerance
Phenylketonuria, cystinuria
Glycogen storage diseases
Lysosomal storage diseases (Gaucher's, Niemann-Pick, Tay-Sachs) except Fabry's disease (X-recessive)

X-linked recessive Inheritance

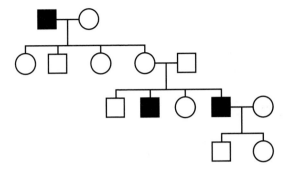

Key Features:
- Usually one generation skipped = Knight's move pattern
- No male-to-male transmission
- Virtually only males affected, females usually carriers only

Risks for offspring:
- Maternal carrier: 1:2 (50%) of <u>sons</u> affected, the others healthy (<u>no male carriers</u>)
  1:2 (50%) of <u>daughters</u> will be carriers
- Affected father   <u>all</u> sons healthy (<u>no male-tomale transmission</u>)
  <u>all</u> daughters carriers (!)
- A woman can only be affected (= homozygous), if her father is affected AND her mother carries at least one abnormal gene (usually consanguinity)

Examples:
Red-green colour blindness
Haemophilia A & B
Idiopathic sideroblastic anaemia
Nephrogenic diabetes insipidus
G6P-dehydrogenase deficiency
Lesch-Nyhan syndrome
Hunter's disease
Fabry's disease
Becker's/Duchenne's muscular dystrophy

X-linked dominant Inheritance

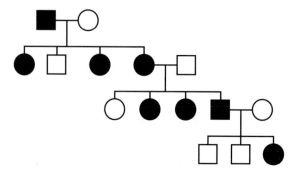

Key Features:
- All generations affected, if daughters present
- No male-to-male transmission
- Most cases will be females

Risks for offspring:
- Affected father

  all sons healthy
  all daughters affected

- Affected mother:

  1:2 children affected if heterozygous
  all children affected if homozygous

Examples:
Pseudohypoparathyroidism
Vitamin D resistant rickets
Chronic granulomatous disease

Sporadic Cases

Key Features
- Short family tree
- Chromosomal pattern usually indicated (i.e. X).XXY)

Risks for offspring
- Usually infertile (!). Rarely mosaic configurations (i.e. X)/XX) may preserve fertility.

Risks of having a further child with the same condition
Not increased (as caused by incidental non-disjunction at meiosis)

Examples:
Turner syndrome (45 XO), incidence 1:3,000–1:5,000
Klinefelter syndrome (47 XXY), incidence 1:750, one of the commonest chromosomal anomalies

HISTOLOGICAL STAINS

Technique	Application
Cresyl blue (supravital stain)	Reticulocytes: blue reticulation Heinz bodies: blue (splenectomy, G-6 PDH def., toxic/met-Hb)
Congo red	Amyloid: red (apple-green under polarised light → positive birefringent)
Gram	Gram-positive cocci: blue (staphylococci = grapes, streptococci = chains, pneumococci = buns) Gram-negative cocci: red (diplococci: Neisseria meningitidis and gonorrhoeae)
Grimelius	APUD-cell tumours (carcinoid, islet cell tumours)
Grocott	See silver
Indian ink	Fungi: pale on black background
Massou-Fontana-Silver	Melanin: black (melanoma)
Periodic acid Schiff (PAS)	Tropheryma whippelii (Whipple's disease): pink bodies within macrophages Fungi: red
Pearl's stain (= Prussian blue)	Iron: dark blue Liver: Haemochromatosis and other causes of iron overload Ring sideroblasts (hereditary, myeloproliferation, toxic/drugs, CTD) Pappenheimer bodies in erythrocytes post-splenectomy
Rose bengal	Mucus: pink (sicca syndrome and Sjögren's)

Romanowsky	<u>Basophilic stippling</u>: dark blue dots in erythrocytes (lead poisoning) <u>Howell-Jolly bodies</u>: blue nuclear fragments (hyposplenism) also a standard bone marrow stain <u>Multiple myeloma</u>: binucleate cells with large amount of blue cytoplasm = 'owl's eyes' appearance (> 8% diagnostic)
Rubeonic acid	<u>Copper</u>: brown (Wilson's disease)
Silver stain	<u>Fungi</u> (incl. histoplasmosis)/yeasts: brown/black, linear <u>Pneumocystis</u>: black, oval
Modified Ziehl-Neelson (Z-N)	Acid fast bacilli (= stain is acid fast, not bacilli; TB, leprosy) cryptosporidium

REFERENCES

1. Whitby L.G., Percy-Robb I.W., Smith A.F. *Lecture notes on clinical chemistry.* 3rd ed. Blackwell scientific publications, Oxford.
2. Zilva J.F., Pannall P.R., Mayne P.D. *Clinical chemistry in diagnosis and treatment.* 5th ed. Edward Arnold, London.
3. Thomas L. *Labor und Diagnose.* 5th ed. TH-Books Verlags- Gesellschaft, Frankfurt
4. Kumar P., Clark M. *Clinical Medicine.* 2nd ed. Bailliere Tindall, London.
5. Herold G. *Innere Medizin.* 1994, Gerd Herold, Köln.
6. Thomson A.D., Cotton R.E. *Lecture notes on pathology.* 3rd ed. Blackwell scientific publications, Oxford.
7. Govan A.D., MacFarlane P.S., Callander R. *Pathology illustrated.* 1st ed. Churchill Livingstone, Edinburgh.
8. Sandritter W., Thomas C. *Histopathologie.* 9th ed. Schattauer, Stuttgart.
9. Oxford textbook of medicine on CD-ROM. Version 1.1, Oxford University Press and Electric Publishing.
10. Firkin, B.G., Whitworth J.A. *Dictionary of Medical Eponyms,* 1st ed. Glaxo/ Parthenon, Carnforth.

INDEX

Numbers given are for pages on which relevant question or answer appear. The word shown may not always be used in the question, but may appear in the explanatory answer. Numbers in bold type are for Major References within the text.

29.99